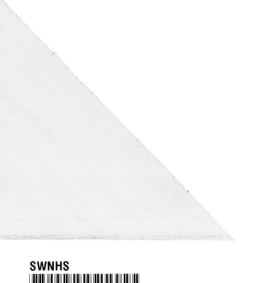

SLEEP AND BRAIN PLASTICITY

SLEEP AND BRAIN PLASTICITY

Edited by

P. MAQUET

Cyclotron Research Centre, University of Liège, Belgium

C. SMITH

Department of Psychology, Trent University, Peterborough, Ontario, Canada

and

R. STICKGOLD

Department of Psychiatry at the Massachusetts Mental Health Center, Harvard Medical School, Boston, Massachusetts, USA

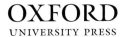

OXFORD
UNIVERSITY PRESS

OXFORD

UNIVERSITY PRESS

Great Clarendon Street, Oxford OX2 6DP

Oxford University Press is a department of the University of Oxford.
It furthers the University's objective of excellence in research, scholarship,
and education by publishing worldwide in

Oxford New York

Auckland Bangkok Buenos Aires Cape Town Chennai
Dar es Salaam Delhi Hong Kong Istanbul Karachi Kolkata
Kuala Lumpur Madrid Melbourne Mexico City Mumbai Nairobi
São Paulo Shanghai Taipei Tokyo Toronto

Oxford is a registered trade mark of Oxford University Press
in the UK and in certain other countries

Published in the United States
by Oxford University Press Inc., New York

A catalogue record for this title is available from the British Library

Library of Congress Cataloging in Publication Data
Data available

ISBN 0 19 857400 2 (Hbk)

10 9 8 7 6 5 4 3 2 1

Typeset by Newgen Imaging Systems (P) Ltd., Chennai, India
Printed in Great Britain
on acid-free paper by
T.J. International Ltd, Padstow, Cornwall

FOREWORD

Poets and physicians have pondered the function of sleep, and neuroscientists have weighed in on this issue for some time as well. However, despite considerable and continuing efforts, no clear and compelling role for sleep has been identified. Yet, we spend so much of our lives asleep, and the motivation to sleep is so powerful, it must have some very important physiological function, right?

One of the most intriguing and lasting proposals is that sleep and, in particular, dreaming, plays a critical role in the consolidation of memories. After all, many of our dreams resurrect distant as well as recent memories. And lack of sleep can result in memory lapses. Is there a critical physiological mechanism of sleep that replays memories and alters their organization or persistence? This book addresses that question through a collection of perspectives on the relationship between sleep, dreaming, and memory. Some chapters pursue the modest hypothesis that sleep is a brain state that facilitates general mechanisms of neural plasticity during development and adulthood, and in so doing impacts representations that underlie memory. Other chapters report evidence consistent with the more bold view that sleep and dreaming organize the specific contents of everyday memory. Within a broad range of experimental programs there is "smoke," that is, strongly suggestive evidence that sleep plays some role in neural plasticity, including that which underlies at least some forms of memory. How should we interpret this evidence?

At a recent US National Institute of Mental Health conference on this topic ("Perspectives on the role of sleep in memory"), I began the meeting by suggesting four comments my mother would offer about sleep, dreams, and memory. I used the metaphor of my mom's critiques to point out that there are issues in the neuroscientific study of this problem that are clarified by a common sense perspective. In this preface, I will summarize those points, and suggest the readers keep them in mind as they consider the scientific evidence: "When I don't sleep, my memory is lousy the next day. But then, most everything else goes to pot, too." Like my mom, everyone has had a sleepless night, and has experienced difficulties with memory the next day. Many neuroscientific studies have documented this observation, and some have further revealed specific alterations in memory function associated with diminution of particular sleep stages. But my mother is concerned that these effects may not identify a fundamental role for sleep in memory *per se*, and instead reflect a general deterioration of cognitive function. We need to determine which effects of sleep deprivation are selective to memory performance and fundamental to memory processing. It is entirely possible that sleep deprivation constitutes a stress state that result in a general metabolic or physiologic dysfunction, and memory performance is simply a very sensitive test of mild cerebral malaise. As you read chapters that consider the effects of sleep deprivation, pay at least as much attention to the controls for memory as to the measures of memory loss. "When something really big happens, I think about it a lot, even when I go to bed that night." The main complementary evidence for an association between sleep and memory involves observations of learning induced alterations in brain activity during sleep, typically recorded in the field potentials reflected in the electroencephalogram or in single neuron firing patterns. Do these brain activity patterns reflect the *consolidation* of memories, that is, does this activity *cause* memories to be fixed? Alternatively, do unique patterns of brain activity during sleep following learning merely reflect the natural *persistence* of memory processing, that is, are these brain activity patterns a *consequence*, rather than a cause, of memory? In simpler terms, my mother suggests sleep may be just a relatively quiescent period when previously established memories dominate our subsequent thoughts both in wakefulness and in sleep. Indeed, the persistence of learning related brain activity would be expected to be especially powerful following strong or unusual recent experiences, those typical of learning that occurs in laboratory experiments. So, as you read chapters that describe neural activity patterns during sleep following learning, consider to what extent the experiment determines whether these patterns reflect the consolidation or the persistence of memories.

"I remember my memories, not my dreams." A problem with the strong claim that the information processing during sleep reflects consolidation of that information is that the contents of the information processed during dreaming is unlike that of the contents of real experiences. My mother distinguished, in her own way, between the defining characterization of dreams during deep sleep as surreal and that of memories as reflecting real events. Often dreams contain elements of recent, as well as remote, real experiences. But the flow of events that occur during dreams is not what we recall. Indeed, except when awakened during a dream, one typically is not able to recall dreams at all. If dreams reflect the replay of experience *per se*, or an integration of recent and remote experience constituting the consolidation process, then why are not our dreams the *best* remembered of events? As you read about the notion of memory replay during sleep, consider the contents of dreams versus those of memories.

"When you came home from school and had a big exam the next day, I told you to study, not to go to bed." Even though my mother wondered about the function of sleep, as we all do, she could not imagine that sleep would be the best way to consolidate memories. Rather, she insisted that the way to improve memory is to study, to think over the material, and to consciously integrate new material with old during wakefulness. So, when you consider the ramifications of evidence of an association between memory and sleep, evaluate whether this is the most important time for consolidation. It is not that memory consolidation cannot occur during sleep, but it may be no more than quiet time for processes that have already been set in motion during wakefulness.

There is one last and potentially quite important question that my mother did not envision: What kind of memories are processed during sleep? Several lines of evidence clearly suggest a connection between sleep and neural plasticity associated with experience-related changes in behavioral performance we call memory. But consider the *kinds of memory* for which this relationship is most evident. It is now well established that there are multiple forms of memory mediated by distinct memory systems (Eichenbaum and Cohen). Consistent with the multiple memory systems notion, there is growing evidence that particular types of memory may be associated with sleep, and others unrelated. In many of the experiments described in this book, the kind of memory dependent on sleep is not "declarative memory," our memory for everyday facts and events that is subject to conscious recollection. Rather, sleep-dependent memories involve perceptual learning, and the acquisition of perceptual-motor routines that are mediated by cortical and motor systems. Even some standard examples of sleep-dependent animal learning, such as conditioned avoidance or approach responses, are now known to be mediated outside the declarative memory system. This does not detract from the potential importance of sleep in memory consolidation, but it may limit its scope.

My (and my mother's) notes should serve not as doom and gloom for sleep and memory research. Rather these points provide cautionary notes for interpreting the new and intriguing evidence about relationships between sleep, neural plasticity, and memory. We should remain as fascinated as ever about the mystery of sleep. But we should enter this new generation of investigations with our eyes wide open.

Laboratory of Cognitive Neurobiology   Howard Eichenbaum
Boston University
Boston, MA 02215
USA

References

Perspectives on the role of sleep in memory. December 2001, Bethesda MD. I. Lederhendler, organizer.

Eichenbaum, H. and Cohen, N. J. (2001). *From conditioning to conscious recollection: memory systems of the brain.* Oxford University Press.

PREFACE

The last 25 years have witnessed a renewed interest in the study of the role of sleep in two main manifestations of brain plasticity: brain development on the one hand, and learning and memory, on the other hand.

At present, the hypothesis has not yet been confirmed and remains debatable. Therefore, we thought that the time had come to provide the general readership with a volume gathering a selected sample of this new material. We believed that this endeavor would be all the more useful because the data are now coming from a wide variety of different disciplines and can easily be overlooked. This book is an attempt to provide an integrated vision of the field. This does not imply that the same mechanisms act in every experimental condition, for example, in different species, in different memory systems, at different age. . . . However, at this stage, it appeared useful to highlight the fact that they all implicate sleep in brain plasticity. We predict that future research will distinguish the characteristic features of each experimental system.

Our basic editorial choice was that the book would be essentially built on hard experimental data, since data can be rationally examined, discussed, or criticized. They are the prerequisite to any sensible and testable hypothesis, and to the eventual characterization of the role of sleep in brain plasticity.

This deliberate choice has obvious consequences. First, the book is edited by researchers having some conviction about the role of sleep in brain plasticity. The findings presented here provide positive evidence in favor of the hypothesis. However, the reader will appreciate the cautious optimism with which the chapters have generally been written. The reader will find a general presentation of the hypothesis in the introduction which also summarizes the main issues raised against the hypothesis and considers the remaining unknowns to be solved by future research.

Second, what the reader will not find in this book is a presentation of general theoretical constructs on the sleep functions, even if they deal with brain plasticity. Once again, they are briefly presented in the introduction. Moreover, these constructs are discussed to various degrees as they relate to the experimental data.

Likewise, computational modeling of the plastic changes during sleep in the brain is not thoroughly covered. The editors are nevertheless convinced that this is an important avenue of research. The interested reader is directed to the Chapters 12–14, as well as to other works (e.g. Destexhe, A. and Sejnowski, T. J. (2000). *Thalamo-cortical assemblies.* Oxford University Press, Oxford).

The plastic changes that occur after a cerebral lesion are not considered in this book. Some references are made to amnesic patients in Chapters 1 and 2, to endogenous depression in Chapter 9 and to the generalized epilepsy in Chapter 14. Once again, although essentially anecdoctal for the moment, we are convinced that the available data warrant a research effort in that direction.

The book is divided in 5 sections. The order of the sections follows an arbitrary but mentally comfortable top-down approach, beginning from behavioral data collected in humans and ending with the evidence of gene transcription during post-training sleep in the animal brain.

The experimental approach to the role of sleep in brain plasticity is multidimensional. This may render the material difficult to comprehend for some readers. Before each section, short introductory texts summarize the main points made in the section as well as the conceptual links, agreements, or disagreements between chapters. We hope these comments will help the reader to better grasp the unifying vision we want to put forward in this book.

Throughout the book, rapid eye movement sleep has been indifferently referred to as REM sleep or paradoxical sleep. Non-REM sleep is mentioned as NREM sleep. In humans, NREM sleep is further split into light sleep (stage 2 sleep) and slow wave sleep (SWS). In contrast, in many animal species (especially rodents), NREM sleep and SWS are synonymous.

We are grateful to Martin Baum and Lisa Catharine Blake, at Oxford University Press for their invaluable help in bringing this text to press. Pierre Maquet (Liège), Carlyle Smith (Peterborough), and Robert Stickgold (Boston).

CONTENTS

CONTRIBUTORS

T. Abel
Department of Biology,
University of Pennsylvania,
Philadelphia PA 19104,
USA

R. L. Ariagno
Division of Neonatal and Developmental
Medicine, Stanford University School of
Medicine, Stanford, California USA

C. A. Barnes
Departments of Psychology, and
Neurology, Arizona Research
Laboratories, Division of Neural Systems,
Memory and Aging, University of
Arizona, Tucson, Arizona, USA

F. P. Battaglia
Arizona Research Laboratories,
Division of Neural Systems,
Memory and Aging,
University of Arizona,
Tucson, Arizona, USA

J. Born
Department of Clinical
Neuroendocrinology, University of
Lübeck, Lübeck, Germany

M. R. Bower
Arizona Research Laboratories Division
of Neural Systems, Memory and Aging,
University of Arizona, Tucson,
Arizona, USA

G. Buzsáki
Center for Molecular and Behavioral
Neuroscience, Rutgers, The State
University of New Jersey, Newark,
New Jersey, USA

D. Carpi
Center for Molecular and Behavioral
Neuroscience, Rutgers, The State
University of New Jersey, Newark,
New Jersey, USA

L. Churchill
Department of Veterinary and
Comparative Anatomy, Pharmacology
and Physiology, Washington State
University, Pullman, Washington, USA

A. Cleeremans
Cognitive Science Research Unit,
Université Libre de Bruxelles, Belgium

S. L. Cowen
Arizona Research Laboratories, Division
of Neural Systems, Memory and Aging,
University of Arizona, Tucson,
Arizona, USA

J. Csicsvari
Center for Molecular and Behavioral
Neuroscience, Rutgers, The State
University of New Jersey, Newark,
New Jersey, USA

S. Datta
Sleep Research Laboratory, Department
of Psychiatry, and Program in Behavioral
Neuroscience, Boston University School
of Medicine, Boston, Massachusetts, USA

G. Dragoi
Center for Molecular and Behavioral
Neuroscience, Rutgers, The State
University of New Jersey, Newark,
New Jersey, USA

A. D. Ekstrom
Arizona Research Laboratories, Division
of Neural Systems, Memory and Aging,
University of Arizona, Tucson,
Arizona, USA

M. G. Frank
Department of Neuroscience, University
of Pennsylvania, School of Medicine,
Philadelphia, Pennsylvania, USA

S. Gais
Department of Clinical
Neuroendocrinology, University of
Lübeck, Lübeck, Germany

J. L. Gerrard
Arizona Research Laboratories, Division
of Neural Systems, Memory and Aging,
University of Arizona, Tucson,
Arizona, USA

A. Giuditta
Dipartimento di Fisiologia Generale ed
Ambientale, Università degli Studi di
Napoli "Federico II", and Interuniversity
Research Center for the Neurosciences,
Napoli, Italy

J. W. Harding
Department of Veterinary and
Comparative Anatomy, Pharmacology
and Physiology, Washington State
University, Pullman, Washington, USA

K. Harris
Center for Molecular and Behavioral
Neuroscience, Rutgers, The State
University of New Jersey, Newark,
New Jersey, USA

K. M. Hellman
Neuroscience Graduate Group University
of Pennsylvania, Philadelphia, USA

E. Hennevin
Laboratoire de Neurobiologie de
l'Apprentissage, de la Mémoire et de la
Communication, UMR CNRS 8620,
Université Paris-Sud, Orsay, France

D. Henze
Center for Molecular and Behavioral
Neuroscience, Rutgers, The State
University of New Jersey, Newark,
New Jersey, USA

H. Hirase
Center for Molecular and Behavioral
Neuroscience, Rutgers, The State
University of New Jersey, Newark,
New Jersey, USA

K. L. Hoffman
Arizona Research Laboratories, Division
of Neural Systems, Memory and Aging,
University of Arizona, Tucson,
Arizona, USA

F. P. Houston
Arizona Research Laboratories, Division
of Neural Systems, Memory and Aging,
University of Arizona, Tucson,
Arizona, USA

Y. Karten
Arizona Research Laboratories, Division
of Neural Systems, Memory and Aging,
University of Arizona, Tucson,
Arizona, USA

J. M. Krueger
Department of Veterinary and
Comparative Anatomy, Pharmacology
and Physiology, Washington State
University, Pullman, Washington, USA

S. Laureys
Cyclotron Research Centre,
University of Liège, Belgium

P. Lipa
Arizona Research Laboratories, Division
of Neural Systems, Memory and Aging,
University of Arizona, Tucson,
Arizona, USA

P. Mandile
Dipartimento di Fisiologia Generale ed
Ambientale, Università degli Studi di
Napoli "Federico II", Napoli, Italy

P. Maquet
Cyclotron Research Centre, University of
Liège, Belgium

B. L. McNaughton
Departments of Psychology, and
Physiology, Arizona Research
Laboratories Division of Neural Systems,
Memory and Aging, University of
Arizona, Tucson, Arizona, USA

M. Mirmiran
Netherlands Institute for Brain Research
and Division of Neonatal and
Developmental Medicine, Stanford
University School of Medicine, Stanford,
California, USA

P. Montagnese
Dipartimento di Fisiologia Generale ed
Ambientale, Università degli Studi di
Napoli "Federico II", Napoli, Italy

R. Nader
Department of Psychology, Trent
University, Peterborough, Ontario,
Canada

F. Obál Jr
Department of Physiology, University of
Szeged, A. Szent-Gyögyi Medical Center,
Szeged, Hungary

E. H. Patterson
Sleep Research Laboratory, Department
of Psychiatry, and Program in Behavioral
Neuroscience, Boston University School
of Medicine, Boston, Massachusetts, USA

C. Pavlides
The Rockefeller University, 1230 York
Avenue, New York, USA

P. Peigneux
Cyclotron Research Centre, University of
Liège, Belgium

C. M. A. Pennartz
The Netherlands Institute of Brain
Research, Amsterdam, Netherlands

S. Piscopo
Dipartimento di Fisiologia Generale ed
Ambientale, Università degli Studi di
Napoli "Federico II", Napoli, Italy

S. Ribeiro
Department of Neurobiology, Duke
University Medical Center, Durham,
North Carolina, USA

C. Smith
Department of Psychology, Trent
University, Peterborough, Ontario,
Canada

M. Steriade
Laboratory of Neurophysiology, School of
Medicine, Laval University, Québec,
Canada

R. Stickgold
Department of Psychiatry at the
Massachusetts Mental Health Center,
Harvard Medical School, Boston,
Massachussetts, USA

G. R. Sutherland
Arizona Research Laboratories, Division
of Neural Systems, Memory and Aging,
University of Arizona, Tucson,
Arizona, USA

M. P. Stryker
W. M. Keck Foundation Center for
Integrative Neuroscience and
Department of Physiology, University of
California, San Francisco, USA

I. Timofeev
Laboratory of Neurophysiology, School of
Medicine, Laval University, Québec,
Canada

S. Vescia
Dipartimento di Scienze Relazionali,
Università degli Studi di Napoli
"Federico II", Napoli, Italy

J. W. Wright
Department of Veterinary and
Comparative Anatomy,
Pharmacology and Physiology,
Washington State University, Pullman,
Washington, USA

INTRODUCTION

PIERRE MAQUET, CARLYLE SMITH, AND
ROBERT STICKGOLD

> It is possible to view [dreams]
> as containing [...] a reminder of a present state.
>
> Artemidorus, *Oneirocritica, 1,1.*

> Porro hominum mentes, magnis quae motibus edunt
> magna, itidem saepe in somnis faciuntque geruntque
> (Again, the minds of mortals which perform
> with mighty motions mighty enterprises,
> often in sleep will do and dare the same in manner like).
>
> Lucretius, *De Natura Rerum, Book IV.*

The hypothesis

The function of sleep remains unknown despite our rapidly increasing understanding of the processes generating and maintaining sleep. A number of nonmutually exclusive hypotheses have been proposed for sleep function: energy conservation (Berger and Phillips 1995), brain thermoregulation (McGinty and Szymusiak 1990), brain detoxification (Inoue *et al.* 1995), tissue "restoration" (Adam and Oswald 1977).... Another hypothesis, with which we are dealing in this book, proposes that *sleep is favorable for brain plasticity.*

Brain plasticity refers to the ability of the brain to persistently change its structure and function according to the genetic information, in response to environmental changes or to comply with the interaction between these two factors (Chen and Tonegawa 1997; Kolb and Whishaw 1998). By facilitating brain plasticity, sleep would allow the organism to adapt its behavior to the circumstances, within the constraints set by species-specific genetic material. Various variants of this hypothesis have been articulated. The first one stressed the importance of sleep for brain development. The large amount of sleep observed during the perinatal period and infancy suggests its involvement in *brain maturation* (Roffwarg *et al.* 1966).

Another version of the hypothesis claims that sleep helps to maintain infrequently used cerebral networks (Krueger and Obal 1993; Kavanau 1997). With the phylogenetic increase in brain complexity, the amount of information necessary to retain both hereditary behavioral traits (Jouvet 1978; Kavanau 1997) and novel behavior acquired through experience (Kavanau 1997) expands. Maintaining the circuitry encoding these two kinds of information would require their "dynamic stabilization" through the reactivation of the corresponding neuronal assemblies. This could not be done during wakefulness because it would interfere with the processing of incoming stimuli and with waking behavior (Krueger and Obal 1993). In contrast, sleep processes would provide the necessary isolation from the external world to permit the dynamic stabilization program. Despite a sound theoretical basis and evidence from comparative biology, this hypothesis is difficult to test experimentally. For practical reasons, infrequently used neuronal networks are not easily isolated. Furthermore, because of the uncertainty about when reactivation might occur, testing this hypothesis would require monitoring them over long periods of time. However, there are neuronal networks that have been infrequently used and can still be efficiently studied, those which have recently been coping with a new waking experience. In this third version of the hypothesis, sleep mechanisms would be involved in learning and memory. This situation is more amenable to experimental testing for two reasons. First, we have now a sufficient knowledge of how memory systems segregate within the brain and, second, the sequence of events is easily controlled. Three main steps may be operationally described: exposure to the new stimulus, processing of memory traces, and performance at retest. In this design, sleep has been primarily involved in processing of memory traces. The usually held view is that *sleep processes participate in the consolidation of the memory traces*. Consolidation refers here to the processing of memory traces during which "the traces may be reactivated, analysed and gradually incorporated into long-term memory" (McGaugh 2000; Sutherland and McNaughton 2000). Following this hypothesis, the memory trace would stay in a fragile state until the first postexposure sleep period has occurred (Fishbein and Gutwein 1977).

The role of sleep in learning and memory: a short historical overview

The early days

The idea that sleep might be involved in memory processes is not new and was undoubtedly suggested by the bits and pieces of memories that are incorporated in our dreams. Although first suggested in the scientific literature by Jackson (1951), the possible relationship between sleep and memory is classically considered to begin with the observation by Ebbinghaus that the rate of forgetting of nonsense syllables is less pronounced in the period from 8 to 24 h after learning, that is, at a time at which the subject slept, than during the initial post-training period (1–8 h after learning) (Ebbinghaus 1885). He originally believed that this observation was an artifact but it was subsequently confirmed. As early as 1914, Heine reported that nonsense syllables learned just before going to bed were better recalled after 24 h than those with a waking period interpolated between learning and sleep (47 percent savings instead of 36 percent, respectively) (Heine 1914). Although sometimes observed only 48 or 144 h after training (Graves

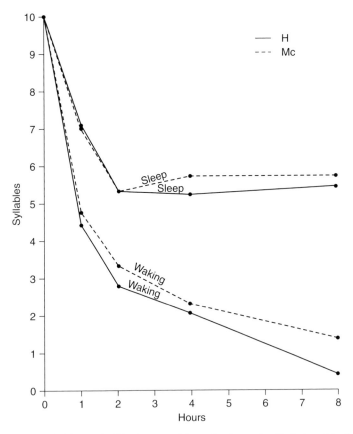

Figure 1 Number of syllables retained by the two subjects after intervals of 1, 2, 4, or 8 h of waking or sleep. (Original figure from Jenkins and Dallenbach 1924.)

1937; Richardson and Gough 1963), the favorable effect of sleep on recent memories was reported by a number of authors (Radossawljewitsch 1907; Foucault 1913; Jenkins and Dallenbach 1924; van Ormer 1932; Lovatt and Warr 1968; Fig. 1). The same effect was observed by Nicolai for the memory of objects (Nicolai 1922).

Several of these observations were made on very few subjects, one of the subjects being the author him/her-self in a number of reports (Ebbinghaus, Heine, Graves, Jenkins, and Dallenbach, and others), and of course, without any check on sleep structure. However, their contribution was important for two reasons. First, they revealed the fundamental effect of sleep on memory. Second, they already spotted several basic experimental difficulties in the study of the effect of sleep on memory such as the circadian fluctuation in learning and performance (Finkenbinder 1913; Lovatt and Warr 1968).

Because sleep was seen as a state of cerebral quiescence, the interpretation of these results was essentially that sleep hampered any significant interference between the recently encoded material and the continuous flow of external inputs.

A period of doubt

In the 1950s, with the discovery of rapid eye movement (REM) sleep, sleep was no longer a homogeneous state of passive rest for the brain. On the contrary, sleep, and especially REM sleep, appeared as an active condition of intense cerebral activity. The experiments were refined and looked for specific effects of the different newly described sleep stages on recent memory traces using various experimental designs. At this time, much of the research effort was put on REM sleep, because (i) it was easily recognized on polygraphic recordings, (ii) selective deprivation of REM sleep was relatively easy in animals, (iii) as an active brain state, it was more likely to modify memory traces, and (iv) it was related to dreaming in humans.

It was quickly discovered that the ontogenetic development of sleep was characterized by a large amount of sleep, especially REM sleep in neonate and infants (Roffwarg *et al.* 1966). The hypothesis was proposed that REM sleep would provide an endogenous source of activation, possibly critical for structural maturation of the central nervous system. This proposal led to a series of experiments looking at the role of sleep in brain development (see Section III).

In adults unfortunately, for the following 20 years, the situation far from being clarified with the description of sleep heterogeneity, became very confusing. A number of divergent results were published, which cast some doubts on the functional role of sleep in memory. For instance, while some groups reported that pre-training and post-training sleep deprivation alters respectively the acquisition or the retention of new material, negative results were simultaneously published, using the same species, the same task, and apparently the same experimental design (McGrath and Cohen 1978; Smith 1985).

The reasons for these discrepant results were different in human studies than in animal experiments. The animal literature has already been extensively reviewed in a number of papers and books (Drucker-Colin and McGaugh 1977; Fishbein and Gutwein 1977; Pearlman 1979; Fishbein 1981; Smith 1985; Hennevin *et al.* 1995; Smith 1995; Maquet 2001; Peigneux *et al.* 2001). We focus here the main experimental factors that were put forward to explain this confusing situation. This will help the reader to position the data summarized in subsequent chapters in relation to these debates.

First, it was suggested that tasks which rely on pre-existing species-specific skills were insensitive to post-training sleep deprivation. This "prepared learning" (Seligman 1970; Pearlman 1979) was thought to be hard-wired in the brain. Learning these tasks would not need any major post-training adjustment in brain circuitry. In contrast, tasks requiring assimilation of unusual information and leading to important modification of behavior could not be acquired if the animal was sleep-deprived after training. These tasks were usually difficult to learn and needed many trials before performance significantly improved. The gain in performance in these tasks was thought to rely on plastic changes in the brain. These brain changes would take time and sleep would provide favorable conditions to these modifications to occur.

Second, different species were used. Tasks that were sensitive to sleep deprivation in one species were not necessarily so in another species. For instance, the retention of a two-way avoidance task is disturbed by post-training REM sleep deprivation in rats (for instance in Leconte and Bloch 1970) but not in mice (Sagales and Domino 1973; Fishbein and Gutwein 1977). This can even be observed in different strains of the same species. In mice of the C57 brown strain, an increase in the amount of REM sleep is observed within a few days after the beginning of the training period, in parallel with an improvement of performance. In contrast, training C57 black mice to the same task is not followed by any change in behavior or of sleep structure in the same time frame (Smith *et al.* 1972). The latter observation indicates the importance of the genetic background in learning, memory and sleep rather than infirming the hypothesis.

Third, the temporal organization of the experiment is critical. For instance, post-training REM sleep deprivation deteriorates the performance of rats on the two-way shuttle avoidance task only if administered right after the training session (Leconte *et al.* 1974). Post-training REM sleep deprivation delayed by an hour after training has no detrimental effect on subsequent performance. Critical periods at which REM sleep deprivation has been shown to significantly alter the retention of the material not only occur right after training but also several hours, and days afterwards (Smith 1985). These so-called REM sleep windows are placed in time differently, depending on the strain of animals, the task, and the temporal distribution of training sessions. REM sleep deprivation outside these windows does not deteriorate learning.

Fourth, the validity of the method for REM sleep deprivation was questioned. The most popular technique used an inverted flower pot emerging in the middle of a pool of water. Placed on the platform, the animal could sustain near normal periods of non-REM (NREM) sleep, but could get very little REM sleep because the muscular atonia would let it fall in the water and wake it up. Control animals were usually put on larger platforms, allowing near normal amounts of sleep. It was realized that the optimal platform size to obtain a significant reduction of REM sleep duration was dependent on the weight of the animal. In most studies failing to report the detrimental effect of REM sleep deprivation on a recent learning, the ratio of the animal weight to the platform area was not different enough between experimental and control animals to allow any clear-cut distinction between the groups (McGrath and Cohen 1978).

Finally, it was argued that the deleterious effects of sleep deprivation on learning was due to nonspecific effects, and especially to the associated stress response. Because stress is an important confound, we delay its discussion to a later section of this chapter on remaining issues.

In humans, the influence of sleep on memory remained uncertain because the respective role of NREM sleep and REM sleep in memory processing was, and is still, unclear. As a rule, tasks such as learning syllables, paired associates, sentences, or prose passages were extensively used to investigate this issue. The favorable effect of sleep on retention was first observed by Ekstrand (1967). However, it has never been clear which sleep stage was most intimately linked to this effect. Deprivation of slow wave sleep (SWS) was shown to be more deleterious than REM sleep deprivation for the learning of paired associates (Barrett and Ekstrand 1972; Fowler *et al.* 1973). REM sleep deprivation had also a negative effect on retention (Empson and Clarke 1970), although a more moderate one, on learning this task (Barrett and Ekstrand 1972; Fowler *et al.* 1973). In keeping with these results, Yaroush *et al.* (1971) showed that the retention of paired associates was better after the early night sleep than after late night sleep. Because of the physiological predominance of SWS in the first part of the night and of REM sleep on the second part of the night, these results suggested again that the retention of the material was facilitated by SWS. However, there were conflicting results reporting the absence of effect of sleep deprivation on the learning of paired associates (Chernik 1972; Castaldo *et al.* 1974) or that REM sleep deprivation had more impact on retention of stories than SWS deprivation (Tilley and Empson 1978).

In the same time, increases in REM sleep have been reported following training in various experiments: conditioning in infants (Paul and Dittrichova 1974), trampolining (Buchegger and Meier-Koll 1988), intensive learning of a foreign language (De Koninck *et al.* 1989), Morse code learning (Mandai *et al.* 1989) and visual field inversion (De Koninck and Prevost 1991; but see Allen *et al.* 1972).

One possible explanation of these discrepancies is that NREM sleep and REM sleep act differently on different memory systems (dual process hypothesis). Unfortunately, the distinction of the main memory systems took some time to transpire into the field of sleep research. The tasks mentioned above involve a variable proportion of implicit and explicit processes, depending on the task and the experimental protocol (material to be learned, depth of encoding, type of retention test, etc.). Another possibility, suggested recently, is that the effect of sleep on memory depends on the temporal sequence of NREM sleep and REM sleep phases (double-step hypothesis, see Chapters 2, 3, and 8).

Finally, many of these experiments were criticized because the effect of circadian rhythms was confounding the results (Barrett and Ekstrand 1972; Hockey *et al.* 1972). The discussion on this potential confound is reported in the last section of this chapter.

The new data

More recently, the positive effects of sleep on recent memory traces were confirmed by an increasing number of publications using refined experimental designs and new techniques of investigations, at several levels of descriptions. They form the bulk of this book. In humans, the clever choice of cognitive tasks has allowed a better characterization of the respective role of NREM sleep and REM sleep in the learning of explicit and implicit memory tasks, respectively (Chapters 2 and 3). Light NREM sleep (stage 2 sleep) has now been shown to be also involved in certain types of memory (Chapters 2 and 4). The possible importance of the succession of NREM sleep and REM sleep has recently been emphasized (Chapters 2 and 3). Recent research has also reinvigorated the study of dreams, especially in relation to memory processes (Chapter 1). At the macroscopic systems levels, experience-dependent brain activities were described by positron emission tomography (Chapter 11).

In animals, further evidence for the importance of REM sleep has been reported during brain development (Chapter 9) and for learning and memory in adults (Chapters 5 and 6). Phasic activities such as the pontine waves were suggested to play an important role in the processing of memory traces in REM sleep (Chapter 7). Likewise, the observation of hippocampal ensembles replaying similar sequences of firing to those observed during previous waking periods suggests a mechanism that might be operating at the microscopic systems level (Louie and Wilson 2001). At the cellular level, an experience-dependent genetic transcription has now been observed during REM sleep in the rat brain (Chapter 16).

The importance of NREM sleep has also been emphasized. During brain development in kittens, SWS seems critical to the plastic reorganization which follows monocular deprivation (Chapter 10). In adults, hippocampal ensembles were shown to fire in an experience-dependent manner during NREM sleep, replaying sequences present during previous waking activity (Chapters 12 and 13). Plastic changes in neuronal firing patterns were also characterized in thalamo-cortical networks during spindles (Chapter 14). At the cellular level, various compounds are released in the brain in task-specific, activity-dependent manner, some of these compounds participating in local cerebral plasticity during sleep (Chapter 17)

Finally, new perspectives are opened by the data suggesting the important role of the temporal succession of NREM sleep and REM sleep periods in the consolidation of recent memory traces (Chapters 2, 3, and 8).

Perspectives

Sleep: definition and scope

Sleep is a physiological, complex, integrated behavior characterized by a significant reduction of the response to the external stimuli, by a characteristic posture, usually in a special environment, by a characteristic change in the neurophysiological recordings of brain acitivity and by a homeostatic increase after its restriction (Tobler 1995). This operational definition is not sufficient to provide a clear answer to the question: "Does sleep play a role in learning and memory?" The question breaks into several different issues. The basic issue is probably whether the patterns of neuronal activity characteristic of sleep are favorable to the consolidation of recently encoded information or, in other words, to the reinforcement of cellular networks recently challenged by new environmental conditions. Equally important is the question asking whether specific neuromodulatory contexts of the sleeping brain influence memory processing. For instance, the importance of the prominent cholinergic drive in REM sleep has been suggested as an important factor favoring plastic brain changes (Hasselmo 1999). Likewise, the role of general (hormones) or local (cytokines, growth factors) humoral contexts prevailing during sleep in brain plasticity remain to be fully understood (see Chapters 3 and 17).

Not only are the answers to these questions fragmentary but the integration of the results at different levels of description is still lacking. For instance, it is not yet known whether the expression of gene transcription products, or the replay of hippocampal firing sequences during sleep entail that memory traces are modified in such a drastic way that the subsequent individual behavior will be detectably and reliably modified.

Remaining issues

The central issue is thus to understand the sequences of events underlying the consolidation of memory traces. This implies the characterization of the time course and functional relationships between various processes including experience-dependent gene transcription, protein synthesis, neuronal firing patterns, and synaptic function, both during the post-training waking period and during the subsequent sleep. The relationships between these processes and subsequent changes in behavior have also to be specified.

Besides this central question, two main issues remain to be thoroughly investigated.

First, the sleep/activity cycle is regulated by the interaction between circadian and homeostatic processes. At present, special care has taken to rule out a circadian effect on the learning phase (Barrett and Ekstrand 1972; Hockey et al. 1972; see Chapters 2 and 3 for recent data). However, the respective role of circadian and homeostatic processes in the reprocessing of memory traces during sleep has yet to be investigated. Up to now, the effect of sleep on recent memory has mainly been investigated in a certain circadian phase (i.e. during the night). It is not yet known if sleep outside this circadian phase will be as effective in consolidating memory traces. Yet, some parameters are known to be both under circadian control and involved in memory consolidation. For instance, the release of cortisol results from the interaction between the output of the circadian pacemaker, light exposure, and the timing of sleep and wakefulness (Czeisler and Klerman 1999). In the same time, cortisol is known to modulate memory consolidation in humans (Plihal and Born 1999; Plihal et al. 1999). Further research should disentangle the respective effects of circadian and sleep factors (or their interaction) on the processing of memory traces.

Second, the issue of stress has been recurrently invoked against the hypothesis of the influence of sleep on memory. The stress argument was raised both in sleep deprivation studies and in studies of the effects of learning on post-training sleep structure. In rodents, the detrimental effects of sleep deprivation on memory was attributed to stress rather than to the lack of sleep (Vertes 2000). As mentioned earlier, this discussion stemmed from the widespread use of the flower pot method for REM sleep deprivation. This technique was indeed shown to be stressful and to modify the post-deprivation activity in rats (Albert et al. 1970). It is fair to say that there are now a number of studies that can rule out this sleep-independent stress effect. For instance, pharmacological REM sleep deprivation, having admittedly its own shortcomings but eschewing the stress effect, was shown to be as effective as mechanical means in altering the retention of a newly learned task (Pearlman and Becker 1974). The demonstration of REM sleep windows is another strong argument against a stress effect. In these studies, although all the animals were submitted to the same amount of stress, the post-deprivation performance was altered or not, depending on the period at which REM sleep deprivation was performed (Smith and Butler 1982; Smith 1985, 1995; see also Chapter 6).

It was also argued that in animals, learning some tasks such as avoidance tasks, would be stressful. In this case, the post-training increase in REM sleep would be due to stress rather than learning. This suggestion is unlikely given that control and slow learning animals did not show any significant REM sleep rebound despite their exposure to the same (or even more) stressful experimental conditions (Hennevin *et al.* 1995).

Despite these experimental arguments, subtle links have been discovered between sleep, learning, memory and stress. First, stress modifies sleep/wakefulness cycles. In rodents, acute immobilization induces a significant increase in REM sleep during the dark period (Rampin *et al.* 1991). A more moderate increase in SWS has also been reported in similar conditions (Vazquez-Palacios and Velazquez-Moctezuma 2000; Koehl *et al.* 2002). The REM sleep increase parallels the secretion of corticotropic peptides (Bonnet *et al.* 2000) and can be induced by their administration (Gonzalez and Valatx 1997). Importantly, in rodents, the dose and time course of corticosterone release may modulate the effect of stress of subsequent sleep. After an initial alerting effect, corticosterone increases SWS at low doses but has the reverse effect at higher doses in rodents (Vazquez-Palacios *et al.* 2001). In humans, the available data indicate that glucocorticoids reduce REM sleep and SWS (Fehm *et al.* 1986; Born *et al.* 1987, 1991).

Second, stress hormones regulate the processing of memory traces. It is usually considered that while persistent stress has deleterious effects on memory, acute stress enhances the formation of new memories (Roozendaal 2000) and glucocorticoids have been involved in the consolidation of recent emotional memories (McGaugh *et al.* 1996). Intriguingly, the favorable influence of late night sleep, rich in REM sleep, has been observed in the formation of emotional memory in humans (Wagner *et al.* 2001).

Although these elements are obviousaly fragmentary, they warrant futher research to disentangle the effects of sleep, stress, and their interaction on recent memory traces.

Conclusions

The role of sleep in memory trace processing remains to be confirmed. The characterization of task-dependent regionally specific brain activities during post-training sleep should be pursued, at different levels of cerebral organization. They should be shown to be related to long-lasting behavioral adaptation. The specific role of sleep (i.e. sleep discharge patterns) in memory processing should be disentangled from other effects like experimentally induced stress or circadian modifications. Finally, the respective influence of SWS and REM sleep on the memory trace should be specified.

References

Adam, K. and **Oswald, I.** (1977). Sleep is for tissue restoration. *Journal of Royal College of Physicians of London*, **11**, 376–388.

Albert, I. B., Cicala, G. A., and **Siegel, J.** (1970). The behavioral effects of REM sleep deprivation in rats. *Psychophysiology*, **6**, 550–560.

Allen, S. R., Oswald, I., Lewis, S., and Tafney, J. (1972). The effects of distorted visual input on sleep. *Psychophysiology*, **9**, 498–504.

Barrett, T. R. and Ekstrand, B. R. (1972). Effect of sleep on memory. 3. Controlling for time-of-day effects. *Journal of Experimental Psychology*, **96**, 321–327.

Berger, R. J. and Phillips, N. H. (1995). Energy conservation and sleep. *Behavioural Brain Research*, **69**, 65–73.

Bonnet, C., Marinesco, S., Debilly, G., Kovalzon, V., and Cespuglio, R. (2000). Influence of a 1-h immobilization stress on sleep and CLIP (ACTH(18–39)) brain contents in adrenalectomized rats. *Brain Research*, **853**, 323–329.

Born, J., Zwick, A., Roth, G., Fehm-Wolfsdorf, G., and Fehm, H. L. (1987). Differential effects of hydrocortisone, fluocortolone, and aldosterone on nocturnal sleep in humans. *Acta Endocrinologica (Copenhagen)*, **116**, 129–137.

Born, J., DeKloet, E. R., Wenz, H., Kern, W., and Fehm, H. L. (1991). Gluco- and antimineralo-corticoid effects on human sleep: a role of central corticosteroid receptors. *American Journal of Physiology*, **260**, E183–188.

Buchegger, J. and Meier-Koll, A. (1988). Motor learning and ultradian sleep cycle: an electroencephalographic study of trampoliners. *Perceptual and Motor Skills*, **67**, 635–645.

Castaldo, V., Krynicki, V., and Goldstein, J. (1974). Sleep stages and verbal memory. *Perceptual and Motor Skills*, **39**, 1023–1030.

Chen, C. and Tonegawa, S. (1997). Molecular genetic analysis of synaptic plasticity, activity-dependent neural development, learning, and memory in the mammalian brain. *Annual Review of Neuroscience*, **20**, 157–184.

Chernik, D. A. (1972). Effect of REM sleep deprivation on learning and recall by humans. *Perceptual Motor Skills*, **34**, 283–294.

Czeisler, C. A. and Klerman, E. B. (1999). Circadian and sleep-dependent regulation of hormone release in humans. *Recent Progress in Hormone Research*, **54**, 97–130; discussion 130–132.

De Koninck, J. and Prevost, F. (1991). Paradoxical sleep and information processing: exploration by inversion of the visual field. *Canadian Journal of Psychology*, **45**, 125–139.

De Koninck, J., Lorrain, D., Christ, G., Proulx, G., and Coulombe, D. (1989). Intensive language learning and increases in rapid eye movement sleep: evidence of a performance factor. *International Journal of Psychophysiology*, **8**, 43–47.

Drucker-Colin, R. R. and McGaugh, J. L. (eds) (1977). *Neurobiology of sleep and memory.* Academic Press, New York.

Ebbinghaus, H. (1885). Über das Gedachtnis.Untersuchungen zur Experimentellen Psychologie. Leipzig: Duncker und Humblot.

Ekstrand, B. R. (1967). Effect of sleep on memory. *Journal of Experimental Psychology*, **75**, 64–72.

Empson, J. A. and Clarke, P. R. (1970). Rapid eye movements and remembering. *Nature*, **227**, 287–288.

Fehm, H. L., Benkowitsch, R., Kern, W., Fehm-Wolfsdorf, G., Pauschinger, P., and Born, J. (1986). Influences of corticosteroids, dexamethasone and hydrocortisone on sleep in humans. *Neuropsychobiology*, **16**, 198–204.

Finkenbinder, E. O. (1913). The curve of forgetting. *American Journal of Psychology*, **24**, 8–32.

Fishbein, W. (ed) (1981). *Sleep, dreaming and memory: advance in sleep research.* Spectrum, New York.

Fishbein, W. and Gutwein, B. M. (1977). Paradoxical sleep and memory storage processes. *Behavioural Biology*, **19**, 425–464.

Foucault, M. M. (1913). Introduction à la psychologie de la perception: Expérience sur l'oubli ou l'inhibition régressive. *Revue des Cours et Conférences 21 série*, **1**, 444–454.

Fowler, M. J., Sullivan, M. J., and Ekstrand, B. R. (1973). Sleep and memory. *Science*, **179**, 302–304.

Gonzalez, M. M. and Valatx, J. L. (1997). Effect of intracerebroventricular administration of alpha-helical CRH (9–41) on the sleep/waking cycle in rats under normal conditions or after subjection to an acute stressful stimulus. *Journal of Sleep Research*, **6**, 164–170.

Graves, E. A. (1937). The effect of sleep upon retention. *Journal of Experimental Psychology*, **19**, 316–322.

Hasselmo, M. E. (1999). Neuromodulation: acetylcholine and memory consolidation. *Trends in Cognitive Sciences*, **3**, 351–359.

Heine, R. (1914). Über der Wiedererkennen und rückwirkende Hemmung. *Zeitschrift für Psychologie*, **68**, 161–236.

Hennevin, E., Hars, B., Maho, C., and Bloch, V. (1995). Processing of learned information in paradoxical sleep: relevance for memory. *Behavioural Brain Research*, **69**, 125–135.

Hockey, G. R. J., Davies, S., and Gray, M. M. (1972). Forgetting as a function of sleep at different times of day. *Quaterly Journal of Experimental Psychology*, **24**, 386–393.

Inoue, S., Honda, K., and Komoda, Y. (1995). Sleep as neuronal detoxification and restitution. *Behavioural Brain Research*, **69**, 91–96.

Jackson, J. H. (1951). *Selected writings of John Hughlings Jackson.* Basic Books, New York.

Jenkins, J. G. and Dallenbach, K. M. (1924). Obliviscence during sleep and waking. *American Journal of Psychology*, **35**, 605–612.

Jouvet, M. (1978). Is paradoxical sleep responsible for a genetic programming of the brain? *Comptes Rendus des Séances de la Sociétié de Biologic et de ses Filiales*, **172**, 9–32.

Kavanau, J. L. (1997). Memory, sleep and the evolution of mechanisms of synaptic efficacy maintenance. *Neuroscience*, **79**, 7–44.

Koehl, M., Bouyer, J. J., Darnaudery, M., Le Moal, M., and Mayo, W. (2002). The effect of restraint stress on paradoxical sleep is influenced by the circadian cycle. *Brain Research*, **937**, 45–50.

Kolb, B. and Whishaw, I. Q. (1998). Brain plasticity and behavior. *Annual Review of Psychology*, **49**, 43–64.

Krueger, J. M. and Obal, F. (1993). A neuronal group theory of sleep function. *Journal of Sleep Research*, **2**, 63–69.

Leconte, P. and Bloch, V. (1970). Déficit de la rétention d'un conditionnement après privation de sommeil paradoxal chez le Rat. *Comptes Rendus de l' Académic Sciences de Paris*, **271**, 226–229.

Leconte, P., Hennevin, E., and Bloch, V. (1974). Duration of paradoxical sleep necessary for the acquisition of conditioned avoidance in the rat. *Physiology and Behaviour*, **13**, 675–681.

Louie, K. and Wilson, M. A. (2001). Temporally structured replay of awake hippocampal ensemble activity during rapid eye movement sleep. *Neuron*, **29**, 145–156.

Lovatt, D. J. and Warr, P. B. (1968). Recall after sleep. *American Journal of Psychology*, **81**, 253–257.

Mandai, O., Guerrien, A., Sockeel, P., Dujardin, K., and Leconte, P. (1989). REM sleep modifications following a Morse code learning session in humans. *Physiology and Behaviour*, **46**, 639–642.

Maquet, P. (2001). The Role of Sleep in Learning and Memory. *Science*, **294**, 1048–1052.

McGaugh, J. L. (2000). Memory—a century of consolidation. *Science*, **287**, 248–251.

McGaugh, J. L., Cahill, L., and Roozendaal, B. (1996). Involvement of the amygdala in memory storage: interaction with other brain systems. *Proceedings of the National Academy of Sciences, USA*, **93**, 13508–13514.

McGinty, D. and Szymusiak, R. (1990). Keeping cool: a hypothesis about the mechanisms and functions of slow-wave sleep. *Trends in Neuroscience*, **13**, 480–487.

McGrath, M. J. and Cohen, D. B. (1978). REM sleep facilitation of adaptive waking behavior: a review of the literature. *Psychology Bulletin*, **85**, 24–57.

Nicolai, F. (1922). Experimentelle Untersuchung über das Haften von Gesicheindrücken und dessen zeitlichen Verlauf. *Archiv für die gesamte Psychologie*, **42**, 132–149.

Paul, K. and Dittrichova, J. (1974). Sleep patterns following learning in infants. In *Sleep*, pp. 388–390. Karger, Basel.

Pearlman, C. (1979). REM sleep and information processing: evidence from animal studies. *Neuroscience and Biobehavioral Reviews*, **3**, 57–68.

Pearlman, C. and Becker, M. (1974). REM sleep deprivation impairs bar-press acquisition in rats. *Physiology and Behaviour*, **13**, 813–817.

Peigneux, P., Laureys, S., Delbeuck, X., and Maquet, P. (2001). Sleeping brain, learning brain. The role of sleep for memory systems. *Neuroreport*, **12**, A111–124.

Plihal, W. and Born, J. (1999). Memory consolidation in human sleep depends on inhibition of glucocorticoid release. *Neuroreport*, **10**, 2741–2747.

Plihal, W., Pietrowsky, R., and Born, J. (1999). Dexamethasone blocks sleep induced improvement of declarative memory. *Psychoneuroendocrinology*, **24**, 313–331.

Radossawljewitsch, P. R. (1907). Das Behalten und Vergessen bei Kindern und Erwachsenen nach Experimentellen Untersuchungen. Otto Nemnich Verlag, Leipzig.

Rampin, C., Cespuglio, R., Chastrette, N., and Jouvet, M. (1991). Immobilisation stress induces a paradoxical sleep rebound in rat. *Neuroscience Letters*, **126**, 113–118.

Richardson, A. and Gough, J. E. (1963). The long range effect of sleep on retention. *Australian Journal of Psychology*, **15**, 37–41.

Roffwarg, H. P., Muzio, J. N., and Dement, W. C. (1966). Ontogenetic development of the human sleep–dream cycle. *Science*, **152**, 604–618.

Roozendaal, B. (2000). 1999 Curt P. Richter award. Glucocorticoids and the regulation of memory consolidation. *Psychoneuroendocrinology*, **25**, 213–238.

Sagales, T. and **Domino, E. F.** (1973). Effects of stress and REM sleep deprivation on the patterns of avoidance learning and brain acetylcholine in the mouse. *Psychopharmacologia*, **29**, 307–315.

Seligman, M. E. P. (1970). On the generality of the laws of learning. *Psychological Review*, **77**, 406–418.

Smith, C. (1985). Sleep states and learning: a review of the animal literature. *Neuroscience and Biobehavioural Reviews*, **9**, 157–168.

Smith, C. (1995). Sleep states and memory processes. *Behavioural Brain Research*, **69**, 137–145.

Smith, C. and **Butler, S.** (1982). Paradoxical sleep at selective times following training is necessary for learning. *Physiology and Behaviour*, **29**, 469–473.

Smith, C. T., Kitahama, K., Valatx, J. L., and **Jouvet, M.** (1972). Sommeil paradoxal et apprentissage chez deux souches consanguines de souris. *Comptes Rendus de l' Académie des Sciences de Paris 275 série*, **D**, 1283–1286.

Sutherland, G. R. and **McNaughton, B.** (2000). Memory trace reactivation in hippocampal and neocortical neuronal ensembles. *Current Opinion in Neurobiology*, **10**, 180–186.

Tilley, A. J. and **Empson, J. A.** (1978). REM sleep and memory consolidation. *Biological Psychology*, **6**, 293–300.

Tobler, I. (1995). Is sleep fundamentally different between mammalian species? *Behavioural Brain Research*, **69**, 35–41.

van Ormer, E. B. (1932). Retention after intervals of sleep and of waking. *Archives of Psychology*, **21**, 5–49.

Vazquez-Palacios, G. and **Velazquez-Moctezuma, J.** (2000). Effect of electric foot shocks, immobilization, and corticosterone administration on the sleep-wake pattern in the rat. *Physiology and Behaviour*, **71**, 23–28.

Vazquez-Palacios, G., Retana-Marquez, S., Bonilla-Jaime, H., and **Velazquez-Moctezuma, J.** (2001). Further definition of the effect of corticosterone on the sleep–wake pattern in the male rat. *Pharmacology, Biochemistry and Behaviour*, **70**, 305–310.

Vertes, R. (2000). The case against memory consolidation in REM sleep. *Behavioural Brain Science*, **23**, 867–876.

Wagner, U., Gais, S., and **Born, J.** (2001). Emotional memory formation is enhanced across sleep intervals with high amounts of rapid eye movement sleep. *Learning and Memory*, **8**, 112–119.

Yaroush, R., Sullivan, M. J., and **Ekstrand, B. R.** (1971). Effect of sleep on memory. II. Differential effect of the first and second half of the night. *Journal of Experimental Psychology*, **88**, 361–366.

HUMAN BEHAVIOR

The chapters of this section are concerned with the evidence relating memory processes to sleep states using human subjects. Understanding this relationship is probably the greatest and most interesting challenge of all. It is the greatest challenge because it is here that we must deal not only with the states of sleep, but also with their mental content. It is the most interesting challenge because it applies directly to our own lives. Robert Stickgold from Harvard University (USA) begins the section with a fascinating chapter on sleep mentation and its possible relationship to memory processes (Chapter 1). He provides a review of the studies that have attempted to relate waking activity to subsequent sleep mentation, differentiating between non-rapid eye movement (NREM) and rapid eye movement (REM) sleep mental activity. Among the numerous methodological problems involved in doing this research, it is clear that getting consistent incorporation of waking events into subsequent dreams and being able to identify these incorporations rank among the most serious. However, a new approach, involving hypnagogic dreaming is introduced. This sleep onset mental imagery following task acquisition results in a much higher rate of incorporation and provides a first step to understanding how mental activity eventually appears during subsequent REM sleep periods.

In Chapter 2, the same author examines the relationship between sleep states and memory for a visual search task. Results implicate both NREM sleep and REM sleep as being involved in off-line memory processing. In more recent work, it was found that Stage 2 sleep was related to memory for a recently learned finger tapping task.

Chapter 3 is provided by Drs Born and Gais of the University of Lübeck (Germany). They bring an interesting research paradigm to the area. They examine the degree of memory processing following the first half of the night (the bulk of which is deep NREM sleep) compared to the memory processing in the second half of the night (which is composed mostly of REM sleep). They compare the memory for various types of acquired tasks after these two time intervals. They have found that declarative or episodic material is enhanced after a session of NREM sleep, while procedural/implicit or emotional material is not. On the other hand, memory for procedural/implicit and emotional material is enhanced after a session of REM sleep, but not after NREM sleep. The role of neuroendocrine and neurotransmitter processes is examined.

In Chapter 4 by Rebecca Nader and Carlyle Smith of Trent University (Canada), the focus is on stage 2 sleep. While we spend 50 percent of our nights in this state of sleep, its functions are not well understood. This chapter provides a brief history of the research examining stage 2 sleep, with an emphasis on cognitive studies. This is followed by a number of recent findings that implicate the importance of stage 2 for memory of certain kinds of tasks and the authors focus on the stage 2 spindle. The spindle, a basic component of mammalian sleep, may indeed be a perfect time for synaptic plasticity to take place.

CHAPTER 1

MEMORY, COGNITION, AND DREAMS

ROBERT STICKGOLD

Recent developments in the fields of molecular genetics, neurophysiology, and the cognitive neurosciences, have produced a striking body of research, involving humans, rats, mice, and birds, that provide converging evidence for a fundamental role of sleep in the reprocessing of memories (Smith 1985, 1995; Hennevin *et al.* 1995; Stickgold 1998; Maquet 2001; Stickgold *et al.* 2001). One approach, which seeks to identify waking tasks that are modified by sleep, has provided strong evidence that sleep plays an important role in the consolidation of procedural learning, as measured with both perceptual and motor tasks. In addition, a more clinically oriented literature suggests that sleep also plays an important role in coping with emotional stress (Cartwright *et al.* 1969, 1984, 1998a,b, 2001; Grieser *et al.* 1972; Greenberg and Pearlman 1974; van der Kolk *et al.* 1984; Kramer *et al.* 1987; Lauer *et al.* 1987; Berger *et al.* 1988; Cartwright 1991; Kramer 1993; Reynolds *et al.* 1993; Hartmann 1998; Newell and Cartwright 2000; Rothbaum and Mellman, 2001). A second approach has been to characterize neurophysiological functioning during sleep (Table 1.1).

Table 1.1 Physiological correlates of sleep states. Some of the changes in brain physiology and chemistry seen across the REM sleep–NREM sleep cycle are listed

Physiological correlates of sleep	REM sleep	Stage 2	SWS
Synchronous brain electrical activity	theta, PGO	beta	delta, SWP
Hippocampal–neocortical dialog	NC→HC	?	HC→NC
Cholinergic modulation (ACh)	↑↑	↓	↓
Aminergic modulation (NE & 5-HT)	↓↓	↓	↓
Glucocorticoids	(↓)	—	(↑)
Frontal activation (DLPFC)	↓↓	?	↓
Limbic activation (ACC, OFC, etc.)	↑	?	↓
Sensory cortices	↑	?	↓

Note: PGO: ponto-occipito-geniculate waves; SWP: sharp wave potentials; NC: neocortex; HC: hippocampus; ACh: acetylcholine; NE: norepinephrine; 5-HT: serotonin; DLPFC: dorsolateral prefrontal cortex; ACC: anterior cingulate cortex; OFC: medial orbitofrontal cortex.

Less common has been to look at changes in cognitive (Stickgold *et al.* 1999; Walker *et al.* 2002) and emotional processing (Grieser *et al.* 1972; Cartwright 1991; Kramer 1993; Cartwright *et al.* 1998*a,b*; Hartmann 1998; Newell and Cartwright 2000) *during* sleep. We have hypothesized (Stickgold 1998; Stickgold *et al.* 2001) that evolution assigned sleep a critical role in selectively consolidating, translocating, integrating, and, in some cases, weakening memories encoded over prior periods of waking, and that the complex and richly varying architecture of sleep evolved in part to facilitate these processes. From this perspective, dreaming can be seen as a probe into the cognitive brain mechanisms involved in this reprocessing of memories and emotions, and the investigation of dreaming becomes a logical extension of ongoing research into the nature and consequences of sleep-dependent memory reprocessing (Stickgold *et al.* 2001).

We use the term "dreaming" here aware of the fact that it leads to a conflict over the meaning of the term. While most people feel quite confident that they understand the meaning of this term, the dream research community has agreed to disagree on the matter. A recent review of two separate panels convened to identify a consensus definition of dreaming (Pagel *et al.* 2001) concluded that "a single definition for dreaming is most likely impossible given the wide spectrum of fields engaged in the study of dreaming, and the diversity in currently applied definitions" (Pagel *et al.* 2001, p. 195). For our purposes here, we define dreaming as any mental activity during sleep, where mental activity refers to processes occurring within consciousness and hence is equivalent to the term "sleep mentation." Indeed, we will use these two terms interchangeably.

The neurocognitive investigation of conscious experiences remains a daunting task. Neurocognitive function during waking normally occurs within conscious awareness, and one of the most fundamental conclusions of the cognitive neurosciences is that conscious experience, when studied appropriately, can inform us of underlying brain processes. Thus, the mental algorithms subjects consciously perceive themselves using in performing a task (e.g. visual imagery or mental rotation) match the brain algorithms that behavioral and brain imaging studies suggest are being employed (Kosslyn *et al.* 1995, 1997). Although many neurocognitive functions (e.g. motor pattern generation, orienting responses, attention, emotional reactions) can be initiated without conscious intent, even these tend to have conscious sequelae. Carried over into sleep, we hypothesize that what reaches conscious awareness is a reflection of underlying functional brain processes. From this perspective, we propose that studies of sleep mentation are formally similar to studies recording the activity of hippocampal neurons during sleep, in that both provide evidence of the reactivation during sleep of patterns of neuronal activity learned during waking.

Several other chapters in this book review behavioral evidence for the critical role of sleep in memory processing as well as physiological mechanisms that may underlie these sleep-dependent processes. In this chapter, we will review recent findings from our laboratory that investigate cognitive processing during sleep using two distinct approaches. We first describe a series of studies that used standard cognitive testing to determine how these basic cognitive processes are altered during various sleep stages. We then describe a second set of experiments which used actual dream reports to investigate the nature of cognitive processing during sleep. We conclude this chapter with a model of dream construction that suggests the nature of the relationship between dreaming and off-line memory reprocessing.

Cognitive processing in REM sleep

One approach to the study of cognition during sleep is to measure cognitive performance during the first 2–5 min after awakenings from REM sleep and NREM sleep when "sleep inertia" (Lubin *et al.* 1976), allows one to study the brain in a condition where cognitive performance hopefully reflects the behavior of the brain in its pre-awakening sleep state (Dinges 1990). Three separate studies using this approach to investigate cognitive functioning during sleep point toward more flexible associative memory processing during REM sleep.

Semantic priming after REM sleep and NREM sleep awakenings

REM sleep is associated with the appearance of bizarre and hyperassociative dreams (Mamelak and Hobson 1989; Stickgold 1998). One straightforward explanation of this would be that the unique physiology of the brain in REM sleep facilitates the activation of associations normally too weak to reach conscious awareness and which, on awakening, appear unexpected and incongruous. To investigate this possibility, we looked at semantic priming during the period of sleep inertia following awakenings from REM sleep and NREM sleep (Stickgold *et al.* 1999). The semantic priming task measures the increased speed with which a word can be identified when it has been "primed" by presentation of a semantically related word. Priming is measured as the decrease in time required to identify target words when they are preceded by semantically related words. Semantic priming is considered a measure of the automatic spread of activation from a "node" representing one word to nodes representing semantically related words (Meyer and Schvaneveldt 1971). When the extent of priming produced by different classes of primes vary across states, a qualitative shift in the rules governing this spread of activation through semantic networks may be the cause. We obtained such a shift following awakenings from REM sleep, when normally weak primes produced significantly more priming than strong primes (Fig. 1.1; paired t-test, $t(103) = 2.51, p = 0.01$). This suggests that the brain is functionally reorganized during REM sleep to preferentially activate weak associative links. Such a shift could explain the bizarre and hyperassociative nature of dreaming during REM sleep.

At the level of off-line memory reprocessing, such a shift would appear to favor the identification, activation, and perhaps strengthening of previously weak associations. Such a shift could facilitate the discovery of novel solutions to pre-existing problems. Indeed, creativity can be thought of as the process of identifying new and useful associations among pre-existing memories. In this sense, one could argue that REM

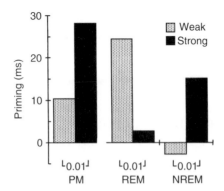

Figure 1.1 Semantic priming. The amount of priming is defined as the difference in reaction times for related (weak or strong) and unrelated target words.

sleep dreaming reflects the activity of the brain as it seeks out such novel and creative associations.

Semantic priming of word associates, as measured in this study, would appear to be a relatively low level for such creativity to be expressed. While this might fit with Freud's fascination with puns as a source of dream bizarreness and meaning (Freud 1900), such word plays do not appear to explain the bizarre transformations seen in actual dreams (Rittenhouse *et al.* 1994). Instead, we suggest that this hyperassociativity within REM sleep generally functions at a higher level of conceptual associations.

Solving anagrams after REM sleep and NREM sleep awakenings

A slightly higher level of associative processing may be seen in the solving of anagrams. Walker *et al.* (2002) have reported that subjects can solve 32 percent more anagrams after awakenings from REM sleep than after awakenings from NREM sleep ($t(15) = 2.3$, $p = 0.03$), despite similar speeds in solving individual anagrams ($t(15) = 0.66, p > 0.50$). It remains unclear, however, whether subjects were altering the process by which they solved anagrams or merely being more successful. Anagrams appear to be solved both by unconscious, bottom-up processes and by conscious, top-down processes. Thus, some subjects, attempting to unscramble the letter string SERMAD, count the number of vowels and consonants (three each), look for possible consonant blends (e.g. DR), consider the possibility that the letter S reflects a plural, and start searching from the reordered string DR-(E-M-A)-S, while other subjects simply look at the initial string until the solution, DREAMS, "pops out." We suspect that it is this latter, bottom-up unconscious processing that is facilitated by REM sleep physiology.

These findings are in keeping with those of Beversdorf *et al.* (1999), who demonstrated that β-adrenergic agonists inhibit the solving of anagrams while antagonists enhance their solution, and suggest that shifts in neuromodulatory regulation across the REM sleep–NREM sleep cycle can cause a shift to greater cognitive flexibility (Cattell 1987) during REM sleep.

Identifying emotional faces

Emotional processing is also altered during sleep, and during REM sleep in particular. A third study of altered processing following REM sleep and NREM sleep awakenings looked at the identification of emotional faces (Garris 2001). Neutral and emotional faces of the same individual (Ekman 1977) were morphed to produce 3 series of 10 faces each, ranging from neutral to sad, happy, or angry. The order of the faces was randomized and subjects asked to identify each face as either neutral or emotional, with the three series of faces presented sequentially. Subjects were tested before going to bed and again in the morning, as well as after awakenings from REM sleep and NREM sleep. To our surprise, the number of faces in each series identified as emotional showed little variation across wake–sleep states. There was no significant difference for happy (repeated measures ANOVA (subject $\times$ condition) $F(3) = 0.70, p = 0.56$) or sad faces ($F(3) = 2.0, p = 0.13$). Only angry faces produced a significant difference in performance ($F(3) = 4.1, p = 0.01$), and *post hoc* tests only indicated that faces were rated less angry in the pre-sleep condition than in other conditions ($p = 0.022$). No differences were seen between REM sleep and NREM sleep awakenings for this or any other emotion.

But while the mean ratings of faces did not vary across sleep stages, the variability of individual subjects as they scored sets of faces did. Since a set of 10 faces constitutes a continuous morph from neutral to emotional, consistent scoring of a set would have no overlap within the series of neutral and emotional faces. Thus, if Face #1 is the pure neutral face and Face #10 is the original happy face, then one would expect that all faces scored as neutral would have serial positions (1–10) lower than all the faces scored as happy. For example, 1–4 might be scored neutral and 5–10 happy. An inconsistency would arise if a face were placed "out of order." For example, if a subject scored faces 1–4 and 6 as neutral, but 5 and 7–10 as happy, one inconsistency would be scored. When the data were reanalyzed from this perspective, both happy (ANOVA, $F(3) = 2.8$, $p = 0.052$; post hoc REM sleep comparison, $p = 0.045$) and sad (ANOVA, $F(3) = 6.2$, $p = 0.0011$; post hoc REM sleep comparison, $p < 0.0001$) faces showed more inconsistencies in scores after REM sleep awakenings than after NREM sleep awakenings. These initial findings suggest that the identification of emotions in faces is more flexible and less predictable during REM sleep than in NREM sleep, but further studies will be needed to justify this conclusion.

State-dependent cognition

These three studies suggest a pattern of altered cognitive functioning during REM sleep. Whether using associative links to identify words in a semantic priming task, solving anagrams, or identifying the emotions displayed on a face, REM sleep awakenings lead to more unpredictable and flexible cognitive and affective processing. The data further suggest that brain functioning may be altered during REM sleep to facilitate neurocognitive searches for novel interpretations of pre-existing information and could lead to the strengthening of newly identified associations within memory networks. These findings suggest that the REM sleep brain is biased toward the processing of associative memories, both cognitive and affective, rather than toward the simple consolidation of recent memory traces. From this perspective, dreaming can provide a window into the nature of these newly identified associative links. Features of REM sleep dreams, such as their bizarre hyperassociative quality (Mamelak and Hobson 1989), minimal incorporation of episodic memories (Fosse *et al.* 2003), and frequent presence of emotion (Strauch and Meier 1996; Fosse *et al.* 2001*b*), might reflect this shift in underlying cognitive processes.

Dreaming and memory

Although sleep is now strongly implicated in functional memory processing, it remains unclear whether dreaming *per se* serves a similar role. But the characteristics of sleep mentation presumably reflect the nature of underlying neurocognitive processes, including the activation and recombination of information stored in memories, and it seems highly unlikely that such activation and recombination would leave the original memories unchanged. At least, three lines of research have attempted to identify the relationship between dreaming and these underlying brain processes. These include studies of the formal dream properties, the incorporation of emotionally charged memories into REM sleep dreams, and the incorporation of recent events into hypnagogic dreams.

Formal dream properties

We described above how cognitive testing after awakenings from REM sleep and NREM sleep supports the notion that cognitive and affective processing is less predictable during REM sleep, with weak associations and fluid thinking enhanced, and the identification of emotional faces less consistent. Analysis of the formal properties of dreams as described in reports from different sleep states show even greater changes. At the most global level, the *types* of cognition—thoughts, emotions, and perceptions—are differentially active across the wake–sleep cycle. When the brain state progresses from quiet waking to sleep onset, NREM sleep, and finally REM sleep, hallucinations increase sharply in frequency, while thinking gradually decreases (Fosse *et al.* 2001*a*) (Fig. 1.2, center and right). Along with the increase in hallucinations, REM sleep dreams show a parallel increase in bizarre, hyperassociative elements (Hobson *et al.* 2000) and emotions, with emotions found in most REM sleep dream reports (Strauch and Meier 1996; Fosse 2001). The occurrence of hallucinations in dreams stands in a reciprocal relationship to the tendency to reflect and think in a logical, directed way.

The decrease in directed thinking during REM sleep is paralleled by a decrease in the rate at which the sources of dream elements are attributed to prior waking episodic memories. In a recent meta-analysis of source attribution studies (Cicogna *et al.* 1986; Cavallero *et al.* 1988, 1990, 1992; Cavallero and Cicogna 1993), Baylor and Cavallero (2001) found that subjects ascribed the waking sources for their dream elements to episodic memory sources less frequently in REM sleep than in NREM sleep or at sleep

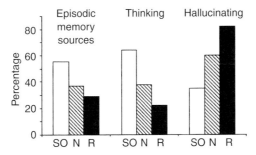

Figure 1.2 Memory sources, thoughts and hallucinations. Percentage of dream elements ("thematic units") with identified episodic memory sources (left) and percentage of dreams containing thoughts (center) and hallucinations (right). SO: sleep onset; N: NREM sleep; R: REM sleep. Data for episodic memory sources are taken from Baylor and Cavallero (2001) and for thinking and hallucinating from Fosse *et al.* (2001*b*).

onset, paralleling the decline in directed thinking capability across these stages (Fig. 1.2, left).

But while the sources in waking of these dream elements appear to be episodic events, this does not mean that the dream elements themselves are episodic memories or even that episodic memories are reactivated in the process of dream construction. Instead, they appear to rise from cortical traces of episodic memory components. The distinction between these two sources is subtle. While the specific elements of an episodic memory are thought to be stored in neocortical networks, their coordinated recall as an episodic memory is dependent on the hippocampus (McClelland *et al.* 1995). In a classic case, Claparede (1951) visited an amnesic patient and, while shaking his hand, stuck him with a pin hidden between two fingers. After leaving the room and returning a few minutes later, the patient, who avowed no memory of ever having met Claparede before, refused to shake hands, stating that "sometimes people hide things in their hands." Thus, he was able to recall a relevant bit of information, presumably stored neocortically, but was unable to identify the event that led to this knowledge. The same appears to occur when we dream.

Dreams fail to incorporate episodic memories

In a descriptive study, we have found that while neocortical memory traces formed during recent waking events frequently contribute to dream scenarios, they only very rarely provide the integrated context of episodic memories. We analyzed 364 dream elements cited in 299 dream reports as having waking antecedents (Table 1.2), and found that only 147 of these referred to waking events, the remaining 217 citing thoughts rather than events (Fosse *et al.* 2003). But only 12 of the 147 elements which cited waking events had the same location, characters, and actions as in the waking event, and only 5–8 of these appeared to judges as reasonable replays of the events, representing only 1–2 percent of the waking citations. Only this 1–2 percent arguably reflect the same

Table 1.2 Sources of dream elements in waking and sleep
(Stickgold *et al.* 2001)

Criterion	Subjects	Reports	Elements
Reports with content	29	299	—
Elements with waking sources	27	194	364 (100%)
Episodic sources	22	104	147 (40%)
+ Conserved location	17	31	38 (10%)
+ Conserved features	9	11	12 (3%)
+ Judged episodic	4–6	5–8	5–8 (1–2%)

presumably hippocampally mediated processes of episodic memory recall that occur in waking. The remaining 98–99 percent of dream elements related to waking thoughts and events appear to result from the priming of neocortical memory systems, in much the same way as implicit memory tasks provide access to often consciously inaccessible cortical memories (Schacter and Tulving 1994), and not from the activation of episodic memories. Thus, we dream *about* what happened, but not what actually occurred.

Interestingly, these reports, collected from spontaneous awakenings in the home, undoubtedly included reports from both REM sleep and NREM sleep. Thus episodic memory replay occurs in neither of these sleep states. This lack of episodic memories might be expected since dorsolateral prefrontal cortex is deactivated in both REM sleep and NREM sleep (Maquet *et al.* 1996; Braun *et al.* 1997; Maquet *et al.* 1997; Nofzinger *et al.* 1997) and the hippocampal formation produces no cortical output in REM sleep (Buzsáki 1996). Both of these structures are central for episodic memory access (Squire 1992*b*; Schacter and Tulving 1994; Squire and Knowlton 1994), and lesions in either of these systems can be sufficient to block episodic memory recall. Thus, the actual episodic memories may be inaccessible and hence irrelevant to the dream construction process (although information stored within the hippocampal formation may still be modified by the recall process).

A similar situation exists at sleep onset, even though hypnagogic dreams (Schacter 1976) appear more tightly associated with recent waking events than do REM sleep dreams. In the following section, we describe experimental studies of sleep onset mentation, including studies of amnesiacs, which confirm this nondeclarative source of dream elements.

Incorporation of emotionally charged memories

There is a rich psychological and psychoanalytic literature which argues that dreaming represents a highly complex analysis and recasting of both memories and emotions (Cartwright *et al.* 1969, 1984, 1998*b*, 2001; Grieser *et al.* 1972; Greenberg and Pearlman 1974; van der Kolk *et al.* 1984; Kramer *et al.* 1987; Lauer *et al.* 1987; Berger *et al.* 1988; Cartwright 1991; Kramer 1993; Reynolds *et al.* 1993; Hartmann 1998; Newell and

Cartwright 2000; Rothbaum and Mellman 2001). Both negatively toned films presented prior to sleep (Lauer *et al.* 1987) and patients' levels of depression (Cartwright *et al.* 1998*a*) have been found to correlate with subjective experience of negative emotion in early night REM sleep periods. Cartwright (1991) found that among recently divorced women, those who were initially depressed dreamt of their ex-spouses more frequently and with stronger emotion than those not depressed, and that those initially depressed women who were in remission at one year had more such dreams than those who remained depressed. In addition, those who showed recovery at a year had more highly developed dreams and fewer reports without recall than those who remained depressed, as well as a shift over time toward more positive affect in dreams that directly incorporated divorce-related elements (Cartwright *et al.* 2001). These findings suggest that sleep can play an important role in processing emotional memories, but it remains unclear whether dreaming affected the process of recovery or vice versa. Such causal relationship are difficult to clarify within the constraints of clinical research.

Various models of emotional processing through dreaming have been proposed. Hartmann's model of contextualized images (Hartmann *et al.* 2001) proposes that traumatic memories are first introduced in dreams through weakly associated images, and then, over time, become more veridical, allowing for the gradual processing of the trauma. Perlis and Nielsen (1993) proposed that dreaming acts as a form of systematic desensitization therapy (Wolpe 1985, pp. 133–180), in which the replay of emotionally charged memories with strong feelings but without motor or sympathetic components, acts to desensitize the affect initially associated with the memory. Both models are relevant to our studies, since, in contrast to Hartmann's model, our findings, described below, suggest that memories are first replayed in near-veridical form and that more weakly related images appear only later. Similarly, these findings suggest that, at sleep onset, the near-veridical images are replayed *without* the expected feelings, perhaps permitting a different form of desensitization from that proposed by Perlis and Nielsen.

The question of the incorporation of stressful waking events into dreams also has been studied intensively in both experimental and clinical studies, but without resolution. Certainly incorporation into REM sleep dreams can and does happen, but the frequency and how it correlates with any of a number of waking parameters remains unclear (for review, see Lauer *et al.* 1987). But these studies often looked at "creative-symbolic" incorporation (Breger *et al.* 1971, p. 184) and involved judges who were blind to neither the condition nor the hypothesis, making judgements of such incorporation difficult to validate.

The special case of post-traumatic stress disorder (PTSD) provides further insight into dream incorporation of emotionally charged waking events, with such incorporation being one of the DSM-IV criteria for the disorder (American Psychological Association 1994). Several studies have confirmed such incorporation (e.g. Esposito *et al.* 1999), and Kramer *et al.* (1987) have presented impressive case histories. A functional role for these dreams in the processing of traumatic events has been proposed (Kramer *et al.* 1987), although whether these nightmares are functional or dysfunctional, has been disputed (e.g. Rothbaum and Mellman 2001).

From these studies it becomes clear that dreaming can incorporate both specific images and loosely associated images and themes from traumatic events in waking life, and also that the form of this incorporation can predict the individual's long-term waking responses to the trauma. But it is still unclear what aspects of the waking event lead to incorporation of specific elements into subsequent dreaming, and what elements are actually incorporated. Indeed, very little work has focused on the effect of attentional or sensorimotor activity on subsequent dream incorporation. Thus, whether the trigger for incorporation is cognitive, emotional, attentional, or sensorimotor (or some complex combination of these features) remains unclear. Much of the difficulty in resolving this question stems from two important obstacles to dream research in general, the inability to reliably get incorporation of waking events or emotions into subsequent dreams and the inability to objectively identify and characterize the nature of this incorporation.

Hypnagogic dreaming

Both of these problems have been resolved using a new sleep onset paradigm for experimental dream research which allows the experimental manipulation of dream content. By collecting sleep onset dream reports from subjects playing the computer game *Tetris*, we have been able to show the robust incorporation of daytime experiences into sleep onset mentation in an experimentally controlled manner (Fig. 1.3; Stickgold *et al.* 2000).

Three groups of subjects were studied—12 subjects with no prior *Tetris* experience ("novices"), 10 subjects with extensive *Tetris* experience ("experts"), and 5 densely amnesic patients with medial temporal lobe damage resulting from anoxia or encephalitis ("amnesiacs"). Subjects played 7–9 h of the computer game over 3–4 days. The game involves manipulating game pieces as they "fall" from the top of a central play window on the computer screen to the bottom. The screen also contains a background picture

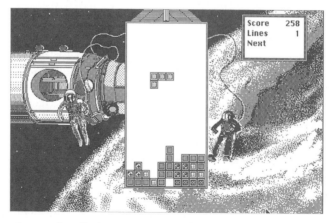

Figure 1.3 Sample screen from Tetris.

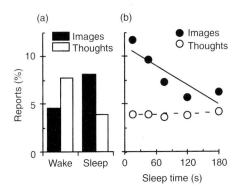

Figure 1.4 Percent of reports with game images or game thoughts without images.

and is in black and white. Players can move pieces to the left or right and rotate them as they fall.

During the first 2 (novices) or 3 (experts and amnesiacs) nights, subjects were automatically and repetitively prompted for mentation reports during the first hour of attempted sleep. Subjects in the three groups all produced an average of 7–8 reports per night. Nine of twelve novices and five of ten experts reported visual images of the game in 9.8 and 4.8 percent of their sleep onset reports, respectively. Taken together, 64 percent of these subjects presented reports with game imagery, amounting to 7.2 percent of the reports from these 22 subjects. Reports of images and of thoughts about *Tetris* were not evenly distributed across the sleep onset period, with the frequency of images being twice as high 15 s into sleep than in either the pre-sleep period (Fig. 1.4(a)) or 2–3 min into sleep (Fig. 1.4(b)).

Several details of the images provide insight into the processes involved:

1. All subjects reported remarkably similar imagery, including seeing *Tetris* pieces falling in front of their eyes, occasionally rotating and fitting into empty spaces at the bottom of the screen. Among the 27 reports of imagery, there were no reports of seeing the larger picture surrounding the play window, the scoreboard, or the keyboard, or of typing on the keyboard. There were only two reports of seeing the computer screen and none of seeing the desk or room. Thus the imagery was limited to those aspects of the experience that were most salient and to which subjects presumably paid the most attention, and none had the characteristics of episodic memories.

2. All but 2 of 19 reports of imagery from novices were obtained on the second night, rather than the first. All told, 2.2 percent of first night reports and 16.8 percent of second night reports contained *Tetris* images. Thus there is normally a 24-h delay after novices start playing before hypnagogic *Tetris* images appear, suggesting that the brain employs a relatively complex algorithm to identify memories for sleep onset reprocessing. This was not the case for the expert players. While it is hard to

explain the delay in novices, many players report that they only become "hooked" on the game on the second day, suggesting that emotional involvement was less on day one. Unfortunately, no measures of engagement were obtained in the study.

3. There is some evidence that hypnagogic game imagery was associated with poorer initial performance. The 3 novices (out of 12) who produced no reports of *Tetris* images performed twice as well as the remaining 9 during their first, 2 h training session (mean scores 2984 vs 1516; unpaired *t*-test: $t(10) = 3.69, p = 0.004$). Similarly, the number of *Tetris* images reported by experts showed a negative correlation with initial performance that approached significance ($r(8) = -0.54, p = 0.11$). However, running each of these analyses with the opposite group produced no significant effects, and it is thus uncertain whether these correlations will hold up with larger sample sizes.

4. Two of the five experts who reported *Tetris* images reported images from earlier versions of the game which they had not played for at least a year, to the exclusion of images of the new version they were playing in this study. Thus, game imagery need not be a simple replay of recent sensory input, but instead can incorporate older, strongly associated memories.

5. One subject reported hypnagogic imagery associated with a nap and a second following a 2 a.m. awakening. These images, which may have been from sleep onset REM sleep periods, were more complex and bizarre than the others in our sample. Thus, the shift in neuromodulation in REM sleep may control the form, as opposed to the content, of the reports.

6. In no case was any affect explicitly or implicitly present in the report.

But the most striking results came from the third group, consisting of the 5 densely amnesic patients. Of the 5 patients tested, 3 reported hypnagogic *Tetris* images despite being unable to recall playing the game before or after the night's sleep. Not only does this represent the same frequency of subjects reporting (60% of amnesiacs vs 64% of normals), but the same percent of all reports (7.4% for amnesiacs vs 7.2% for normals). Even more striking was the similarity in actual report content (Table 1.3). Although unable to recall having played the game (or even recognizing the experimenter from session to session), they nonetheless reported, for example, "little squares coming down on a screen." In the case of DF (Table 1.3), it is clear that she produced dream images of events of which she had no declarative knowledge.

Taken together, these results suggest that hypnagogic images arise exclusively from memories stored in non-hippocampal memory systems and recalled without participation of the hippocampal system. Although the number of amnesiacs does not allow us to confidently conclude that the percent of patients producing such imagery or the percent of reports containing such imagery is identical to that of the normal groups, these results, together with the study of episodic memory replay in dreaming described above and physiological findings of minimal hippocampal outflow through the entorhinal

Table 1.3 Excerpts from reports with *Tetris* imagery. Representative reports of *Tetris* imagery are presented from subjects in each of the study groups

Subjects	Excerpts
Novices	Just seeing TETRIS shapes floating around in my head like they would in the game, falling down, sort of putting them together in my mind (JEG—Night 2)
Experts	. . . seeing in my mind how the game pieces kind of float down and fit into the other pieces, and am also rotating them (TPR—Night 2)
Amnesiacs	I see images that are turned on their side. I don't know what they are from, I wish I could remember, but they are like blocks (DF—Night 1)

cortex during REM sleep (Chrobak and Buzsáki 1994; Buzsáki 1996; Chrobak and Buzsáki 1996), provide converging evidence supporting the hypothesis that the generation of these dream images does not depend materially on the declarative memory system (Squire 1992*a*).

Whether this hypnagogic mentation contributes to processes of memory consolidation and integration remains unknown. Video games are intentionally designed to have non-Gaussian distributions of scores (with frequent catastrophic failures), resulting in very high variances, and making them poor choices for studies of learning. But three findings—the tendency for the appearance of *Tetris* images to be inversely related to initial performance, subjects' reports that they saw the shapes which had the greatest salience for them (Stickgold *et al.* 2000), and the appearance of images from earlier versions of the game in the reports of experts—suggest that these images may reflect the activity of an underlying neurocognitive system acting to alter the strengths, structures or associations among emotionally identified memories. If this were true, the memory processes most likely involved neocortical memory systems with little or no participation by or interference from hippocampal or other medial temporal lobe structures. The studies described here provide tantalizing, if not definitive, support for such a model.

More recent studies using a video arcade downhill skiing simulator, *Alpine Racer II*, provide further support for this model. Game imagery was found in 42 percent of all first night reports (Emberger 2001), with both visual and kinesthetic sensations being reported. Unlike *Tetris*, where 90 percent of images from novices were obtained on the second night, the highest frequency of *Alpine Racer* images were seen on the first night (Fig. 1.5). This robust incorporation of waking imagery into hypnagogic dreams has generated a clearer understanding of the mechanisms controlling this process. First, 14 of 16 subjects reported skiing dreams at sleep onset as did 3 of 3 controls who merely watched other subjects play the game. The two subjects who did not report imagery did not differ from the others in terms of performance or improvement, but did report significantly less overall involvement in the game on the first day (Emberger 2001). Half of the subjects had previous experience with downhill skiing, and half of these (4 of 8)

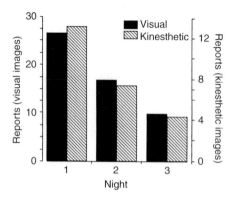

Figure 1.5 Number of visual and kinesthetic images reported on the first 3 nights of Alpine Racer play.

reported images from actual prior skiing experiences, a finding reminiscent of the images of earlier versions of *Tetris* reported by experienced *Tetris* players. Images from *Alpine Racer* were predominantly from scenes with high emotional salience, such as an initial steep hill on one course, or places where subjects tended to crash, matching the *Tetris* reports of preferentially seeing highly salient game pieces. Despite this, subjects reported relatively flat affect during the dreams (Emberger 2001), the opposite of the strong emotions associated with hypnagogic replay of traumatic events in PTSD patients.

If these hypnagogic dreams are functional, rather than simply the residual activity of a neural system shutting down for the night, then one would expect to see functional changes in the memories related to the dreams. We have begun to look at this question by having subjects sleep for 2 h without interruption, and then awakening them and probing their hypnagogic dreaming as they fall back to sleep. We hypothesized that after a complete REM sleep cycle the memories would have been altered such that they would no longer be intrusive at sleep onset. Our initial results suggest something even more interesting. While subjects no longer reported seeing images from the *Alpine Racer* game or from related skiing experiences, they now reported images that appear to represent concepts more weakly related to the game experience, such as "I felt as though I was falling downhill" (unpublished results). These findings suggest that the memories had indeed been altered during the initial REM sleep cycle , so that they were now becoming integrated into wider associative networks within the neocortical semantic memory system. Obviously, more work is needed to confirm this interpretation.

All told, these studies have demonstrated that hypnagogic dreaming involves (i) a high rate of incorporation of memories of events from the day or (ii) from older, strongly related memories, with (iii) a preference for emotionally salient material but (iv) without high dream affect and (v) without hippocampal or medial temporal lobe involvement. In addition, there is now a suggestion that this hypnagogic dreaming initiates a process that ultimately leads to the integration of these new experiences into the individual's broader network of semantic knowledge.

A working model of dreaming

It is our belief that dreaming merely represents one of numerous mechanisms of off-line memory reprocessing occurring during sleep. We propose that dreaming occurs when certain specific brain regions are activated during these processes, and in relation to a specific form of sleep-dependent memory reprocessing. But the function of dreaming in relation to these processes is unclear. The model we present here offers one possible role for dreaming in this off-line memory reprocessing.

The phenomenology of dreaming

One of the most confusing issues surrounding dreaming involves understanding its very nature and its possible function. Like waking consciousness, dreaming is the philosophers' delight and the scientists' despair. Presumably, both result from the activation of specific neural systems in the brain and are, as such, inseparable from them. But it is absolutely clear that there currently are no useful models of how such neural activity gives rise to consciousness or dreaming. While various authors have suggested that consciousness arises as an inherent property of matter (Chalmers 1997), from nerve cell microtubules (Penrose 1989), or from complex neural circuitry (Damasio 1999), none provide any hint of how or why these would give rise to consciousness or dreaming. Given this ignorance, it is hardly surprising that we have no clear scientific evidence that consciousness *per se* might be separate from or influential on the underlying activity of neural systems. Thus we find ourselves currently unable to even properly phrase a question concerning a specific function of dreaming *qua* dreaming. Instead, we can only ask of the function of those brain processes which produce dreaming.

The neurophysiology of dreaming

The study of the neurophysiological basis of dreaming is in its infancy. Solms (1997) has presented data from 332 neuropsychological patients to argue that dreaming (or the recall of dreaming) is lost with either unilateral or bilateral damage to the parieto-temporal-occipital junction (involved in waking visuospatial function) or bilateral lesions in the white matter underlying the frontal lobes. This has led to a widening belief that dreaming arises from these limited brain regions. There is, however, an important caveat which, to our knowledge, has never been raised elsewhere, namely that the brain systems that sub-serve waking consciousness are most likely also critically involved. Obviously, this cannot be easily tested, since when waking consciousness is lost there is no opportunity to inquire about dream activity. But since all participants in the debate over the brain basis of dreaming seem to agree that brain regions are serving very similar, albeit modified, functions in dreaming and waking consciousness, we presume that there would be general agreement that the waking consciousness brain systems are equally critical for dreaming.

Based on neurological examinations, Damasio (1999) has argued for several discrete regions responsible for consciousness, including several brainstem nuclei (e.g. the classical reticular nuclei as well as monoaminergic and cholinergic nuclei), the hypothalamus, superior colliculus, thalamus, somatosensory cortices (including the insula and medial parietal cortex), and the cingulate cortex. Brain imaging studies provide evidence for many, if not all, of the areas proposed by both Solms and Damasio being activated during REM sleep (Hobson *et al.* 1998). We propose that when the fundamental regions defined by Damasio are sufficiently active, consciousness arises in sleep as it does in waking, but that the regions noted by Solms must be additionally active if this consciousness is to take on the more complex hallucinatory and narrative form normally referred to as dreaming.

The functional significance of dreaming

These arguments provide us with a brain that supports the phenomenological experience normally referred to as dreaming. But they fail to explain the form, content or function of dreaming. For such an explanation, one must turn to neurocognitive and neurophysiological data. What we present here is a model of how the brain activity during REM sleep might orchestrate a high level, functional reprocessing of existing memories and associations, accompanied by the phenomenon of dreaming.

Brain imaging and neurophysiological studies during REM sleep have provided evidence of decreased activity in dorsolateral prefrontal cortex (DLPFC) and the locus coeruleus, together with increased activity in the limbic system, including the anterior cingulate cortex (ACC), medial orbitofrontal cortex (OFC), and amygdala. One proposed function of these structures during waking is to act as a closed loop circuit for error detection and correction (Falkenstein *et al.* 1995; Carter *et al.* 1998; Cohen *et al.* 2000; Gehring and Knight 2000).

According to a model proposed by Cohen *et al.* (2000),the left and central portions of the circuit shown in Fig. 1.6 control performance when an individual undertakes a task. As an example, consider a task where the subject must press one key when the letter "A" is displayed, and another when "B" is displayed, doing so as quickly and accurately as possible. As trials are presented, the left-hand pathway, from perception through responses selection to behavior is activated. The task goal is held in mind and conveyed to the response selector by the DLPFC, which not only defines how the selection should be made, but also allocates attentional resources to the task to ensure good performance.

At the same time, performance is monitored by the ACC, which acts to detect mismatches between expected and actual behavioral outcomes (Paus 2001). When errors are detected, Cohen *et al.* (2000) suggest, the ACC activates the locus coeruleus, whose noradrenergic neurons increase their firing. The resulting increase in norepinephrine release in the DLPFC leads to the assignment of additional attentional resources to the task (so the subject tries harder), while norepinephrine release at the response selector leads to a shift its bias to favor accuracy over speed (so the subject slows down). Under such circumstances, the right-hand limbic portion of the circuit, which assesses the emotional significance of the entire process, plays a minimal role, serving only to maintain the motivation, via the DLPFC, for performing the task.

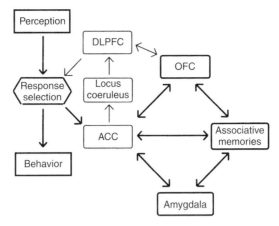

Figure 1.6 An error-detection model of dream construction. The error-detection model of Cohen *et al.* (2000) has been extended. The portion of the system active during REM sleep is highlighted, although the *perception–response selection–behavior* pathway becomes hallucinatory rather than actual. The critical DLPFC–ACC loop, mediated by locus coeruleus input, is shut down in REM sleep. DLPFC: dorsolateral prefrontal cortex, OFC: medial orbitofrontal cortex; ACC: anterior cingulate cortex.

With entry into REM sleep, activity in the DLPFC and locus coeruleus drops to the lowest levels of the day. As a result, the feedback loop, which normally controls the allocation of attentional resources and the shift in bias toward accuracy over speed is disabled. At the same time, activity in the ACC, medial orbitofrontal cortex, and amygdala remain high. As a result, errors in ongoing cognitive processing continue to be detected, but the ACC fails to signal this information to the DLPFC, both because norepinephrine release from the locus coeruleus is blocked and DLPFC activity is already suppressed, and DLPFC therefore fails to allocate additional attentional resources (Cohen *et al.* 2000). Thus, the limbic components continue to analyze potential (i.e. dreamed) behaviors for desired as well as undesired outcomes, with errors detected by the ACC and consciously perceived as negative emotional responses.

The inability of DLPFC to allocate additional attentional resources (and the dreaming brain classically pays little attention to bizarre incongruities in dreams), is compounded by the inability of hippocampally mediated episodic memories to be reactivated in cortex (Buzsáki 1996). As a result, dreamed responses must be constructed from those primarily weak neocortical associations available during REM sleep (Stickgold *et al.* 1999), without the help of the directed (DLPFC) recall of episodic (hippocampal) memories. While the process of incorporation of these weak associates into the dream narrative is unknown, we predict that associated emotions, mediated by both the amygdala and the medial orbitofrontal cortex, play an important role. These responses are then, in turn, reanalyzed by the limbic error-detection circuitry. The consequences of this repeated modification and reanalysis of potential behaviors are twofold. First, at the brain level, we see novel associations being activated within neocortical networks and being tested by an error-detection system that may then adjust the strengths of these associations based on the error-detection system's response to imagined behavioral outcomes. But at the conscious level, we see classic REM sleep dream construction. Situations arise in the dream narrative without the dreamer appearing to participate in directing the course of events (DLPFC inactive). Instead the dreamer appears to merely respond emotionally to each turn of events (ACC, OFC, amygdala), not paying attention (DLPFC) to incongruous or impossible twists in the plot (weak associations). The frequent perplexity that the dreamer experiences surrounding dream behavior suggests that , as in waking, "the ACC seems to come into play when rehearsed actions are not sufficient to guide behavior" (Paus 2001).

Dreams, memory, and cognition

The direct study of dreams represents an important approach to the study of sleep and brain plasticity. Perhaps the most important implication of the studies of hypnagogic dreaming described above is that the sleep onset period allows us, for the first time ever, to objectively monitor the robust incorporation of waking memories into dreams under controlled experimental conditions. An understanding of the rules of incorporation, and the changes that occur with time, will inevitably provide valuable clues as to the brain mechanisms underlying this sleep-dependent memory reprocessing.

This new methodology has already born fruit. For example, it has allowed us to eliminate a major role for the medial temporal lobe's declarative memory system in this process. In addition, by changing the waking experience from *Tetris* to *Alpine Racer*, we dramatically altered both the frequency of reports and their distribution across nights, with *Tetris* images in novices being several time more frequent on night 2 than on night 1, while with *Alpine Racer* images *decreased* by 39 percent from night 1 to night 2. Future experiments can further characterize the factors which affect this and other features of dream construction.

Equally interesting is the shift in hypnagogic dream imagery seen when sleep onset reports are collected later in the night. The related images seen following 2 h of sleep are no longer near-veridical images from the game or strongly related waking memories, but instead appear to be drawn from more distantly related associative memories. These finding suggest that studying dreams will eventually allow us to monitor the progress of these sleep-dependent processes of memory consolidation and integration, although this goal is undoubtedly still some distance away.

References

American Psychological Association. (1994). *Diagnostic and statistical manual of mental disorders, (4th edn, Text revision)*. American Psychiatric Association, Washington DC.

Baylor, G. W. and **Cavallero, C.** (2001). Memory sources associated with REM sleep and NREM sleep dream reports throughout the night: a new look at the data. *Sleep*, **24**(2), 165–170.

Berger, M., Riemann, D., and Lauer, C. (1988). The effect of presleep stress on subsequent sleep EEG and dreams in healthy subjects and the depressed. In *Sleep '86*, (eds W. P. Poella, F. Obál, H. Schulz, and P. Visser), pp. 84–86. Gustav Fischer Verlag, New York.

Beversdorf, D. Q., Hughes, J. D., Steinberg, B. A., Lewis, L. D., and Heilman, K. M. (1999). Noradrenergic modulation of cognitive flexibility in problem solving. *Neuroreport*, **10**(13), 2763–2767.

Braun, A. R., Balkin, T. J., Wesensten, N. J., Carson, R. E., Varga, M., Baldwin, P., Selbie, S., Belenky, G., and Herscovitch, P. (1997). Regional cerebral blood flow throughout the sleep–wake cycle. *Brain*, **120**, 1173–1197.

Breger, L., Hunter, I., and Lane, R. W. (1971). The effects of stress on dreams. *Psychological Issues*, **7**(3) Monograph 27.

Buzsáki, G. (1996). The hippocampo-neocortical dialogue. *Cerebral Cortex*, **6**, 81–92.

Carter, C. S., Braver, T. S., Barch, D. M., Botvinick, M. M., Noll, D., and Cohen, J. D. (1998). Anterior cingulate cortex, error detection, and the online monitoring of performance. *Science*, **280**(5364), 747–749.

Cartwright, R. (1991). Dreams that work: the relation of dream incorporation to adaptation to stressful events. *Dreaming*, **1**, 3–9.

Cartwright, R., Luten, A., Young, M., Mercer, P., and Bears, M. (1998*a*). Role of REM sleep and dream affect in overnight mood regulation: a study of normal volunteers. *Psychiatry Research*, **81**(1), 1–8.

Cartwright, R., Newell, P., and Mercer, P. (2001). Dream incorporation of a sentinel life event and its relation to waking adaptation. *Sleep and Hypnosis*, **3**, 25–32.

Cartwright, R., Young, M. A., Mercer, P., and Bears, M. (1998*b*). Role of REM sleep and dream variables in the prediction of remission from depression. *Psychiatry Research*, **80**, 249–255.

Cartwright, R. D., Bernick, N., Borowitz, G., and Kling, A. (1969). Effect of an erotic movie on the sleep and dreams of young men. *Archives of General Psychiatry*, **20**, 263–271.

Cartwright, R. D., Lloyd, S., Knight, S., and Trenholme, I. (1984). Broken dreams: a study of the effects of divorce and depression on dream content. *Psychiatry*, **47**, 251–259.

Cattell, R. B. (1987). *Intelligence: its structure, growth, and action*. Elsevier, New York.

Cavallero, C. and Cicogna, P. (1993). Memory and dreaming. In *Dreaming as cognition* (eds C. Cavallero and D. Foulkes), Harvester Wheatsheaf, New York.

Cavallero, C., Cicogna, P., and Bosinelli, M. (1988). Mnemonic activation in dream production. In *Sleep '86* (eds W. P. Koella, F. Obal, H. Schulz, and P. Visser), Fisher Verlag, Stuttgart, New York.

Cavallero, C., Cicogna, P., Natale, V., Occhionero, M., and Zito, A. (1992). Slow wave sleep dreaming. *Sleep*, **15**, 562–566.

Cavallero, C., Foulkes, D., Hollifield, M., and Terry, R. (1990). Memory sources of REM sleep and NREM sleep dreams. *Sleep*, **13**, 449–455.

Chalmers, D. (1997). *The conscious mind: in search of a fundamental theory*. Oxford University Press, New York.

Chrobak, J. J. and **Buzsáki, G.** (1996). High frequency oscillations in the output networks of the hippocampal–entorhinal axis of the freely behaving rat. *Journal of Neuroscience*, **16**, 3056–3066.

Chrobak, J. J. and **Buzsáki, G.** (1994). Selective activation of deep layer (V–VI) retrohippocampal cortical neurons during hippocampal sharp waves in the behaving rat. *Journal of Neuroscience*, **14**, 1660–1670.

Cicogna, P., Cavallero, C., and **Bosinelli, M.** (1986). Differential access to memory traces in the production of mental experience. *International Journal of Psychophysiology*, **4**, 209–216.

Claparede, E. (1951). Recognition and 'me-ness'. In *Organization and pathology of thought* (ed. D. Rapaport), pp. 58–75 (Reprinted from Archives de Psychologie, 1911, 1911, 1979–1990), Columbia University Press, New York.

Cohen, J. D., Botvinick, M., and **Carter, C. S.** (2000). Anterior cingulate and prefrontal cortex: who's in control? *Nature Neuroscience*, **3**(5), 421–423.

Damasio, A. R. (1999). *The feeling of what happens*. Harcourt Brace, New York.

Dinges, D. F. (1990). Are you awake? Cognitive performance and reverie during the hypnopompic state. In *Sleep and cognition* (eds R. Bootzin, J. Kihlstrom, and D. Schacter), pp. 159–178, American Psychological Association, Washington, DC.

Ekman, R. (1977). *Emotion in the human face*. Cambridge University Press, Cambridge.

Emberger, K. M. (2001). *To sleep perchance to ski: the involuntary appearance of visual and kinesthetic imagery at sleep onset following play on the Alpine Racer II.* Unpublished Undergraduate Honors Thesis, Harvard University, Cambridge, MA.

Esposito, K., Benitez, A., Barza, L., and **Mellman, T.** (1999). Evaluation of dream content in combat-related PTSD. *Journal of Traumatic Stress*, **12**(4), 681–687.

Falkenstein, M., Hohnsbein, J., and **Hoorman, J.** (1995). Perspectives of event-related potentials research. In *Perspectives of event-related potentials research* (eds G. Karmos, M. Molnar, V. Csepe, I. Czigler, and J. E. Desmedt), pp. 287–296, Elsevier, Amsterdam.

Fosse, M.J., Fosse, R., Hobson, J.A., and **Stickgold, R.** (2003). Dreaming and episodic memory: a functional dissociation? *Journal of Cognitive Neuroscience*, **15**, 1–9.

Fosse, R. (2001). REM sleep: a window into altered emotional functioning. *Sleep*, **24** (Suppl.), 179.

Fosse, R., Stickgold, R., and **Hobson, J. A.** (2001a). Brain mind states: reciprocal variation in thoughts and hallucinations. *Psychological Science*, **12**(1), 30–36.

Fosse, R., Stickgold, R., and **Hobson, J. A.** (2001b). Thoughts and hallucinations in NREM sleep and REM sleep across the night. *Sleep*, **24**, A178.

Freud, S. (1900). *The interpretation of dreams* (trans. J. Strachey). Basic Books, New York.

Garris, K. R. (2001). *Emotional perception in rapid eye movement sleep and dreaming.* Harvard University, Cambridge, MA.

Gehring, W. J. and **Knight, R. T.** (2000). The anterior cingulate cortex lends a hand in response selection. *Nature Neuroscience*, **3**, 516–520.

Greenberg, R. and **Pearlman, C. A.** (1974). Cutting the REM sleep nerve: an approach to the adaptive function of REM sleep. *Perspectives in Biological Medicine*, **17**, 513–521.

Grieser, C., Greenberg, R., and Harrison, R. H. (1972). The adaptive function of sleep: The differential effects of sleep and dreaming on recall. *Journal of Abnormal Psychology*, **80**, 280–286.

Hartmann, E. (1998). Nightmare after trauma as paradigm for all dreams: a new approach to the nature and functions of dreaming. *Psychiatry*, **61**(3), 223–238.

Hartmann, E., Kunzendorf, R., Rosen, R., and Grace, N. G. (2001). Contextualizing images in dreams and daydreams. *Dreaming*, **11**, 97–104.

Hennevin, E., Hars, B., Maho, C., and Bloch, V. (1995). Processing of learned information in paradoxical sleep: relevance for memory. *Behavioural Brain Research*, **69**, 125–135.

Hobson, J. A., Pace-Schott, E. F., and Stickgold, R. (2000). Dreaming and the brain: toward a cognitive neuroscience of conscious states. *Behavioral Brain Sciences*, **23**, 793–842.

Hobson, J. A., Stickgold, R., and Pace-Schott, E. F. (1998). The neuropsychology of REM sleep dreaming. *Neuroreport*, **9**, R1–R14.

Kosslyn, S. M., Thompson, W. L., and Alpert, N. M. (1997). Neural systems shared by visual imagery and visual perception: a positron emission tomography study. *Neuroimage*, **6**, 320–334.

Kosslyn, S. M., Thompson, W. L., Kim, I. J., and Alpert, N. M. (1995). Topographical representations of mental images in primary visual cortex. *Nature*, **378**(6556), 496–498.

Kramer, M. (1993). The selective mood regulatory function of dreaming: an update and revision. In *The functions of dreaming* (eds A. Moffitt, M. Kramer, and R. Hoffman), State University of New York Press, Albany.

Kramer, M., Schoen, L. S., and Kinney, L. (1987). Nightmares in Vietnam veterans. *Journal of the American Academy of Psychoanalysis*, **15**(1), 67–81.

Lauer, C., Riemann, D., Lund, R., and Berger, M. (1987). Shortened REM sleep latency: a consequence of psychological strain. *Psychophysiology*, **24**, 263–271.

Lubin, A., Hord, D., Tracy, M. L., and Johnson, L. C. (1976). Effects of exercise, bedrest, and napping on performance decrement during 40 hours. *Psychophysiology*, **13**, 334–339.

Mamelak, A. N. and Hobson, J. A. (1989). Dream bizarreness as the cognitive correlate of altered neuronal behavior in REM sleep. *Journal of Cognitive Neuroscience*, **1**, 201–222.

Maquet, P. (2001). The role of sleep in learning and memory. *Science*, **294**, 1048–1052.

Maquet, P., Degueldre, C., Delfiore, G., Aerts, J., Peters, J.-M., Luxen, A., and Franck, G. (1997). Functional neuroanatomy of human slow wave sleep. *Journal of Neuroscience*, **17**, 2807–2812.

Maquet, P., Peters, J.-M., Aerts, J., Delfiore, G., Degueldre, C., Luxen, A., and Franck, G. (1996). Functional neuroanatomy of human rapid-eye-movement sleep and dreaming. *Nature*, **383**, 163.

McClelland, J. L., McNaughton, B. L., and O'Reilly, R. C. (1995). Why there are complementary learning systems in the hippocampus and neocortex: insights from the successes and failures of connectionist models of learning and memory. *Psychological Review*, **102**, 419–457.

Meyer, D. E. and Schvaneveldt, R. W. (1971). Facilitation in recognizing pairs of words: evidence of a dependence between retrieval operations. *Journal of Experimental Psychology*, **90**, 227–234.

Newell, P. T. and **Cartwright, R. D.** (2000). Affect and cognition in dreams: a critique of the cognitive role in adaptive dream functioning and support for associative models. *Psychiatry*, **63**(1), 34–44.

Nofzinger, E. A., Mintun, M. A., Wiseman, M. B., Kupfer, D. J., and **Moore, R. Y.** (1997). Forebrain activation in REM sleep: an FDG PET study. *Brain Research*, **770**, 192–201.

Pagel, J. F., Blagrove, M., Levin, R., States, B., Stickgold, R., and **White, S.** (2001). Definitions of Dream: a paradigm for comparing field descriptive specific studies of dream. *Dreaming*, **11**, 195–202.

Paus, T. (2001). Primate anterior cingulate cortex: where motor control, drive and cognition interface. *Nature Reviews Neuroscience*, **2**, 417–424.

Penrose, R. (1989). *The emperor's new mind*. Oxford University Press, Oxford, New York.

Perlis, L. and **Nielsen, T. A.** (1993). Mood regulation, dreaming and nightmares: evaluation of a desensitization function. *Dreaming*, **3**, 243–257.

Reynolds, C. F. I., Hoch, C. C., Buysse, D. J., Houck, P. R., Schlernitzauer, M., Pasternak, R. E., Frank, E., Mazumdar, S., and **Kupfer, D. J.** (1993). Sleep after spousal bereavement: a study of recovery from stress. *Biological Psychiatry*, **34**, 791–797.

Rittenhouse, C. D., Stickgold, R., and **Hobson, J. A.** (1994). Constraint on the transformation of characters and objects in dream reports. *Consciousness and Cognition*, **3**, 100–113.

Rothbaum, B. O. and **Mellman, T. A.** (2001). Dreams and exposure therapy in PTSD. *Journal of Traumatic Stress*, **14**(3), 481–490.

Schacter, D. L. (1976). The hypnagogic state: a critical review of the literature. *Psychological Bulletin*, **83**, 452–481.

Schacter, D. L. and **Tulving, E.** (1994). *Memory systems 1994*. MIT Press, Cambridge, MA.

Smith, C. (1985). Sleep states and learning: a review of the animal literature. *Neuroscience and Biobehavioral Reviews*, **9**(2), 157–168.

Smith, C. (1995). Sleep states and memory processes. *Behavioral Brain Research*, **69**(1–2), 137–145.

Solms, M. (1997). *The neuropsychology of dreams: a clinico-anatomical study*. Lawrence Erlbaum Associates, Mahwah, N J.

Squire, L. R. (1992*a*). Declarative and nondeclarative memory: multiple brain systems supporting learning and memory. *Journal of Cognitive Neuroscience*, **4**, 231–243.

Squire, L. R. (1992*b*). Memory and the hippocampus: a synthesis from findings with rats, monkeys, and humans. *Psychological Review*, **99**, 191–231.

Squire, L. R. and **Knowlton, B. J.** (1994). Memory hippocampus and brain systems. In *The cognitive neurosciences* (ed. M. Gazzaniga), MIT Press.

Stickgold, R. (1998). Sleep: off-line memory reprocessing. *Trends in Cognitive Sciences*, **2**(12), 484–492.

Stickgold, R., Hobson, J. A., Fosse, R., and **Fosse, M.** (2001). Sleep, learning and dreams: off-line memory reprocessing. *Science*, **294**, 1052–1057.

Stickgold, R., Malia, A., Maguire, D., Roddenberry, D., and **O'Connor, M.** (2000). Replaying the game: hypnagogic images in normals and amnesiacs. *Science*, **290**, 350–353.

Stickgold, R., Scott, L., Rittenhouse, C., and **Hobson, J. A.** (1999). Sleep induced changes in associative memory. *Journal of Cognitive Neuroscience,* **11,** 182–193.

Strauch, I. and **Meier, B.** (1996). *In search of dreams: results of experimental dream research.* State University of New York Press, Albany.

van der Kolk, B., Blitz, R., Burr, W., Sherry, S., and **Hartmann, E.** (1984). Nightmares and trauma: a comparison of nightmares after combat with lifelong nightmares in veterans. *American Journal of Psychiatry,* **141**(2), 187–190.

Walker, M., Brakefield, T., Morgan, A., Hobson, J. A., and **Stickgold, R.** (2002). Practice with sleep makes perfect: sleep dependent motor skill learning. *Neuron,* **35,** 205–211.

Wolpe, J. (1985). *The practice of behavior therapy* (3rd edn). Pergamon Press, New York.

CHAPTER 2

HUMAN STUDIES OF SLEEP AND OFF-LINE MEMORY REPROCESSING

ROBERT STICKGOLD

Recent studies in molecular genetics, neurophysiology, and the cognitive neurosciences have produced an extensive body of research that provides converging evidence for an important role of sleep in learning and memory (Smith 1993, 1995; Stickgold 1998; Maquet 2001; Stickgold *et al.* 2001), although the extent of this role remains hotly debated (Horne 2000; Vertes and Eastman 2000; Siegel 2001). Supportive findings include behavioral studies in humans and other animals, neurochemical and neurophysiological studies of the brain basis of sleep-dependent memory processing, and neurocognitive studies of information processing during sleep. In humans and other mammals, sleep is divided into several stages, based on patterns of brain electrical activity measured in the electroencephalogram (EEG) as well as in eye movements, and muscle tone (Rechtschaffen and Kales 1968). These stages can be broadly categorized as rapid eye movement (REM) sleep and non-rapid eye movement (NREM) sleep. During sleep, mammals cycle through these sleep stages, with the human REM sleep–NREM sleep cycle typically having a 90-min period. Recent evidence strengthens the hypothesis that sleep plays a role in learning and memory processing at several levels, including such diverse processes as memory consolidation-related gene inductions (Ribeiro *et al.* 1999; Graves *et al.* 2001), sleep-dependent developmental plasticity of binocular cells in visual cortex (Shaffery *et al.* 1999; Frank *et al.* 2001), procedural learning of a visual discrimination task (Karni *et al.* 1994; Gais *et al.* 2000; Stickgold *et al.* 2000a,b), the learning of problem-solving skills (Smith 1993), and sleep state dependent shifts in cognitive performance (Stickgold *et al.* 1999; Walker *et al.* 2002c).

This chapter focuses on human behavioral studies of sleep, learning, and memory. Ignoring for the most part mechanistic questions, it is possible to ask simply (!) how sleep impacts on learning and memory. This is, of course, just a subset of the larger questions of how learning and memory formation take place in general. Particularly relevant to this chapter are questions of the time course of learning—how much of the learning process occurs after the completion of actual training? What is the time course of slow changes in learning and memory that develop after training? How does additional training interact with this time course? How does sleep contribute to these slow changes? But even when we limit ourselves to the last of these questions, we find that it

Box 2.1   How does sleep affect learning and memory?

1.   Sleep occurring when, relative to training?

    1.1.   Prior to training

    1.2.   After training

2.   Which aspects of learning or memory?

    2.1.   Encoding

    2.2.   Stabilization

    2.3.   Strengthening

    2.4.   Integration

3.   What stages of sleep?

    3.1.   Stage 1 sleep (sleep onset)

    3.2.   Stage 2 sleep (light NREM sleep)

    3.3.   Stages 3 and 4 sleep (SWS)

    3.4.   REM sleep

4.   Over what time period?

    4.1.   Same-day naps

    4.2.   First night

        4.2.1.   Early night

        4.2.2.   Late night

    4.3.   More distant nights

5.   What types of memory are affected?

    5.1.   Declarative

        5.1.1.   Episodic

            5.1.1.1.   Simple

            5.1.1.2.   Emotional

        5.1.2.   Semantic

            5.1.2.1.   Simple

            5.1.2.2.   Complex

    5.2.   Procedural

        5.2.1.   Perceptual

        5.2.2.   Motor

        5.2.3.   Complex cognitive

Since each of the major headings in this list is independent of the others, we have a total of $2 \times 4 \times 4 \times 4 \times 7$, or about 900 distinct questions, such as whether SWS in naps taken after perceptual skill training (but on the same day) affects stabilization of the memory of the task. Even with all this separate questions, we have not begun to ask more subtle questions, such as whether, for each of these 900 possible effects of sleep on learning and memory, sleep is necessary or sufficient or both. It is one thing to say that a given form of memory consolidation *can* occur during sleep, but a very different one to say that it can *only* occur during sleep.

quickly branches into numerous questions, based on what kind of sleep we are talking about, and what kind of learning or memory. Overall, we can develop a hierarchy of questions (Box 2.1) that simply tries to specify what we mean when we refer to the role of sleep in learning and memory.

Visual texture discrimination learning

Obviously, this chapter can only focus on a small fraction of these questions. Since most of our work has looked at the effects of post-training sleep on procedural learning, this will be the focus of the chapter. But we shall return to questions of episodic and semantic declarative memory at the end of the chapter. The majority of our work has used a visual texture discrimination task (TDT; Box 2.2) originally developed by Karni and Sagi (1991), and modified in our laboratory (Stickgold *et al.* 2000).

Independence of task from medial temporal lobe function

Pure procedural learning tasks can be successfully accomplished by amnesic patients for whom damage to medial temporal lobe structures has made the acquisition of declarative knowledge impossible (Schacter and Tulving 1994). Improvement on the TDT is also possible in such patients. This was shown using a group of five densely amnesic patients. All five had extensive medial temporal lobe damage, including the

Box 2.2 The visual texture discrimination task (TDT)

Figure 2.1 shows two sample target screens (a, b) and a sample mask screen (c). Each target screen consists of a rotated "T," as in Fig. 2.1(a), or "L," as in Fig. 2.1(b), at the fixation point and a horizontal, as in Fig. 2.1(a), or vertical, as in Fig. 2.1(b), array of three diagonal bars in the lower left quadrant of the visual field against a background of horizontal bars. The exact positions of both the horizontal and diagonal bars vary slightly from trial to trial.

The target screen is displayed for 16 ms, followed by a blank screen, which is displayed for a variable length of time. After this interstimulus interval (ISI), a mask screen, such as that shown in Fig. 2.1(c), is displayed for 16 ms, after which the screen is again blanked, and subjects report both the letter seen at the fixation point and the orientation of the diagonal bar array (either horizontal as in Fig. 2.1(a) or vertical as in Fig. 2.1(b)), entering their responses on a keyboard. A session normally consists of 25 blocks of 50 trials each. Each block had a fixed ISI, but which decreases monotonically from block to block across the session.

Performance is defined as the interpolated threshold ISI at which subjects can correctly determine the orientation of the diagonal array in 80 percent of trials (Fig. 2.2). Learning is measured as the improvement in performance between sessions, that is, the decrease in threshold ISI between two session. For example, the improvement shown in Fig. 2.2 is the difference between the two thresholds, 53.8 − 35.6, or 18.2 ms.

For amnesic patients, a simpler form of the task was used, in which the array of diagonal bars was either present, in a vertical column, or absent. Thus patients responded "yes" or "no" to the question, "Were the diagonal bars present?" rather than responding "vertical" or "horizontal" to the question, "How were the diagonal bars arranged?"

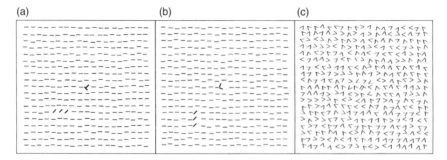

Figure 2.1 Sample screens for the visual texture discrimination task (TDT). See text for explanation.

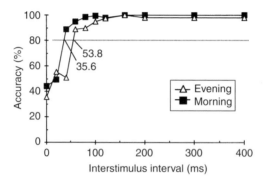

Figure 2.2 Accuracy in horizontal–vertical discrimination. Accuracy is plotted against ISI for the training session (triangles) and the retest session (squares). Points at 0–120 ms reflect averages of three blocks.

hippocampal formation. Three suffered lesions secondary to anoxia, one to Herpes simplex encephalitis, and one to a cerebrovascular accident. Patients had 12–20 years of education (15.2 ± 3.6 year), normal IQs (Wechsler Adult Intelligence Scale-III, Full Scale Intelligence Quotient (FSIQ) = 94 ± 11) but severely impaired memory functions (Wechsler Memory Scale III—General Memory Index: 48.6 ± 3.2). Because of their age (21–62 years old; mean = 42.8 ± 14.9 (SD)), a simpler version of the TDT was used (Box 2.2). Patients were trained on day 1 and retested on days 2 and 5. A repeated measures ANOVA showed significant learning ($F(4, 2) = 8.43, p = 0.04$) despite the small sample size. Post hoc tests (single-tailed paired t-tests) show significant or almost significant improvement from sessions 1 to 2 ($p = 0.056$), from 2 to 3 ($p = 0.048$) and from 1 to 3 ($p = 0.047$). On days 2 and 5, patients evidenced no conscious recollection of having taken the test before. Thus, the TDT appears to be a virtually pure procedural task, with no role for the medial temporal lobe in the learning and consolidation of the task.

Cortical changes accompanying learning

Brain regions altered by TDT training can be visualized using functional magnetic resonance imaging (fMRI). Two groups have reported specific, localized activation increases in regions of visual cortex following training. Karni *et al.* (1995) reported increased activation in both primary and secondary visual cortex when subjects were presented with target stimuli after several days of training on the task. More recently, Schwartz *et al.* (2002) found similar increases just 24 h after a single training session, and demonstrated that the location of the increased activity was indistinguishable from the region activated by visual stimuli in the same region of visual space. Unfortunately, neither study successfully distinguished between rapid changes, that might have taken place during training, and slower ones that might be sleep-dependent.

Maquet *et al.* (2000) have also looked at changes in regional brain activation after procedural task training. Using a procedural "serial reaction time" task with both visual and motor components, they found that regions of cortex activated during task rehearsal were reactivated, in the absence of overt rehearsal, during subsequent REM sleep. But how this relates to the fMRI changes seen with the TDT during retesting remains unclear.

Time course of improvement

Improvement on the TDT develops slowly after training (Karni and Sagi 1993; Stickgold *et al.* 2000), with no improvement when retesting occurs on the same day as training. Instead, improvement is only observed after a night of sleep. When 32 subjects were trained and retested on the same day, no significant improvement was seen (Fig. 2.3(a), open circles; Student's t-test; mean improvement $= -0.5$ ms, df $= 31$, $t = -0.49$, $p = 0.63$), even with 12 h between training and retesting. This is in apparent contradiction with results reported earlier by Karni and Sagi (1993), who concluded that there was a 6–8 h delay before improved performance could be observed, and that same-day improvement did occur. But in fact, only two of their subjects showed improvement prior to a night's sleep, and one of these only showed the improvement in a second retesting session. A third subject retested in this same time interval showed no improvement at all. Since there is considerable intersubject variability (e.g. see standard error (SE) bar for daytime subjects at 9 h in Fig. 2.3(a)), it seems reasonable to conclude that the apparent same-day improvement shown by the two subjects in the earlier study (Karni and Sagi 1993) reflected statistical variability and not actual learning. In contrast to the results with same day retesting, subjects retested after a night's sleep showed significant improvement (Fig. 2.3(a), filled circles; mean improvement $= 12.3$ ms, df $= 37$, $t = 5.55$, $p < 0.0001$). This was true even for the group of subjects retested only 9 h after training. Importantly, there was not even a trend to greater improvement when the training–retest interval was increased from 9 to 22.5 h (regression analysis, df $= 34$, $t = 1.12$, $p = 0.55$). Thus, additional wake time after the night of sleep provided no additional benefit. While further wake time provided no benefit, additional nights of sleep did produce incremental improvement. When subjects were retested 2–7 days after training, 50 percent greater

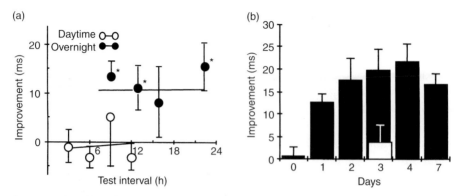

Figure 2.3 Sleep-dependent improvement on the TDT. All subjects were trained and then retested only a single time. Each point in (a) and each bar in (b) represents a separate group of subjects. Error bars in (a) and (b) are SEMs (from Stickgold *et al.* 2000*a*,*b*).

improvement was observed than after a single night of sleep (Fig. 2.3(b), solid bars; 18.9 vs 12.6 ms; unpaired *t*-test, df $= 88, t = 2.26, p < 0.05$).

The slow improvement that occurs over time is clearly sleep-dependent. This fact is shown by the open bar at day 3 in Fig. 2.3(b). These subjects, like those reflected in the filled bar behind it, were trained on day 0 and retested 3 days later. But unlike the subjects in the filled bars, these subjects were sleep-deprived the night after training. After a night of sleep deprivation and two nights of recovery sleep, no residual learning was evident (mean $= 3.9$ ms; df $= 10, t = 1.06, p > 0.30$).

There are two important methodological details that should be noted in these studies. First, subjects were never retested on more than one occasion. This was done to avoid conflating the consequences of sleep and the passage of time with those of rehearsal. While repeated testing allows for more powerful statistical testing, it leaves unclear whether improvement seen over time results from repeated training sessions or the simple passage of time (with or without sleep). Other studies, described below, point out the complexity of interpreting results from multiple retest sessions.

The second detail has to do with the process of determining the initial level of performance (see Box 2.2). Under normal conditions, the threshold interstimulus interval (ISI) at training is in the vicinity of 50 ms. In such cases, the actual threshold is obtained by interpolating between the values obtained for ISIs of 40 and 60 ms. But because the stimulus blocks are presented in order of descending ISI, 13 blocks of trials are completed before the critical blocks are run, and then 3 blocks are run at each of the two critical ISIs. Since each block contains 50 trials, 650 trials are completed before determination of the threshold begins, and another 300 before it is completed. Thus, we are effectively blind to any improvement that occurs during the first 650–900 trials. As a result, our statements that *no* improvement occurs before a night's sleep would more accurately be stated as that there is no improvement between the end of training and the end of subsequent retesting.

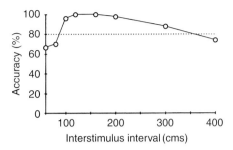

Figure 2.4 Rapid learning of TDT. The increase in accuracy from the 400-ms ISI block to the 200-ms block reflects an increase in performance over the first 100–150 trials of the 1250-trial block. This example is taken from an amnesic patient. These patients generally showed a larger rapid learning component, although the difference did not reach significance.

Indeed, some improvement does appear to develop during the initial portion of the training session. This is seen as an actual *improvement* in accuracy over the first two or three blocks of trials, as the ISI decreases from 400 to 300 or 200 ms (Fig. 2.4). Nevertheless, this rapid learning does not appear to be relevant to the perceptual learning being studied, since the characteristics of learning seen with the sleep-dependent phase is not seen with this rapid phase. Specifically, the slow improvement in TDT performance has been shown to be (i) eye-dependent, not transferring from one eye to the other, (ii) retinotopically specific, not transferring to other quadrants of visual space, and (iii) orientation-specific, not transferring to stimuli in which the background bar are rotated from their horizontal orientation to a vertical orientation (Karni and Sagi 1991). None of these features appear to hold for the rapid phase of learning, which can transfer between eyes, visual quadrants, and orientations (Karni and Sagi 1991).

Time versus rehearsal

Another variable to be considered is the relative effects of time and rehearsal on TDT learning. The results presented above all involved subjects who were trained in one session and then tested in a second. What effect would repeated training sessions have? Would this hasten or increase the amount of learning? The answer to these questions are not what one might expect. In a series of experiments (Luskin 2001), we found that additional training sessions had no apparent effect on learning at all. In the first experiment, three groups of subjects were trained on the TDT and retested the next day (Fig. 2.5(a)). Two of these groups (1-1A and 1-1B) received one training session on day 1 and one test session on day 2. The third group (3-1) received three training sessions on day 1. Despite this additional training, no increase in improvement (measured relative to the first training session) was observed on day 2. In a second experiment (Fig. 2.5(b)), subjects were either trained in one session on day 1 and retested on day 4(1001), trained once each on days 1, 2, and 3 and then tested on day 4(1111), or trained with three sessions on day 1 and then tested on day 4(3001). The improvement seen after 3 days did

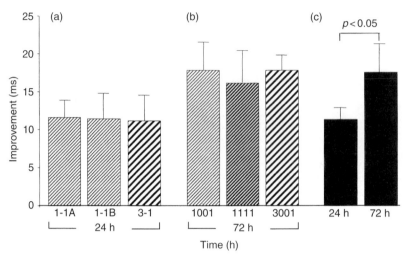

Figure 2.5 Effects of time and practice on TDT improvement. Labels indicate number of training/test sessions on each of four days. For 24 h groups, the numbers in parentheses reflect subject group, but are irrelevant to 24 h improvement values.

not differ significantly between the groups. The results demonstrate that the amount and timing of training beyond a single sessions does not affect the final level of performance reached either 24 or 72 h after the first training session. In contrast to this lack of effect of rehearsal, the extra 48 h before retesting in the 72-h groups produced 53 percent more improvement beyond that seen at 24 h (df $= 55, t = 2.2, p = 0.03$; Fig. 2.5(c)).

These findings resolve an interesting conflict in the literature. Schoups and Orban (1996) reported that, contrary to the reported findings of Karni and Sagi (1991), they found no evidence of monocular improvement on the TDT. To look for the transfer of learning between eyes, they first trained each eye monocularly on day 1, and then retrained the "experimental" eye daily for 13–27 days. When they retested each eye monocularly on the last day, they found equal improvement in the two eyes, and concluded that learning must have transferred. Their mistake was in the conclusion that the slow improvement they saw in the trained eye demonstrated that "performances improved as a function of practice" (Schoups and Orban 1996, p. 7360). In fact, our data suggests that performance was improving as a function of *time* and not *practice*. As a result, both eyes would be expected to show similar levels of final performance (e.g. Fig. 2.5(b), 1001 and 1111), even without transfer between the eyes.

Rehearsal and performance deterioration

Not only does additional practice appear to offer no advantage to the subject, but we have recently shown that repeated, same-day testing on the TDT leads to an actual deterioration in performance (Mednick *et al.* 2002). When subjects are trained on the TDT and then retested once on the same day, no improvement is seen (Fig. 2.3(a)).

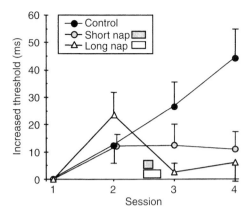

Figure 2.6 Deterioration in TDT performance with repeated same-day testing and recovery following napping. Note that the ordinate reflects changes in ISI threshold and, hence, higher values indicate worse performance (from Mednick *et al.* 2002).

But, with repeated testing on the same day, there was a progressive *deterioration* in TDT performance (Fig. 2.6, filled circles; $p = 0.0003$, repeated measures ANOVA and post hoc tests). In this study, subjects were tested on the task four times in one day (9 a.m., 12, 4, and 7 p.m.), and on each successive test session, performance worsened significantly, demonstrating a 52 percent slowing in perceptual processing across the four test sessions.

Since nocturnal sleep is known to both enhance alertness and consolidate TDT learning, we asked whether a mid-day nap might stop or even reverse the process of deterioration seen with repeated within-day testing. When subjects were allowed a nap with 30 or 60 min of sleep time after the second session, their performance improved ($p = 0.001$, group by session interaction, mixed-model ANOVA), with 30-min naps preventing the normal deterioration seen during sessions 3 and 4 (Fig. 2.6, gray circles), and 60-min naps reversing the deterioration evident in the second session (Fig. 2.6, open triangles). Thus, while controls showed a 14.1 ms increase in threshold between the second and third sessions, the short nap group showed *no* change (<1 ms), and the long nap group showed a 20.9 ms *decrease* ($p = 0.03$, paired t-test). The short nap group showed no significant change in thresholds across the last three sessions ($p = 0.94$), but significantly lower threshold than controls in the fourth session ($p = 0.01$). Further- more, the long nap group showed significantly better performance on both the third and fourth session ($p = 0.03$) than controls.

This represents the first finding of training induced decreases in cognitive performance following perceptual training, a deficit which lasts for up to 10 h. The finding that a brief, 30-min nap can halt the continued deterioration with further practice, and that a 60-min nap can actually reverse the observed deterioration raises important theoretical questions concerning how the level of cognitive performance is regulated. For example, does the decrease in performance simply reflect a decrease in motivation and effort? Does it reflect a global attentional deterioration? Similarly, one can ask whether the napping effect is actually a consequence of sleep, or, alternatively, might it simply result from a period of time with no active visual input?

That the recovery is actually sleep-dependent was shown by a group of subjects who repeat the long nap protocol, but with the naps replaced by quiet rest with blindfolding. Wake–sleep states were continuously monitored polysomnographically (Rechtschaffen and Kales 1968) to ensure maintained wakefulness. Despite an hour of rest without visual input, subjects showed additional performance decrements at 4 and 7 p.m. Thresholds increased by an average of 29.0 ms between the second and fourth sessions ($p < 0.05$), a decrement nearly identical ($p = 0.31$) to the 32 ms seen in controls (Fig. 2.6, filled circles). Thus, quiet rest failed to produce the improved performance seen with even 30 min of sleep.

Nor did the deterioration appear to be due to decreased motivation. When subjects were informed after their second session that their performance had worsened, and were told they would receive a cash bonus if they subsequently returned to their baseline performance, none of the subjects regained baseline performance levels during the third or fourth sessions, and mean thresholds were 32.2 ms slower on the fourth session compared to the first ($p = 0.001$), a decrement nearly identical to the 32 ms seen in matched controls.

TDT performance deterioration is retinotopically specific

Several mechanisms might underlie this performance deterioration. One would be a generalized fatigue effect, mediated by a decrease in alertness or attentional resources. Alternatively, specific neural networks in primary visual cortex may gradually become saturated with information through repeated testing, interfering with further perceptual processing. This would be seen behaviorally as a training-specific deterioration in perceptual processing. In such a case, the performance decrements should be restricted to behaviors mediated by the specific neural networks previously involved in processing the target stimuli. Since learning of the TDT does not transfer to untrained portions of the visual field (Karni and Sagi 1991), there would be no training-specific deterioration if stimuli were presented to an untrained region of the visual cortex, and hence late-day task performance should return to baseline values.

To test this hypothesis, subjects were trained and tested four times on one day, but with the target stimuli switched to the contralateral visual field for the final test, presumably eliminating any retinotopic effects. Indeed, while performance of the switch group did not differ significantly from the control group during the first three sessions, the switch group showed significant recovery in the fourth session (Fig. 2.7; $p = 0.002$, ANOVA group × session interaction and post hoc test on the fourth session). Since performance during the switch condition was not significantly worse than during the first session, the behavioral deterioration observed in the trained visual quadrant did not transfer to the untrained, contralateral visual quadrant. These results provide strong support for

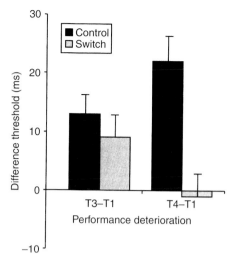

Figure 2.7 Retinotopic deterioration in texture discrimination. Both groups showed deterioration in session 3 (T3–T1), but in the fourth session (T4–T1), the controls deteriorated further while the switch group recovered to baseline levels of performance (from Mednick *et al.* 2002).

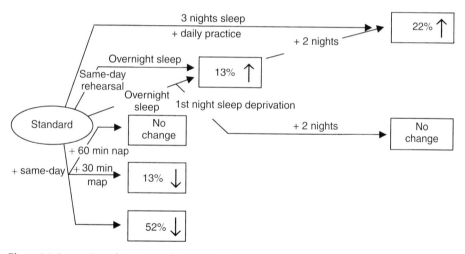

Figure 2.8 Interaction of training and sleep on TDT performance. Boxes show results from actual experiments described above.

the training-specific deterioration hypothesis, and are contrary to the predictions of a generalized fatigue hypothesis.

Interactions of practice and sleep

Figure 2.8 summarizes the four main findings of these studies. (i) Repeated testing on the same day causes a retinotopically specific deterioration in performance that can be stopped or reversed by a midday nap. The additional training does not, however, appear to have any significant effect on improvement measured after a nights sleep; there is neither a carry-over of the deterioration nor a benefit of the additional training. (ii) Additional training, whether on the same day as the initial training or spread over several days, provides no benefit to learning. (iii) Additional days between training and testing results in increased improvement, despite the lack of any additional practice. (iv) Improvement at 3 days after training is absolutely dependent on sleep during the first night after training. But beyond these findings, there is also a sleep stage dependence of overnight improvement.

Sleep stage correlates of improvement

The data in Fig. 2.3(b) demonstrated that time alone is not enough to produce long-term benefits from TDT training; sleep is also required. These sleep requirements actually appear to be quite specific. When subjects were trained and their subsequent sleep monitored in the sleep laboratory, the amount of improvement was proportional to the amount of SWS during the first quarter of the night (Fig. 2.9(a); $r = 0.70$, df $= 10$, $p = 0.012$) as well as to the amount of REM sleep in the last quarter (Fig. 2.9(b); $r = 0.76$, df $= 10$, $p = 0.004$). No significant correlations were found for either sleep stage during other parts of the night (Fig. 2.9(c)) or for the amount of stage 2 sleep at

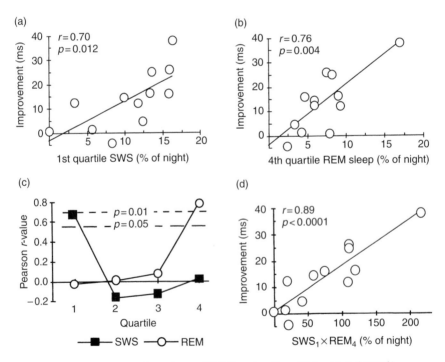

Figure 2.9 REM sleep and SWS dependence of TDT learning (from Stickgold *et al.* 2000*b*).

any time during the night. Thus, improved performance on the TDT appears to require not only training, but subsequent events occurring during SWS early the following night and REM sleep later that same night. Thus, the amount of improvement should be approximated by the formula:

$$\text{Improvement} = E \times \text{SWS}_1 \times \text{REM}_4$$

where E represents the amount of encoding occurring during task training, SWS_1 is the amount of SWS during the first quarter of the night and REM_4 is the amount of REM sleep in the last quarter. In this case, improvement should be proportional to $\text{SWS}_1 \times \text{REM}_4$, as confirmed by Fig. 2.9(d). The correlation between improvement and this combined parameter is a surprising 0.89, explaining over 80 percent of the intersubject variance.

Gais *et al.* (2000), have come to a similar conclusion. They looked at improvement after 3 h of sleep either early or late in the night, and concluded that both SWS and REM sleep contribute to optimal consolidation of learning. Thus, while 3 h of sleep early in the night and rich is SWS produced 8 ms improvement, a full night of sleep adding REM sleep-rich late sleep, produced a 26 ms improvement, three times that seen with just early sleep. Interestingly, 3 h of sleep late in the night actually resulted in a deterioration in performance, similar to what might be expected based on the work of Mednick *et al.* (2002)(Table 2.1). By comparison 12 h of waking produced no detectable change in performance, even though retesting occurred at approximately the same time of the morning, a result similar to one that we have recently obtained (unpublished data). While Gais and Born concluded that either SWS or neurohormonal changes associated with the early portion of the night were critical for consolidation, a third study, by Karni *et al.* (1994) came to the opposite conclusion. Comparing nights with selective REM sleep or SWS deprivation, they found that total REM sleep deprivation prevented overnight improvement while SWS deprivation did not. Taking the three studies together, perhaps the best conclusion would be that both SWS and REM sleep play roles in the sleep-dependent consolidation of learning on this task. but another interpretation is that the sleep dependency is actually more complex than these studies have been able to determine. Hopefully, future studies will resolve this question.

Table 2.1 TDT and partial sleep. SWS, and REM sleep times for the full night of sleep assumed to be sums of early and late sleep

	SWS (min)	REM sleep (min)	Sleep effect (ms)	Wake effect (ms)
Early	73.8	24.3	8.1	−11.0
Late	31.6	58.1	−17.0	−23.5
Early + Late	(105.4)	(82.4)	25.6	−1.8

Note: Performance actually decreases after late sleep (from Gais *et al.* 2000).

Motor finger-tapping

The sleep effects found for the TDT are striking in that they display an absolute improvement across a night of sleep. This is different from the bulk of the sleep and learning data which tends to show that sleep prevents the deterioration of performance. Thus, subjects might show a 40 percent decrease in performance after sleep deprivation and no change or only a 10 percent decrease after a night of sleep. But they rarely show actual improvement after sleep. This raises the question of whether the TDT is an anomaly.

Evidence that this is anything but an anomaly comes from studies at the other end of the procedural learning domain, namely motor task learning. The task itself is a finger-tapping task (FTT). Karni *et al.* (1998) demonstrated that, as with the TDT, there is improvement in performance on the FTT 24 h after training without further practice. He used these findings to argue for the existence of both fast and slow components of motor skill learning. Walker *et al.* (2002) asked whether this slow improvement was in fact sleep-dependent. Task training consisted of typing the numeric sequence "4–1–3–2–4" as quickly and accurately as possible (Box 2.3). Training consisted of twelve 30-s trials, separated by 30-s rest periods. Subjects show considerable (59%) improvement during the 12 trials of the training session (Box 2.3). When trained in the morning and retested 12 h later, only an additional 3.9 percent improvement was seen ($t(14) = 1.5, p = 0.13$; Fig. 2.11(a)). But when tested again the next morning, a large (14.4%) and robust ($t(14) = 5.4, p < 0.0001$) improvement was seen. The failure to improve during the daytime was not due to interference from related motor activity during this time, since subjects required to wear mittens and refrain from fine motor actions for 11 of the 12 h showed a similar pattern of wake/sleep improvement (Fig. 2.11(b)).

In contrast, when subjects were trained in the evening, improvement was seen overnight, 12 h after training, but not across an additional 12 h of wake (Fig. 2.11(c)). Thus it was the night of sleep and not the simple passage of time which produced the improved performance. Curiously, unlike the findings for the visual TDT, overnight improvement on this task correlated with the amount of Stage 2 NREM sleep during

Box 2.3 The finger-tapping task (FTT)

Right-handed subjects placed four fingers of the left hand on the keyboard keys for the numbers 1–4, and typed the sequence "4–1–3–2–4" as quickly and as accurately as possible. The sequence was displayed on a computer monitor at all times to eliminate any declarative memory component of the task. The timing of all trials was controlled by the computer.

Subjects trained in the morning (Fig. 2.10, triangles) and evening (squares) showed nearly identical learning curves, demonstrating a lack of circadian effects at these two times. When tested 12 h after morning training (circles), subjects showed no significant increase, and an amount similar to that expected from rehearsal effects (dotted line) alone.

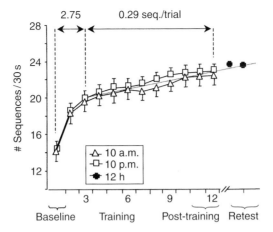

Figure 2.10 Rapid learning of finger tapping task (from Walker *et al.* 2002).

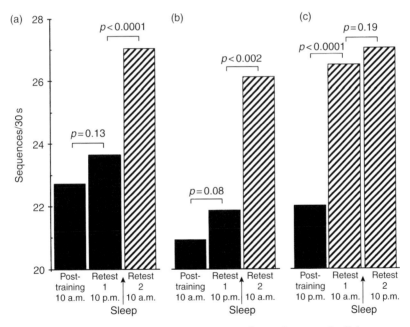

Figure 2.11 Sleep-dependent motor learning. Improvement in speed was seen in all three groups over a night of sleep, but not over 12 h of daytime wake (from Walker *et al.* 2002).

the night ($r(10) = 0.66, p = 0.01$), and especially during the last quarter of the night ($r(10) = 0.72, p = 0.008$). These findings are in agreement with those of Smith *et al.* (Smith and MacNeill 1994; Tweed *et al.* 1999; Fogel *et al.* 2001), who concluded that stage 2 sleep, and possibly the spindles which are most frequent during late night stage 2 sleep, are critical for simple motor task learning.

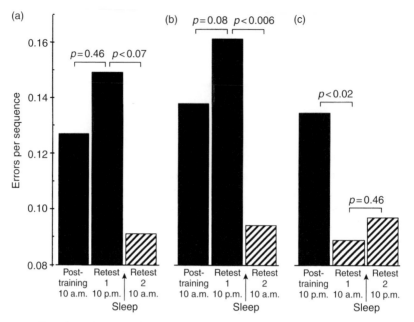

Figure 2.12 Sleep-dependent motor learning. Improvement in accuracy was seen in all three groups over a night of sleep, but not over 12 h of daytime wake.

The overnight improvement was not due to a speed-accuracy trade-off. When the number of errors per 30-s trial was compared between evening and morning, the number of errors actually decreased, although not significantly (Walker *et al.* 2002). However, when error rates (i.e. errors per sequence) were calculated, a highly significant 43 percent decrease in error rate was seen overnight (df $= 39, t = 4.63, p < 0.0001$; Fig. 2.12).

In contrast, a 20 percent *increase* in error rate was seen across 12 h of wake (df $= 39$, $t = 2.1, p = 0.04$), although this was seen mostly in the mittens condition, and may reflect residual motor slowness after wearing mittens. It should be noted that the evening slowing is not just a simple circadian effect, since subjects trained in the evening (Fig. 2.12(c)) showed evening error rates 43 percent lower than for the mitten group (df $= 23, t = 2.48, p = 0.02$; Fig. 2.12(b)). In addition, the 24-h retest data showed a robust (df $= 39, t = 3.23, p = 0.002$) 32 percent decrease in the error rate.

Thus, sleep provides benefits for both speed and accuracy. Whether these two sleep-dependent effects reflect a single process or two distinct processes remains to be seen, although preliminary data (unpublished) suggest that they may in fact be dissociable.

Sleep and "simple" declarative memory formation

Early studies found relatively little evidence for sleep, or REM sleep in particular, playing a role in declarative memory consolidation. This early literature has been reviewed by

Smith (1996). He found that studies of declarative memory based on simple recall of word lists or paired-associate lists reported no effects of total or REM sleep deprivation (Empson and Clarke 1970; Ekstrand *et al.* 1971; Ekstrand 1972; Lewin and Glaubman 1975; McGrath and Cohen 1978; Smith 1993). A nonverbal declarative memory task, the Rey–Osterrieth task, similarly showed no sleep dependence (Conway and Smith 1994).

More recently, these findings have been challenged by Plihal and Born (1997, 1999*a*), who have suggested that SWS may mediate declarative memory consolidation. Using two distinct declarative memory tasks—a verbal paired-associates task and a visuospatial memory rotation task—they showed that early night sleep, rich in SWS, preferentially enhanced declarative memory. Thus, on the paired-associates task, subjects trained at 10 p.m. and allowed to sleep for 3 h recalled 32 percent more paired associates than they had at the end of training. This increase was three times that seen when subjects were allowed to sleep for 3 h, were then trained on the task and allowed another 3 h of sleep before retesting. In contrast to these results, simultaneous testing on a procedural motor task (mirror tracing) showed twice as much improvement over 3 h of late, REM sleep-rich, sleep than after earlier, SWS-rich sleep.

Interestingly, Plihal and Born have argued that it is not SWS *per se*, but the decrease in cortisol levels during the early portion of the night that is responsible for the declarative memory consolidation, showing effects of dexamethasone and cortisol that affect learning while not affecting SWS (Plihal and Born 1999*b*; Plihal *et al.* 1999). This may or may not be a question of "false concreteness." When we say that a particular phenomenon, be it growth hormone secretion (Van Cauter *et al.* 1998) or declarative memory formation, is "dependent on SWS," we are not suggesting that SWS causes the phenomenon, but some biological process strongly associated with the sleep state causes it. For example, it is probably not slow cortical oscillations that cause growth hormone secretion, since secretion during SWS is modulated by sex independent of changes in SWS. But, at the same time, secretion is generally linearly related to the amount of SWS an individual has, decreases with age in parallel with decreases in SWS, and is altered pharmacologically by drugs that alter SWS (Van Cauter and Copinschi 2000). Thus the linkage with SWS is clearly stronger for growth hormone secretion than for declarative memory consolidation.

Sleep and "emotional" declarative memory formation

The situation appears to change when declarative memories with strongly associated affect are considered. Wagner *et al.* (2001), using the same early-night late-night paradigm of Plihal and Born (1997), have argued that while early sleep is overall better for simple declarative memory retention, REM sleep augments recall of emotionally charged memories. They have also presented data suggesting that REM sleep might increase the negative reaction to previously viewed pictures with negative content (Wagner *et al.* 2002).

These newer reports are in keeping with a long history of evidence suggesting that REM sleep, and possibly REM sleep dreaming in specific, can contribute to the processing of affective memories (Greenberg *et al.* 1972; Grieser *et al.* 1972; Lewin and Gombosh 1973; Cartwright *et al.* 1975; McGrath and Cohen 1978). In addition, shortenings of REM sleep latencies and increases in REM densities have been reported in major depression (Kupfer and Foster 1972; Cartwright 1983), the state of bereavement (Cartwright 1983; Reynolds *et al.* 1993), war-related anxiety (Greenberg *et al.* 1972), and, more generally in post traumatic stress disorder (Ross *et al.* 1989). All of these findings suggest that REM sleep processes emotional memories and that changes in REM sleep might lead to dysfunctional processing of traumatic memories during sleep, which might in turn contribute to PTSD (Stickgold 2002).

Sleep and "complex cognitive procedural" memory formation

Perhaps the most intriguing aspect of sleep-dependent memory processing is that related to what Smith has called complex "cognitive procedural" learning (Smith 2001). Greenberg and Pearlman proposed that "habitual reactions, which are closely linked with survival, are REM sleep independent; but activities involving assimilation of unusual information require REM sleep for optimal consolidation" (Greenberg and Pearlman 1974, p. 516). Subsequently, Pearlman suggested that simpler tasks were learned without a REM sleep dependency, while the learning of more complex tasks was dependent on post-training REM sleep (Pearlman 1979). Behavioral evidence in support of this view is seen in studies demonstrating interactions between learning and REM sleep after training on complex logic games (Smith 1993) and foreign language acquisition (DeKoninck *et al.* 1989), as well as after intensive studying in general (Smith and Lapp 1987).

These findings suggest that sleep-dependent reprocessing in humans can consolidate and integrate not only procedural and motor learning, but complex conceptual knowledge as well. The distinction between "complex" and "simple" learning is suggestive of the dichotomy between prepared and unprepared learning proposed by Seligman (1970). He argued that tasks that could be carried out within an animal's existing behavioral repertoire were learned rapidly, while tasks that required modification of this repertoire were learned more slowly. Such suggestions are reminiscent of the distinction between assimilation and accommodation made by Piaget, in describing how children learn about the world around them (Piaget 1952). Assimilation, according to Piaget, is the process by which the brain/mind "incorporates all the given data of experience within its framework" (Piaget 1952, p. 6). This "framework" consists of a collection of models or "schemas" which the child develops to explain the external world. Insofar as the brain/mind views the world through these schemas, assimilation consists of pigeon-holing new information into existing schemas. In contrast, when these prove inadequate for explaining novel information, the schemas are modified to encompass the new information, a process that he called "accommodation." From this perspective, REM sleep would be necessary for the accommodation of existing schemas to explain novel data, but not for the simple assimilation of new data into pre-existing schemas.

Conclusion

This volume provides what appears to be an incontrovertible wealth of evidence that sleep plays not one, but several roles in the processing of learning and memories. Findings from human studies, reviewed in this chapter, suggest distinct roles for SWS, stage 2 NREM sleep, and REM sleep in these processes, and suggest that sleep may help to consolidate both perceptual and motor skill learning, simple declarative memory, emotional memories, and complex cognitive learning. Of the various sleep stages, evidence is undoubtedly the strongest for a role of REM sleep, and of the various forms of learning and memory, there is more convincing evidence for sleep's role in procedural and complex cognitive learning. Further studies will certainly clarify those areas that still remain in doubt.

Despite the immense advances that have occurred over the last 5–10 years, one is left with the sense, at least in regard to human learning and memory, that we still "don't get it," that there is a fundamental process or function here that we have not yet successfully attacked. One thinks of the concept of "sleeping on a problem," which often seems to involve weighing various options and selecting a preferred alternative, or of the phenomenon of going to bed with a "jumble of facts" in ones head and awakening the next morning with them all sorted out into a logical, organized framework.

Are these processes the same as those which enhance simple perceptual skills, or has sleep evolved to serve many conceptually similar functions but using totally distinct mechanisms? Will an understanding of the developmental processes described in this volume by Frank and Stryker (Chapter 10) and the hippocampal replay patterns (Chapters 12 and 13; see also Louie and Wilson 2001) provide the cellular basis of these more complex human phenomena, or is something more required? And how does dreaming fit into these questions? Is dreaming simply an epiphenomenon, or does the process of dreaming actually contribute to sleep-dependent memory reprocessing? It will most likely take another volume to even begin to answer these questions.

References

Cartwright, R. (1983). Rapid eye movement sleep characteristics during and after mood-disturbing events. *Archives of General Psychiatry*, **40**, 197–201.

Cartwright, R. D., Lloyd, S., Butters, E., Weiner, L., McCarthy, L., and Hancock, J. (1975). Effects of REM sleep time on what is recalled. *Psychophysiology*, **12**, 561–568.

Conway, J. and Smith, C. (1994, May 22–27). REM sleep and learning in humans: a sensitivity to specific types of learning tasks. Paper presented at the 12th Congress of the European Sleep Research Society, Florence, Italy.

DeKoninck, J., Lorrain, D., Christ, G., Proulx, G., and Coulombe, D. (1989). Intensive language learning and increases in rapid eye movement sleep: evidence of a performance factor. *International Journal of Psychophysiology*, **8**, 43–47.

Ekstrand, B. R. (1972). To sleep, perchance to dream (about why we forget). In *Human memory: Festchrift in honor of Benton J. Underwood* (eds C. P. Duncan and L. Sechrest), pp. 59–82, Appleton-Century-Crofts, New York.

Ekstrand, B. R., Sullivan, M. J., Parker, D. F., and West, J. N. (1971). Spontaneous recovery and sleep. *Journal of Experimental Psychology*, **88**, 142–144.

Empson, J. A. C. and Clarke, P. R. F. (1970). Rapid eye movements and remembering. *Nature*, **227**, 287–288.

Fogel, S., Jacob, J., and Smith, C. (2001). Increased sleep spindle activity following simple motor procedural learning in humans. *Actas de Fisiología*, **7**, 123.

Frank, M. G., Issa, N. P., and Stryker, M. P. (2001). Sleep enhances plasticity in the developing visual cortex. *Neuron*, **30**, 275–287.

Gais, S., Plihal, W., Wagner, U., and Born, J. (2000). Early sleep triggers memory for early visual discrimination skills. *Nature Neuroscience*, **3**, 1335–1339.

Graves, L., Pack, A., and Abel, T. (2001). Sleep and memory: a molecular perspective. *Trends in Neurosciences*, **24**, 237–243.

Greenberg, R. and Pearlman, C. A. (1974). Cutting the REM sleep nerve: an approach to the adaptive function of REM sleep. *Perspectives in Biological Medicine*, **17**, 513–521.

Greenberg, R., Pearlman, C. A., and Gampel, D. (1972). War neuroses and the adaptive function of REM sleep. *British Journal of Medical Psychology*, **45**(1), 27–33.

Greenberg, R., Pillard, R., and Pearlman, C. (1972). The effect of dream (stage REM sleep) deprivation on adaptation to stress. *Psychosomatic Medicine*, **34**, 257–262.

Grieser, C., Greenberg, R., and Harrison, R. H. (1972). The adaptive function of sleep: The differential effects of sleep and dreaming on recall. *Journal of Abnormal Psychology*, **80**, 280–286.

Horne, J. A. (2000). REM sleep—by default? *Neuroscience and Biobehavioral Reviews*, **24**, 777–797.

Karni, A., Meyer, G., Rey-Hipolito, C., Jezzard, P., Adams, M. M., Turner, R., and Ungerleider, L. G. (1998). The acquisition of skilled motor performance: Fast and slow experience-driven changes in primary motor cortex. *Proceedings of the National Academy of Sciences, USA*, **95**, 861–868.

Karni, A. and Sagi, D. (1991). Where practice makes perfect in texture discrimination: evidence for primary visual cortex plasticity. *Proceedings of the National Academy of Sciences, USA*, **88**, 4966–4970.

Karni, A. and Sagi, D. (1993). The time course of learning a visual skill. *Nature*, **365**, 250–252.

Karni, A., Tanne, D., Rubenstein, B. S., Askenasy, J. J. M., and Sagi, D. (1994). Dependence on REM sleep Sleep of overnight improvement of a perceptual skill. *Science*, **265**, 679–682.

Karni, A., Weisberg, J., Lalonde, F., and Ungerleider, L. G. (1995). Slow changes in primary and secondary visual cortex associated with perceptual skill learning: an fMRI study. *Neuroimage*, **3**, S543.

Kupfer, D. J. and Foster, F. G. (1972). Interval between onset of sleep and rapid eye movement sleep as an indicator of depression. *Lancet*, **2**, 648–649.

Lewin, I. and **Glaubman, H.** (1975). The effect of REM sleep deprivation: is it detrimental, beneficial or neutral? *Psychophysiology*, **12**, 349–353.

Lewin, I. and **Gombosh, D.** (1973). Increase in REM sleep time as a function of the need for divergent thinking. In *Sleep: Physiology, biochemistry, psychology, pharmacology, clinical implications*, (eds W. P. Koella and P. Levin), Karger, Basel, Switzerland.

Louie, K. and **Wilson, M. A.** (2001). Temporally structured replay of awake hippocampal ensemble activity during rapid eye movement sleep. *Neuron*, **29**, 145–156.

Luskin, D. (2001). *Practice does not make perfect: the time-course of change in performance on a sleep-dependent perceptual learning task.* Unpublished Undergraduate honors thesis, Harvard University, Cambridge, MA.

Maquet, P. (2001). The role of sleep in learning and memory. *Science*, **294**, 1048–1052.

Maquet, P., Laureys, S., Peigneux, P., Fuchs, S., Petiau, C., Phillips, C., Aerts, J., Del Fiore, G., Degueldre, C., Meulemans, T., Luxen, A., Franck, G., Van Der Linden, M., Smith, C., and **Cleeremans, A.** (2000). Experience-dependent changes in cerebral activation during human REM sleep. *Nature Neuroscience*, **3**(8), 831–836.

McGrath, M. H. and **Cohen, D. B.** (1978). REM sleep facilitation of adaptive waking behavior: a review of the literature. *Psychiatric Bulletin*, **85**, 24–57.

Mednick, S. C., Nakayama, K., Cantero, J. L., Atienza, M., Levin, A. A., Pathak, N., and **Stickgold, R.** (2002). The restorative effect of naps on perceptual deterioration. *Nature Neuroscience*, **5**, 677–681.

Pearlman, C. (1979). REM sleep Sleep and information processing: Evidence from animal studies. *Neuroscience and Biobehavioral Reviews*, **3**, 57–68.

Piaget, J. (1952). *The origins of intelligence in children* (trans. M. Cook). International Universities Press, Inc, New York.

Plihal, W. and **Born, J.** (1997). Effects of early and late nocturnal sleep on declarative and procedural memory. *Journal of Cognitive Neuroscience*, **9**(4), 534–547.

Plihal, W. and **Born, J.** (1999*a*). Effects of early and late nocturnal sleep on priming and spatial memory. *Psychophysiology*, **36**, 571–582.

Plihal, W. and **Born, J.** (1999*b*). Memory consolidation in human sleep depends on inhibition of glucocorticoid release. *Neuroreport*, **10**(13), 2741–2747.

Plihal, W., Pietrowsky, R., and **Born, J.** (1999). Dexamethasone blocks sleep induced improvement of declarative memory. *Psychoneuroendocrinology*, **24**, 313–331.

Rechtschaffen, A. and **Kales, A.** (1968). *A manual of standardized terminology, techniques and scoring system for sleep stages of human subjects.* Brain Information Service, University of California, Los Angeles.

Reynolds, C. F. I., Hoch, C. C., Buysse, D. J., Houck, P. R., Schlernitzauer, M., Pasternak, R. E., Frank, E., Mazumdar, S., and **Kupfer, D. J.** (1993). Sleep after spousal bereavement: a study of recovery from stress. *Biological Psychiatry*, **34**, 791–797.

Ribeiro, S., Goyal, V., Mello, C., and **Pavlides, C.** (1999). Brain gene expression during REM sleep depends on prior waking experience. *Learning and Memory*, **6**, 500–508.

Ross, R. J., Ball, W. A., Sullivan, K. A., and Caroff, S. N. (1989). Sleep disturbance as the hallmark of posttraumatic stress disorder. *American Journal of Psychiatry*, **146**(6), 697–707 (see comments).

Schacter, D. L., and Tulving, E. (1994). *Memory systems 1994*. MIT Press, Cambridge, MA.

Schoups, A. A. and Orban, G. A. (1996). Interocular transfer in perceptual learning of a pop-out discrimination task. *Proceedings of the National Academy of Sciences, USA*, **93**, 7358–7362.

Schwartz, S., Maquet, P., and Frith, C. (2002). Overnight experience-dependent plasticity in human early visual areas revealed by fMRI. *Journal of Cognitive Neuroscience*, **14**, S94.

Seligman, M. E. P. (1970). On the generality of the laws of learning. *Psychological Reviews*, **77**, 406–418.

Shaffery, J. P., Roffwarg, H. P., Speciale, S. G., and Marks, G. A. (1999). Ponto-geniculo-occipital-wave suppression amplifies lateral geniculate nucleus cell-size changes in monocularly deprived kittens. *Brain Research*, **114**(1), 109–119.

Siegel, J. M. (2001). The REM sleep-memory consolidation hypothesis. *Science*, **294**, 1058–1063.

Smith, C. (1993). REM sleep and learning: some recent findings. In *The functions of dreaming* (eds M. K. A. Moffitt, M. and R. Hoffman), pp. 341–361. SUNY Press, New York.

Smith, C. (1995). Sleep states and memory processes. *Behavioural Brain Research*, **69**(1–2), 137–145.

Smith, C. (1996). Sleep states, memory processes and synaptic plasticity. *Behavioural Brain Research*, **78**(1), 49–56.

Smith, C. (2001). Sleep states and memory processes in humans: procedural vs. declarative memory systems. *Sleep Medicine Reviews*, **5**, 491–506.

Smith, C. and Lapp, L. (1987). Increased number of REMs following an intensive learning experience in college students. *Sleep Research*, **16**, 211.

Smith, C. and MacNeill, C. (1994). Impaired motor memory for a pursuit rotor task following Stage 2 sleep loss in college students. *Journal of Sleep Research*, **3**, 206–213.

Stickgold, R. (1998). Sleep: off-line memory reprocessing. *Trends in Cognitive Sciences*, **2**(12), 484–492.

Stickgold, R. (2002). EMDR: a putative neurobiological mechanism of action. *Journal of Clinical Psychology*, **58**, 61–75.

Stickgold, R., Hobson, J. A., Fosse, R., and Fosse, M. (2001). Sleep, learning and dreams: off-line memory reprocessing. *Science*, **294**, 1052–1057.

Stickgold, R., James, L., and Hobson, J. A. (2000a). Visual discrimination learning requires post-training sleep. *Nature Neuroscience*, **2**(12), 1237–1238.

Stickgold, R., Scott, L., Rittenhouse, C., and Hobson, J. A. (1999). Sleep induced changes in associative memory. *Journal of Cognitive Neuroscience*, **11**, 182–193.

Stickgold, R., Whidbee, D., Schirmer, B., Patel, V., and Hobson, J. A. (2000b). Visual discrimination task improvement: a multi-step process occurring during sleep. *Journal of Cognitive Neuroscience*, **12**, 246–254.

Tweed, S., Aubrey, J. B., Nader, R., and **Smith, C. T.** (1999). Deprivation of REM sleep or stage 2 sleep differentially affects cognitive procedural and motor procedural memory. *Sleep,* **22,** S241.

Van Cauter, E. and **Copinschi, G.** (2000). Interrelationships between growth hormone and sleep. *Growth Hormone and IGF Research,* **10** (Suppl. B), S57–S62.

Van Cauter, E., Plat, L., and **Copinschi, G.** (1998). Interrelations between sleep and the somatotropic axis. *Sleep,* **21**(6), 553–566.

Vertes, R. P. and **Eastman, K. E.** (2000). The case against memory consolidation in REM sleep. *Behavioral Brain Sciences,* **23,** 867–876.

Wagner, U., Fischer, S., and **Born, J.** (2002). Changes in emotional responses to aversive pictures across periods rich in slow-wave sleep versus rapid eye movement sleep. *Psychosomatic Medicine,* **64**(4), 627–634.

Wagner, U., Gais, S., and **Born, J.** (2001). Emotional memory formation is enhanced across sleep intervals with high amounts of rapid eye movement sleep. *Learning and Memory,* **8,** 112–119.

Walker, M., Brakefield, T., Morgan, A., Hobson, J. A., and **Stickgold, R.** (2002*b*). Practice with sleep makes perfect: Sleep dependent motor skill learning. *Neuron,* **35,** 205–211.

Walker, M. P., Liston, C., Hobson, J. A., and **Stickgold, R.** (2002*c*). To sleep perchance to solve an anagram: cognitive flexibility across the sleep–wake cycle. *Cognitive Brain Research,* **14,** 317–324.

CHAPTER 3

ROLES OF EARLY AND LATE NOCTURNAL SLEEP FOR THE CONSOLIDATION OF HUMAN MEMORIES

JAN BORN AND STEFFEN GAIS

For almost a century, numerous studies demonstrated an improving effect of sleep on memory function in animals and humans for different retention intervals and different types of learning materials (e.g. Heine 1914; Jenkins and Dallenbach 1924; Newman 1939; Lovatt and Warr 1968; Smith 1995; Peigneux *et al.* 2002). However, it is still poorly understood which aspect of memory function is affected by sleep and which processes are mediating the consolidation. An ongoing discussion is whether memory consolidation is linked to a particular sleep stage and whether different types of memory (e.g. declarative and procedural memory) are differentially influenced by the sleep stages. Because sleep comprises a highly complex array of neurotransmitter and neuroendocrine changes, any attempt to associate the assumed memory function of sleep with the classically defined sleep stages, which represent only the phenotype of this dynamic pattern, might be misleading. Moreover, due to its covert nature, the consolidation process probably cannot be characterized appropriately with a purely behavioral approach. Studies are required to identify the electrophysiological and neurochemical processes relevant for the consolidation process in humans as well. This chapter will concentrate on some of our own studies, done in humans, examining the influence of different types of sleep on different memory systems and some of the underlying mechanisms.

Behavioral indicators of memory

Sleep as an obligatory prerequisite for memory formation

Many studies in humans have supported the notion that memory consolidation is facilitated during sleep as compared to the effects of retention intervals of wakefulness. However, if it can be shown that sleep is necessary for the formation of certain types of memories, this would strongly support the view that the role of sleep is going beyond a mere permissive action. In fact, this type of evidence derives from a series of recent studies testing procedural memory for visual discrimination skills (Gais *et al.* 2000; Stickgold *et al.* 2000a,b). A basic texture discrimination task was used in these experiments, which

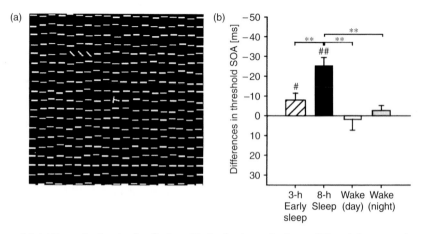

Figure 3.1 (a) Example of a stimulus display with the fixation point (rotated T) and the target stimulus (three oblique lines in the upper left quadrant). The stimulus display was presented with progressively shorter exposure times (360–60 ms). Subjects had to report the fixation stimulus letter (T or L) and the alignment of the target stimulus (horizontal or vertical). (b) Changes in discrimination threshold. Increased discrimination performance at retrieval testing (indicating memory formation) could only be seen when subjects got at least 3 h of early sleep (hatched bar). Performance further increased when subjects were allowed to sleep for 8 h (black bar). Note that late sleep did not enhance performance if it was not preceded by early sleep (data not shown). Time awake had also no effect, regardless of time of day (**: $p < 0.01$ for comparisons between conditions; #: $p < 0.05$, ##: $p < 0.01$ for difference from zero; modified after Gais *et al.* 2001).

requires the subject to discriminate a target texture (three parallel diagonal lines) within a large square array of irregular lines at very short exposure times (Karni and Sagi 1991; Fig. 3.1). Previous studies have shown that memory for this discrimination skill as indicated by a persistent performance improvement occurs several hours later, rather than during or immediately after practicing the task (Karni and Sagi 1991). This finding indicated a slow, latent process of learning continuing after training. However, this latent learning process also requires sleep. If subjects were trained on the task in the morning, and were retested the same day after periods of 3–12 h of wakefulness, no memory formation occurred (Fig. 3.1). Also, no memory formation was indicated when subjects were retested after a night spent awake. A significant and persistent increase in discrimination skills was observed only after subjects had at least 3 h of nocturnal sleep (Gais *et al.* 2000), with the improvement increasing in magnitude in step with increasing time asleep (Stickgold *et al.* 2000*b*). Explanations related to circadian rhythm, attention, and arousal as possible sources for the improvement after sleep could be excluded, because supplementary testing showed that the improvement in discrimination performance is limited to that region of the visual field, in which the target stimulus appeared during learning.

Also, because of this regional confinement of learning, texture discrimination is considered to take place at a rather early stage during visual processing in the primary visual cortex and closely associated areas. Moreover, the improving effect of sleep suggests sleep does more than stabilize respective memories. Since perceptual performance after sleep starts at a level significantly higher than at the end of training before sleep, the consolidation presumably involves active processing of memory traces, thereby increasing their efficacy.

In an attempt to generalize the concept of a critical dependence of memory formation on sleep, recent experiments have focused on the effects of sleep on motor skill learning rather than sensory skills (Fischer *et al.* 2002). For different motor skill tasks, it had been shown that aside from an improvement in performance during training, an additional performance gain can be observed at retesting some time after practice has ended (Brashers-Krug *et al.* 1996; Shadmehr and Brashers-Krug 1997; Karni *et al.* 1998). Practice is assumed to generate an internal model of the required motor sequence, which continues to develop after practice has ended. Within about 5 h, a recently acquired motor skill became resistant to behavioral interference, indicating a latent consolidation of the internal model, although at that time no further behavioral improvement was observed. However, performance gains were found with task recall 24 h after initial training (Brashers-Krug *et al.* 1996). Employing a simple motor task where subjects had to oppose the fingers (of the nondominant hand) to the thumb in certain sequences (e.g. 4–1–3–2–4), Karni *et al.* (1998) showed a 30 percent increase in the number of correct sequences at retesting on the next day in the absence of any intervening training. Potential effects of intervening sleep were not considered.

Using the same finger-to-thumb opposition task,[1] Fischer *et al.* (2002) compared recall of motor skills after 8-h nocturnal retention periods of sleep and wakefulness. Sleep induced a distinct increase in motor speed, averaging 31 percent in comparison with performance at training before sleep (Fig. 3.2). Also, the number of errors decreased across nocturnal sleep but not across nocturnal wakefulness. The effect of sleep at retesting was specific to the learned task, since performance after retention sleep on a novel finger-to-thumb sequence was closely comparable to that in naïve subjects. Also, confounding effects of diminished alertness after nocturnal deprivation of sleep were excluded. When subjects had two nights of regular sleep, the improvement in performance was still distinctly superior to that seen when one night of wakefulness and a succeeding night of recovery sleep followed initial training.

To control for circadian influences, Fischer *et al.* also examined effects of corresponding retention intervals of sleep and wakefulness during the daytime. Daytime sleep induced an increase in motor speed and accuracy similar to that of nighttime sleep. However, although much smaller, there was also a significant improvement of motor speed over daytime retention intervals filled with wakefulness, whereas error rates did not decrease across this interval. These data indicate a circadian influence, which allows for weak but significant latent consolidation of motor skills to occur during wakefulness depending on the circadian phase. This view is consonant with results of increased resistance

---

1   This task is nearly identical to the finger-tapping task (FTT) described in Chapter 2.

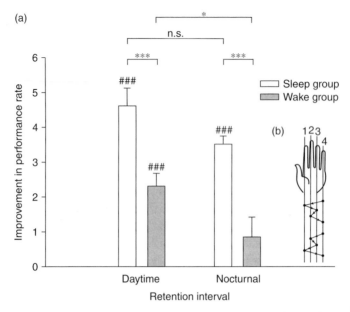

Figure 3.2 (a) Improvement in motor skill performance (number of correctly completed sequences per 30 s). Mean differences (±SEM) are shown for sleep (empty bars) and wake conditions (filled bars). Sleep groups show significantly greater improvement than respective control groups (*: $p < 0.05$, ***: $p < 0.001$ for comparisons between conditions; ###: $p < 0.001$ for difference from zero; n.s.: non-significant). (b) Illustration of two different sequences of finger movement (4–1–3–2–4 and 4–2–3–1–4). Subjects had to do finger-to-thumb movements with the finger indicated by the sequence. (Fischer *et al.* 2002.)

to interference and of changes in the neural representation of motor skills observable within hours after completion of practice under conditions of wakefulness (Shadmehr and Holcomb 1997). Studies in animals as well as in humans indicate that the consolidation process involves distinct changes in the skills' central nervous representation as it continues for hours and perhaps even days after practicing simple motor skills. These changes pertain to the primary motor cortex, associated premotor cortical areas, and cerebellar structures (Shadmehr and Holcomb 1997; Karni *et al.* 1998; Hund-Georgiadis and von Cramon 1999; Sanes and Donoghue 2000; Giraux *et al.* 2001). Moreover, some of the structures activated when practicing a serial motor task before sleep, such as the left premotor cortex and the cuneus have been found to be selectively reactivated during subsequent rapid eye movement (REM) sleep. This suggests the occurrence of reprocessing that underlies memory formation during sleep (Maquet *et al.* 2000). Unlike perceptual memory consolidation, however, consolidation of procedural motor skills, although strongly benefiting from sleep, appears not to occur solely during sleep.

Declarative memory, which stores facts and events, is fundamentally different from procedural memory (Squire 1993; Schacter and Tulving 1994). While procedural memory shows little generalization to apparently similar behaviors (e.g. when shifting performance to the contralateral hand), declarative memory is characterized by a greater spread to related associations and contextual stimuli (Squire and Zola-Morgan 1991; Squire 1992; Karni and Bertini 1997; Karni *et al.* 1998; Eichenbaum 2001). Also, acquisition of declarative memories appears to be faster and may take place after a single salient event. The retention of declarative memories initially is critically dependent on the hippocampal formation (Schacter and Tulving 1994). However, over the long term, memories become independent of the hippocampus due to the development of neuronal interconnections between the more distant parts of the representational network within the neocortex (Winocur 1990; Kim *et al.* 1995; Riedel *et al.* 1999; Teng and Squire 1999).

Consolidation of declarative memories has been shown, so far, to be facilitated, but not restricted to sleep. This may be due to the "fast," hippocampal component of declarative learning and its fast rate of decay, masking a presumed "slower" process of consolidation, represented by a hippocampo-neocortical transfer of information. It is reasonable to assume that this reiterative process of declarative memory formation extends over several sleep periods. Manipulation of sleep in a single post-learning night may thus be insufficient to detect significant differences in long-term recall. It cannot be excluded that sleep may provide not only optimal but even necessary conditions for a reprocessing of memories that allows for gradual integration of new experience with old memories (McClelland *et al.* 1995). In summary, evidence that sleep is obligatory for consolidation of long-term memories has been provided so far for procedural material only. However, a distinctly facilitating influence of sleep on the consolidation has been established for hippocampus-dependent declarative memories as well. This picture clearly implies a functional advantage of sleep over the wake state for memory preserving processes.

Early SWS versus late REM sleep

Traditionally, REM sleep has been believed to represent the essential sleep stage in which memories are formed, accompanied more or less systematically by dreaming activity. This "REM sleep memory hypothesis" is based mainly on data from studies employing REM sleep deprivation. However, REM sleep deprivation studies show mixed results, indicating impaired recall in some cases (e.g. Empson and Clarke 1970; Grieser *et al.* 1972; Lewin and Glaubman 1975; Tilley and Empson 1978; Karni *et al.* 1994), and unchanged performance in others (e.g. Feldman and Dement 1968; Muzio *et al.* 1972; Castaldo *et al.* 1974; Lewin and Glaubman 1975; Tilley and Empson 1981; Greenberg *et al.* 1983). This heterogeneous outcome, has been repeatedly attributed to the effects being more distinct for complex than simple tasks (e.g. Greenberg and Pearlman 1974; Hennevin and Leconte 1977; Smith and Wong 1991). Also, in humans, vulnerability to REM sleep deprivation was supposed to be greater for emotionally loaded materials than for neutral and nonsemantic material (Empson and Clarke 1970; Dujardin *et al.* 1990). Another explanation for the failure of REM sleep-deprivation studies to find uniform results is that the procedural and the declarative memory systems could also be differentially influenced by sleep stages such as REM sleep and slow wave sleep (SWS).

Box 3.1

> The "early vs late sleep comparison" developed by Ekstrand and co-workers in the 1970s (Yaroush *et al.* 1971; Barrett and Ekstrand 1972; Fowler *et al.* 1973; Ekstrand *et al.* 1977) takes advantage of the circadian variation in the distribution of sleep stages. Retention rates are compared across sleep periods of equal length, but placed at different times of the night, that is, across early and late sleep. In humans, both parts of the night contain comparable amounts of sleep stages 1 and 2. However, they differ with respect to SWS and REM sleep, with the amount of SWS more than threefold higher during early than late sleep, and the amount of REM sleep more than threefold higher during late than early sleep. In fact, since REM sleep during early sleep only comes to around 10 percent, the early sleep condition in this respect is comparable with a REM sleep-deprivation condition that usually suppresses REM sleep to similar levels. However, this strategy is not hampered by the typical flaws of sleep-deprivation procedures (see *Sleep deprivation*). Nevertheless, the "early vs late sleep comparison" is not free form confounds, since there are many factors for which circadian rhythms have been demonstrated, such as body temperature and the release of glucocorticoids and growth hormone (Aschoff *et al.* 1974; Born and Fehm 1998). To control for such circadian confounds, the early vs late comparison has been combined in most studies with wake control conditions in which subjects stay awake during the early and late retention intervals (Fig. 3.3).

Smith (1995) concluded from a review predominantly of animal studies that REM sleep might be critical in the consolidation of procedural skills, but not of declarative memory.

A strategy that appears appropriate to compare effects of REM sleep with those of SWS was adopted by Ekstrand and co-workers (Yaroush *et al.* 1971; Barrett and Ekstrand 1972; Fowler *et al.* 1973; Ekstrand *et al.* 1977). Those experiments compared retention rates following undisturbed periods of early and late nocturnal sleep, which differ with respect to the architecture of sleep stages only in the proportions of SWS and REM sleep (Box 3.1). If learning was followed by a 4-h retention interval placed in the early, SWS-rich period of nocturnal sleep, recall of word pairs was markedly superior to recall after a 4-h retention interval placed in the late, REM sleep-rich part of nocturnal sleep. The findings were explained by the authors in terms of the decay theory of forgetting, assuming that the decay of memory traces is more rapid during high levels of central nervous arousal, that is, during REM sleep, than during states of low arousal as in SWS. It is to note, however, that recall of the word pairs following the late REM sleep-rich interval was still improved if compared with a retention interval of wakefulness.

While the work of Ekstrand and co-workers was restricted to declarative memory tasks, in two more recent studies we extended the comparison between undisturbed periods of early and late nocturnal sleep to procedural memory tasks (Plihal and Born 1997, 1999*a*). In the first of these studies, before the critical 3-h retention intervals, subjects were trained to a criterion on recall of paired-associate words, a typical task of declarative memory, and on a mirror tracing task. Mirror tracing is a typical procedural task, which requires the subject to trace (with an electronic stylus) a line drawn figure as fast and as accurately as possible while visual feedback is only given in a mirror. Confirming the results of Ekstrand's group, recall of paired-associate words improved more across an interval covering early sleep than across late sleep and corresponding

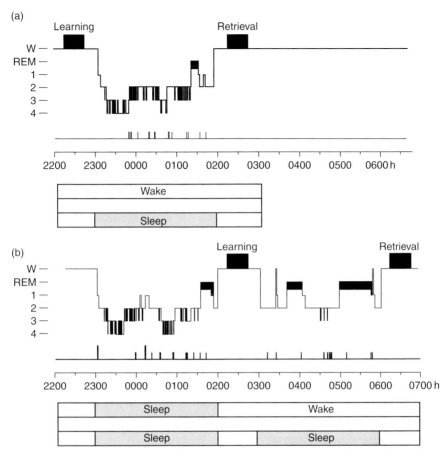

Figure 3.3 Representative hypnograms from two subjects in an experimental design used to study the influence of early and late sleep on memory consolidation. Sleep and wake groups were tested both on early and late nights, with the order of nights balanced across subjects. (a) Early night. Subjects learned the tasks to a criterion at 2215 h and were tested at 0215 h. Between 2300 h and 0200 h the sleep group was allowed to sleep, while the wake control group stayed awake. (b) Late night. All subjects slept during the first half of the night to reduce propensity for SWS. They learned the tasks to a criterion at 0215 h and were tested at 0615 h. From 0300 h to 0600 h the sleep group was allowed to sleep. Note the high amount of SWS during early sleep and the high amount of REM sleep during late sleep.

intervals of wakefulness (Fig. 3.4). In contrast, recall of mirror tracing skills, reflected by increased speed and less errors, was improved most after periods of late sleep intervals predominated by REM sleep, compared with the early sleep retention or with equivalent wake retention intervals.

Since the procedural task in this experiment was nonverbal and the declarative task was verbal, a subsequent study aimed to exclude selective effects of the type of material used (Plihal and Born 1999a). Here, a spatial rotation task was employed for testing

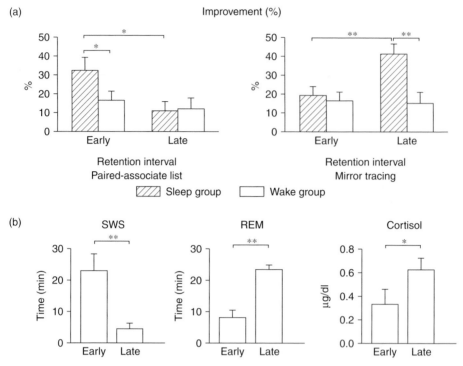

Figure 3.4 (a) Mean improvement (±SEM) in performance after early and late sleep (hatched bars) and respective wake control conditions (empty bars) for a declarative (paired-associate word list) and a procedural (mirror tracing) memory task. There is a double dissociation between memory system and time of night. While declarative memory benefits from early, SWS rich sleep, procedural memory is enhanced after late, REM sleep-rich sleep. (b) Amounts of SWS and REM sleep and cortisol levels during the early and late half of the night. While early sleep is accompanied by high amounts of SWS and low levels of cortisol, late sleep shows a marked increase in REM sleep ($*$: $p < 0.05$, $**$: $p < 0.01$ for comparisons between conditions; data from Plihal and Born 1997).

declarative memory, and a verbal word stem priming task was used to test a type of nondeclarative memory with certain features resembling procedural learning (Baylis and Rolls 1987; Squire *et al.* 1992). The mental rotation task required subjects to recall spatial locations. For the word stem priming, subjects rated the melodical pleasantness of nouns. After the 3-h retention intervals, subjects were asked to complete word stems with the first matching word to come into their minds. Word stems were derived from the previously presented and from novel words. Priming is demonstrated by the increased completion probability of previously presented words in comparison to novel words. On this task, amnesiacs with proven hippocampal damage regularly perform as well as healthy controls, which is characteristic for nondeclarative types of tasks (Squire 1992). Consistent with the hypothesis, subjects displayed enhanced priming following late sleep in comparison with early sleep and wake control intervals. In contrast, the number of correctly recalled spatial locations was selectively improved following early sleep, compared to late retention sleep and wake retention intervals. Together, these results indicate a selective facilitation of declarative memory consolidation by early, SWS-rich periods of sleep, and conversely, a selective facilitation of consolidation of nondeclarative procedural types of memory during late, REM sleep-rich periods of sleep. These findings contrast with studies showing an impaired recall of declarative memories following selective deprivation of REM sleep in comparison with arousals during SWS (e.g. Tilley and Empson 1978). Based on our results, the greater nonspecific disturbances of recall following arousals from REM sleep than SWS have to be held responsible for this discrepancy.

Circadian factors can hardly explain the differential pattern of benefits for declarative and procedural memories during, respectively, early and late retention sleep, since such an effect should have appeared also in the wake control conditions of these experiments. Generally, recall on the wake control conditions did not differ between the early and late part of the night in these experiments. Time of day effects have been likewise excluded in foregoing experiments as a possible explanation for the differential effects of early and late periods of sleep (Barrett and Ekstrand 1972). It has been also argued that differences in memory performance between the early and late sleep conditions may reflect differences already present during learning, since learning before the late condition was preceded by a 3-h period of sleep whereas learning on the early condition was not. There are some hints that prior sleep can indeed influence subsequent learning (Stones 1973; Ekstrand *et al.* 1977). Nevertheless, it is very unlikely that this factor contributed to the differential effects of early and late sleep, because the tasks were trained until a certain criterion was reached, and performance at acquisition was well comparable between the early and late conditions. Moreover, to avoid proactive negative effects on learning that have been observed after awakenings from SWS and REM sleep (Stones 1973, 1977), in our experiments subjects were not awakened until reaching stage 2 or stage 1 sleep, and a 15-min interval separated awakening from performance testing.

Grosvenor and Lack (1984) argued that sleep prior to learning due to lower arousal could impair recall of declarative material after sleep even in the absence of any difference at the time of acquisition. It may indeed be that memory performance in the late retention conditions is generally at a lower level. However, since both late sleep and late wake retention conditions are similarly influenced by prior sleep, this cannot account for the differential effects of early and late sleep assessed with reference to the effects of the respective wake control condition. Other factors that may confound the influence of early and late retention sleep include the length of the sleep period, task difficulty, and the emotionality of the material (Schoen and Badia 1984).

Emotional memory

Convergent evidence exists that within the declarative memory system, processing of emotional materials involves neurophysiological mechanisms and structures separable from those involved in the processing of neutral stimuli. Specifically, in addition to the hippocampal formation, declarative memory for emotional material essentially relies on the integrity of the amygdala (Markowitsch *et al.* 1994; Cahill *et al.* 1995, 1996; Adolphs *et al.* 1997, 2000). Human positron emission tomographic (PET) studies revealed an increased activation of the amygdala selectively during periods of REM sleep (Maquet *et al.* 1996; Nofzinger *et al.* 1997).

To assess whether the benefit of declarative memory consolidation from REM sleep is greater for emotionally aversive than for neutral material, we compared recall of emotional and neutral texts following early and late nocturnal retention periods filled with sleep or wakefulness (Wagner *et al.* 2001). The procedure was otherwise identical to that used in the study of Plihal and Born (1997). In line with these foregoing studies, the neutral texts did not benefit from late sleep. But, a pronounced increase in recall performance after late sleep for the highly emotional texts (one describing in detail the murder of a child, the other sexual problems of a paraplegic man) was found. The early retention periods did not differentially affect subsequent recall of neutral and highly emotional material. This may be due to ceiling effects observed in this part of the night. In fact, recall performance was generally superior on the early compared to the late conditions of this study, which could reflect circadian influences, or, as discussed above, an impairing effect of the sleep preceding the acquisition of material on the late conditions (Grosvenor and Lack 1984). Ceiling effects would clearly limit the interpretation of these data with regard to the role of early sleep in emotional memory consolidation. However, initial learning of the texts did not differ before early and late periods of sleep, and the increase in retention of emotional texts during late sleep was found to be highly significant not only in comparison with the late wake condition but also in comparison with the early sleep condition. This latter observation argues strongly against a critical influence of a ceiling effect during early sleep preventing the emergence differential effects on neutral and emotional texts in these conditions.

In line with Freud's "Interpretation of Dreams," it is a widely held view that sleep and especially REM sleep plays a cathartic role for emotions. Accordingly, the formation of emotional memories in REM sleep should be accompanied by reduced emotional reactivity to the memorized stimuli. Contrary to this assumption, emotional reactivity to aversive pictures was found to be increased following sleep during the late, REM sleep-rich part of the night (Wagner *et al.* 2002). In this study, subjects rated the aversiveness and arousal (low vs high) of pictures, taken from the International Affective Picture System (Lang *et al.* 1988). Each picture was rated before and after 3-h periods of sleep or wakefulness. The second rating was compared with ratings of similar pictures that had not been presented before. Emotional reactivity was defined as the difference between after sleep ratings of old and novel pictures. In comparison with the effects of early sleep and wake periods, following late sleep emotional reactivity was increased, that is, the previously presented pictures were rated more aversive than novel pictures (Fig. 3.5). Interestingly, after a 7-h period of sleep, the enhancement in emotional reactivity was even more pronounced. Taken together, the data point to an aggravating influence of REM sleep on the valence of emotional stimuli in conjunction with improved emotional

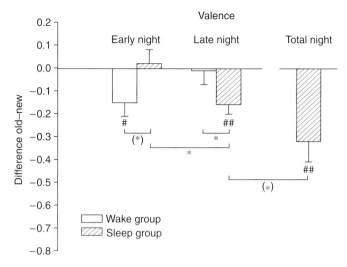

Figure 3.5 Difference in valence ratings for old (familiar) and new (unfamiliar) aversive pictures obtained at retrieval time after 3-h intervals of sleep (hatched bars) and wakefulness (empty bars) during the early and late night. The rightmost bar shows the results of a supplementary condition, in which ratings were obtained before and after a period of sleep across an entire night (2300–0600 h). Note the enhanced negativity for old–new differences (i.e. increased emotional reactivity to the previously presented pictures) after late sleep compared to late wakefulness and early sleep. The 7-h period of sleep likewise revealed enhanced aversive reactivity, which was also significant in comparison to the effects of early sleep and late wakefulness (significances not shown) and tended to be more pronounced than after late sleep (*: $p < 0.05$, (*): $p < 0.10$ for comparisons between conditions; #: $p < 0.05$, ##: $p < 0.01$ for differences from zero, Wagner *et al.* 2002).

memory formation during the REM sleep-rich part of the night, and argue against an emotionally cathartic function of sleep.

Sequential processes of memory consolidation

In summary, the comparison of retention rates over periods of early, SWS-rich sleep and late, REM sleep-rich sleep indicates specific facilitating effects of late sleep for procedural skill memory and of early sleep for declarative memories, if emotionally neutral. These results are consonant with a *dual-process* hypothesis that REM sleep and SWS act differently on memory traces depending on the memory system (Peigneux *et al.* 2002). However, it cannot be excluded that residual amounts of REM sleep and SWS during early and late sleep, respectively, contribute to the observed consolidation effects. There are distinct hints that aside from a particular sleep stage, the succession of SWS and REM sleep is relevant for memories to become consolidated (Giuditta *et al.* 1995; Ficca *et al.* 2000). Stickgold *et al.* (2000*b*) found that the improvement in procedural visual texture discrimination skills over an 8-h period of nocturnal sleep was proportional to the amount of SWS in the first quarter of the night, as well as to the amount REM sleep in the last quarter. The effects of early SWS and late REM sleep were statistically independent, which led those authors to propose a two-step model of procedural memory consolidation. This view was confirmed by a study done by Gais *et al.* (2000) where only early sleep triggered visual discrimination memory formation, but late sleep further tripled this effect.

In addition, although declarative and procedural memory, as well as emotional memory, are conceptualized as separate memory systems they mutually interact (Kim *et al.* 1999; Poldrack *et al.* 2001), and during learning are probably activated in parallel. Probably, there are no pure tasks of procedural or declarative memory, and each task is also more or less emotional. Thus, while their relative contributions can vary extremely, these memory systems for a given task benefit from the SWS–REM sleep sequence at different times.

Electrophysiological conditions of memory formation

It is assumed that the consolidation of memories during sleep is based on some kind of reactivation of neuronal networks that are involved in the prior encoding of the experience. Analysis of the human sleep electroencephalogram (EEG) provided confirmatory evidence with respect to two aspects central for this concept. To assess changes in cortical excitability occurring with sleep onset and during sleep, Marshall and co-workers (Marshall *et al.* 1996, 1998) examined the time course of the scalp recorded direct current (DC) potential in healthy humans. Potential shifts of negative polarity in the DC recordings typically originate from a synchronized wide spread depolarization of the apical dendrites that may coincide with hyperpolarization around the soma, whereas DC positivity can indicate decreased apical depolarization in conjunction with synchronized depolarization around the soma (Birbaumer *et al.* 1990). During human sleep, the DC potential was revealed to shift strongly toward negative polarity at the transition from sleep stage 2 to SWS, reaching maximum negativity at about the onset of actual SWS. With proceeding SWS, the DC negativity gradually decreased again. This temporal pattern was most pronounced for the first sleep cycle typically showing the highest amount of SWS. Notably, the period of the steepest negative DC potential shift coincided with a maximum in spindle activity (Fig. 3.6). This pattern of electrical activity in humans fits remarkably well with the concept proposed by Sejnowski and Destexhe (2000) that during spindle activity an intracortical dipole is generated, characterized by strong depolarization in the apical dendrites of the pyramidal cells and hyperpolarization of their somata, which by triggering strong calcium influx prepares the pyramidal cells for subsequent memory consolidation.

SWS in healthy young humans is dominated by slow synchronized delta activity and usually at visual inspection there is little evidence for intervening periods of fast oscillatory activity as conceptualized by Sejnowski and Destexhe (2000). However, each slow wave oscillation represents a systematic variation of excitability of thalamo-neocortical circuits, which, depending on the phase, allows for or prevents the occurrence of fast

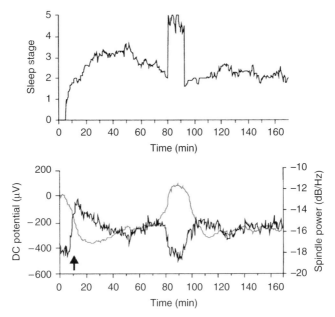

Figure 3.6 Sleep stages and related changes in DC potentials and spindle power. *Top*: Mean sleep stage averaged over 15 subjects (0: wake, 1–4: sleep stages 1–4, 5: REM sleep). Recording started 5 min before sleep onset and profiles were synchronized across subjects to the common length of the NREM sleep-REM sleep cycle. *Bottom*: Changes in DC potential and spindle power (12–15 Hz). Note the sharp rise in spindle power concurrent to the increasing DC negativity (arrow) preceding the occurrence of SWS. DC negativity reaches a maximum at the beginning of SWS (Marshall *et al.* unpublished). (See Plate 1.)

activity (Steriade 1999). Comparing the negative half wave and the positive half wave of slow delta oscillations in human EEG recordings we found the surface-negative half wave to be associated with a suppression and a subsequent increase in fast oscillatory activity in the 12–15 Hz range (Mölle *et al.* 2001). This observation corresponds with findings based on cortical recordings in cats, which likewise showed that extracellularly recorded neurons fire in coincidence with the depth-negative (surface-positive) EEG component of slow-wave complexes, whereas the depth-positive (surface-negative) component is associated with neuronal silence (Steriade *et al.* 1996; Destexhe *et al.* 1999). They suggest that embedded in SWS, phases of fast oscillatory activity occur that might reflect a more or less fragmented reprocessing of previously encoded representation.

Together these findings support the notion that SWS enables a reactivation of previously encoded representations within neocortical networks. Moreover, assuming that the pronounced surface-negative cortical DC potential shift developing at the transition to SWS causes a strong intracellular accumulation of calcium, SWS may represent a condition in which reprocessing effectively induces more permanent synaptic changes necessary for the long-term consolidation of memory representations in cortical networks. However, it still has to be proved that fast oscillatory activity present during the positive part of slow waves indeed represent the reprocessing of prior experience.

Neurochemical conditions of memory formation

Aside from the differences in EEG activity, SWS and REM sleep are characterized by a specific regulation of neurochemical processes including neurotransmitter and neuroendocrine activity. While this concept is based centrally on findings in animals, surprisingly few neuropharmacological studies have been performed to identify those transmitters and neuroendocrine factors critically involved in sleep-associated memory formation. Here, we give two examples to illustrate the relevance of this approach. A distinct neuroendocrine feature of early, SWS-rich sleep in humans is a strong suppression of the hypothlamo-pituitary-adrenal (HPA) system (Born and Fehm 1998). Accordingly, the release of adrenal cortisol reaches an absolute minimum during this time. In the presence of SWS, this suppression is maximal (Spath-Schwalbe *et al.* 1993; Bierwolf *et al.* 1997). Cortisol exerts multiple functions in the periphery and the central nervous system. Aside from the hypothalamus, the most important central target structure is the hippocampal formation, which shows highest expression of corticosteroid receptors (de Kloet *et al.* 1998). In order to test whether the inhibition of cortisol release during early sleep enhances declarative memory formation, we compared memory for word pairs across periods of early sleep under a "placebo" and a "cortisol" condition. During the latter, cortisol was intravenously infused at moderate doses (mimicking physiological stress) for a 3-h sleep period (Plihal and Born 1999*b*). While under placebo conditions, recall performance increased as expected, the infusion of cortisol completely blocked this increase. Procedural memory was not affected by cortisol. Also, the effect cannot be attributed to influences of the substance during learning or retrieval, since the cortisol infusion started with sleep onset and was stopped half an hour before awakening, so that cortisol concentrations differed between the experimental conditions only during the period of retention, but were closely comparable at the time of acquisition and recall testing. The results show that the decrease in cortisol release as it naturally occurs in the 24-h cycle only during the period of early nocturnal sleep is obviously a prerequisite for the effective consolidation of declarative memories.

Cortisol regulates hippocampal excitability via binding two different receptor types, the mineralocorticoid receptors (MR) and the glucocorticoid receptors (GR) (de Kloet *et al.* 1998). While GR show a widespread distribution in the brain, the distribution of MR is more focused on the hippocampal formation and associated limbic and temporal cortical structures. Experiments assessing effects of GR agonist and MR antagonists in humans provided evidence that the impairing effect of cortisol on declarative memory results mainly from an activation of GR, which during SWS are usually in a state of inactivation (Plihal *et al.* 1999; Plihal and Born 1999*b*). Accordingly, administration of the GR agonist dexamethasone prior to early retention sleep impaired post-sleep recall of declarative word pairs in the same way as cortisol. In contrast, administration of the

MR-blocker canrenoate left declarative memory recall performance unaffected. However, to exclude any contribution of MR to declarative memory consolidation during early sleep might be premature based on these data, since ceiling effects of memory performance in the student subjects might have prevented additional gains in recall performance. Collectively, these data indicate deactivation of GR as an essential prerequisite for declarative memory consolidation during early sleep. These observations corroborate results of *in vitro* and animal studies, which revealed diverse mechanisms that could mediate detrimental effects of GR activation on hippocampally dependent declarative memory consolidation. For example, GR activation by selective agonists and during high levels of endogenous glucocorticoid suppressed long-term potentiation (LTP) in hippocampal cells but stimulated long-term synaptic depression and depotentiation (Pavlides *et al.* 1995a,b). Also, GR activation was found to suppress hippocampal glutamatergic neurotransmission and output of hippocampal CA1 neurons (Horner *et al.* 1990; de Kloet *et al.* 1998).

Recent observations have also indicated an involvement of glutamatergic neurotransmission in memory formation during human sleep. LTP is the most fundamental neurophysiological mechanism commonly regarded to underlie memory formation at the neuronal level. It has been shown to occur in various brain regions at excitatory glutamatergic synapses via activation of N-methyl-D-aspartate (NMDA) and alpha-amino-3-hydroxy-5-methyl-4-isoxazone-proprionic acid (AMPA) receptors (Malenka and Nicoll 1999). It appears that initially, activation of the NMDA receptor is essential for inducing LTP and that subsequently the expression of AMPA receptors, mediated via NMDA receptor activation dependent induction of CaMKII, serves to maintain and stabilize the LTP. With this background, we tested the effects of caroverine, a quinoxaline derivative, that at low concentrations is a fairly selective blocker of the AMPA receptor (Honore *et al.* 1988; Ehrenberger and Felix 1992). Intravenous infusion of caroverine during the first 7.5 h of an 8-h period of nocturnal sleep, compared to placebo, strongly reduced the overnight improvement in procedural visual texture discrimination skills (Gais *et al.*, unpublished). The effect was not accompanied by any distinct changes in sleep architecture. Though preliminary, these data provide the first evidence for an involvement of glutamatergic neurotransmission in the sleep associated consolidation of procedural skills within neocortical networks.

Conclusions

Here, we concentrated on studies in humans exploring an assumed memory function of sleep. While most of the individual experiments can be criticized on the bases of possible confounds, related, for example, to circadian oscillations, nonspecific effects of sleep deprivation, or the type of memory task, collectively the available data justify several conclusions. (i) There are tasks of procedural learning which require sleep as a necessary condition for their long-term consolidation. Declarative memory consolidation also benefits from sleep, although sleep has not been shown to be critical for this type of memory. (ii) Although both SWS and REM sleep may normally act cooperatively on memory consolidation, the strength of the influence of each of these sleep stages depends on the type of memory. Declarative memory benefits more from SWS, predominant during early sleep, while procedural memory as well as emotional declarative memory receives great benefit from REM sleep, predominant during late nocturnal sleep. (iii) Electrophysiological evidence has been provided, that neocortical reprocessing of memory representations assumed to underlie the consolidation process, can take place not only during REM sleep but also during SWS in humans. (iv) Neurotransmitter (glutamatergic) and neuroendocrine (cortisol) processes have been identified in humans, which do not appear to be strictly linked to one of the classically defined sleep stages, but essentially contribute to memory consolidation during sleep.

References

Adolphs, R., Cahill, L., Schul, R., and Babinsky, R. (1997). Impaired declarative memory for emotional material following bilateral amygdala damage in humans. *Learning and Memory*, **4**, 291–300.

Adolphs, R., Tranel, D., and Denburg, N. (2000). Impaired emotional declarative memory following unilateral amygdala damage. *Learning and Memory*, **7**, 180–186.

Aschoff, J., Fatranska, M., Gerecke, U., and Giedke, H. (1974). Twenty-four-hour rhythms of rectal temperature in humans: effects of sleep-interruptions and of test-sessions. *Pflügers Archiv European Journal of Physiology*, **346**, 215–222.

Barrett, T. R. and Ekstrand, B. R. (1972). Effect of sleep on memory. 3. Controlling for time-of-day effects. *Journal of Experimental Psychology*, **96**, 321–327.

Baylis, G. C. and Rolls, E. T. (1987). Responses of neurons in the inferior temporal cortex in short term and serial recognition memory tasks. *Experimental Brain Research*, **65**, 614–622.

Bierwolf, C., Struve, K., Marshall, L., Born, J., and Fehm, H. L. (1997). Slow wave sleep drives inhibition of pituitary-adrenal secretion in humans. *Journal of Neuroendocrinology*, **9**, 479–484.

Birbaumer, N., Elbert, T., Canavan, A. G., and Rockstroh, B. (1990). Slow potentials of the cerebral cortex and behavior. *Physiological Reviews*, **70**, 1–41.

Born, J. and Fehm, H. L. (1998). Hypothalamus-pituitary-adrenal activity during human sleep: a coordinating role for the limbic hippocampal system. *Experimental Clinical Endocrinology and Diabetes*, **106**, 153–163.

Brashers-Krug, T., Shadmehr, R., and Bizzi, E. (1996). Consolidation in human motor memory. *Nature*, **382**, 252–255.

Cahill, L., Babinsky, R., Markowitsch, H. J., and McGaugh, J. L. (1995). The amygdala and emotional memory. *Nature*, **377**, 295–296.

Cahill, L., Haier, R. J., Fallon, J., Alkire, M. T., Tang, C., Keator, D., Wu, J., and McGaugh, J. L. (1996). Amygdala activity at encoding correlated with long-term, free recall of emotional information. *Proceedings of the National Academy of Sciences, USA*, **93**, 8016–8021.

Castaldo, V., Krynicki, V., and **Goldstein, J.** (1974). Sleep stages and verbal memory. *Perceptual and Motor Skills*, **39**, 1023–1030.

de Kloet, E. R., Vreugdenhil, E., Oitzl, M. S., and **Joels, M.** (1998). Brain corticosteroid receptor balance in health and disease. *Endocrine Reviews*, **19**, 269–301.

Destexhe, A., Contreras, D., and **Steriade, M.** (1999). Spatiotemporal analysis of local field potentials and unit discharges in cat cerebral cortex during natural wake and sleep states. *Journal of Neuroscience*, **19**, 4595–4608.

Dujardin, K., Guerrien, A., and **Leconte, P.** (1990). Sleep, brain activation and cognition. *Physiology and Behavior*, **47**, 1271–1278.

Ehrenberger, K. and **Felix, D.** (1992). Caroverine depresses the activity of cochlear glutamate receptors in guinea pigs: in vivo model for drug-induced neuroprotection? *Neuropharmacology*, **31**, 1259–1263.

Eichenbaum, H. (2001). The hippocampus and declarative memory: cognitive mechanisms and neural codes. *Behavioural Brain Research*, **127**, 199–207.

Ekstrand, B. R., Barrett, T. R., West, J. N., and **Meier, W. G.** (1977). The effect of sleep on human long-term memory. In *Neurobiology of Sleep and Memory* (eds R. R. Drucker-Colin and J. L. McGaugh), pp. 419–438. Academic Press, New York.

Empson, J. A. and **Clarke, P. R.** (1970). Rapid eye movements and remembering. *Nature*, **227**, 287–288.

Feldman, R. and **Dement, W.** (1968). Possible relationships between REM sleep and memory consolidation. *Psychophysiology*, **5**, 243.

Ficca, G., Lombardo, P., Rossi, L., and **Salzarulo, P.** (2000). Morning recall of verbal material depends on prior sleep organization. *Behavioural Brain Research*, **112**, 159–163.

Fowler, M. J., Sullivan, M. J., and **Ekstrand, B. R.** (1973). Sleep and memory. *Science*, **179**, 302–304.

Fischer S, Hallschmid M, Elsner AL, Born J. (2002). Sleep forms memory for finger skills. *Proceedings of the National Academy of Sciences, USA*, **99**, 11987–11991.

Gais, S., Plihal, W., Wagner, U., and **Born, J.** (2000). Early sleep triggers memory for early visual discrimination skills. *Nature Neuroscience*, **3**, 1335–1339.

Giraux, P., Sirigu, A., Schneider, F., and **Dubernard, J. M.** (2001). Cortical reorganization in motor cortex after graft of both hands. *Nature Neuroscience*, **4**, 691–692.

Giuditta, A., Ambrosini, M. V., Montagnese, P., Mandile, P., Cotugno, M., Grassi, Z. G., and **Vescia, S.** (1995). The sequential hypothesis of the function of sleep. *Behavioural Brain Research*, **69**, 157–166.

Greenberg, R. and **Pearlman, C.** (1974). Cutting the REM nerve: an approach to the adaptive role of REM sleep. *Perspectives in Biology and Medicine*, **17**, 513–521.

Greenberg, R., Pearlman, C., Schwartz, W. R., and **Grossman, H. Y.** (1983). Memory, emotion, and REM sleep. *Journal of Abnormal Psychology*, **92**, 378–381.

Grieser, C., Greenberg, R., and **Harrison, R. H.** (1972). The adaptive function of sleep: the differential effects of sleep and dreaming on recall. *Journal of Abnormal Psychology*, **80**, 280–286.

Grosvenor, A. and Lack, L. C. (1984). The effect of sleep before or after learning on memory. *Sleep*, 7, 155–167.

Heine, R. (1914). Über Wiedererkennen und rückwirkende Hemmung. *Zeitschrift fur Psychologie mit Zeitschrift fur Angewandte Psychologie*, 68, 161–236.

Hennevin, E. and Leconte, P. (1977). Study of the relations between paradoxical sleep and learning processes. *Physiology and Behavior*, 18, 307–319.

Honore, T., Davies, S. N., Drejer, J., Fletcher, E. J., Jacobsen, P., Lodge, D., and Nielsen, F. E. (1988). Quinoxalinediones: potent competitive non-NMDA glutamate receptor antagonists. *Science*, 241, 701–703.

Horner, H. C., Packan, D. R., and Sapolsky, R. M. (1990). Glucocorticoids inhibit glucose transport in cultured hippocampal neurons and glia. *Neuroendocrinology*, 52, 57–64.

Hund-Georgiadis, M. and von Cramon, D. Y. (1999). Motor-learning-related changes in piano players and non-musicians revealed by functional magnetic-resonance signals. *Experimental Brain Research*, 125, 417–425.

Jenkins, J. G. and Dallenbach, K. M. (1924). Obliviscence during sleep and waking. *American Journal of Psychology*, 35, 605–612.

Karni, A. and Bertini, G. (1997). Learning perceptual skills: behavioral probes into adult cortical plasticity. *Current Opinion in Neurobiology*, 7, 530–535.

Karni, A., Meyer, G., Rey-Hipolito, C., Jezzard, P., Adams, M. M., Turner, R., and Ungerleider, L. G. (1998). The acquisition of skilled motor performance: fast and slow experience-driven changes in primary motor cortex. *Proceedings of the National Academy of Sciences, USA*, 95, 861–868.

Karni, A. and Sagi, D. (1991). Where practice makes perfect in texture discrimination: evidence for primary visual cortex plasticity. *Proceedings of the National Academy of Sciences, USA*, 88, 4966–4970.

Karni, A., Tanne, D., Rubenstein, B. S., Askenasy, J. J., and Sagi, D. (1994). Dependence on REM sleep of overnight improvement of a perceptual skill. *Science*, 265, 679–682.

Kim, J. J., Andreasen, N. C., O'Leary, D. S., Wiser, A. K., Ponto, L. L., Watkins, G. L., and Hichwa, R. D. (1999). Direct comparison of the neural substrates of recognition memory for words and faces. *Brain*, 122 (Pt 6), 1069–1083.

Kim, J. J., Clark, R. E., and Thompson, R. F. (1995). Hippocampectomy impairs the memory of recently, but not remotely, acquired trace eyeblink conditioned responses. *Behavioral Neuroscience*, 109, 195–203.

Kopell, B. S., Zarcone, V., De la, P. A., and Dement, W. C. (1972). Changes in selective attention as measured by the visual averaged evoked potential following REM deprivation in man. *Electroencephalography and Clinical Neurophysiology*, 32, 322–325.

Lang, P. J., Ohman, A., and Vaitl, D. (1988). *The international affective picture system [photographic slides]*. Center for Research in Psychophysiology, University of Florida, Gainesville., Gainesville, FL.

Lewin, I. and Glaubman, H. (1975). The effect of REM deprivation: is it detrimental, beneficial, or neutral? *Psychophysiology*, 12, 349–353.

Lovatt, D. J. and **Warr, P. B.** (1968). Recall after sleep. *American Journal of Psychology*, **81**, 253–257.

Malenka, R. C. and **Nicoll, R. A.** (1999). Long-term potentiation—a decade of progress? *Science*, **285**, 1870–1874.

Maquet, P., Laureys, S., Peigneux, P., Fuchs, S., Petiau, C., Phillips, C., Aerts, J., Del Fiore, G., Degueldre, C., Meulemans, T., Luxen, A., Franck, G., van der, L. M., Smith, C., and **Cleeremans, A.** (2000). Experience-dependent changes in cerebral activation during human REM sleep. *Nature Neuroscience*, **3**, 831–836.

Maquet, P., Peters, J., Aerts, J., Delfiore, G., Degueldre, C., Luxen, A., and **Franck, G.** (1996). Functional neuroanatomy of human rapid-eye-movement sleep and dreaming. *Nature*, **383**, 163–166.

Markowitsch, H. J., Calabrese, P., Wurker, M., Durwen, H. F., Kessler, J., Babinsky, R., Brechtelsbauer, D., Heuser, L., and **Gehlen, W.** (1994). The amygdala's contribution to memory—a study on two patients with Urbach-Wiethe disease. *Neuroreport*, **5**, 1349–1352.

Marshall, L., Mölle, M., Michaelsen, S., Fehm, H. L., and **Born, J.** (1996). Slow potential shifts at sleep—wake transitions and shifts between NREM sleep and REM sleep. *Sleep*, **19**, 145–151.

Marshall, L., Mölle, M., Fehm, H. L., and **Born, J.** (1998). Scalp recorded direct current brain potentials during human sleep. *European Journal of Neuroscience*, **10**, 1167–1178.

McClelland, J. L., McNaughton, B. L., and **O'Reilly, R. C.** (1995). Why there are complementary learning systems in the hippocampus and neocortex: insights from the successes and failures of connectionist models of learning and memory. *Psychological Review*, **102**, 419–457.

Mölle, M., Marshall, L., Gais, S., and **Born J.** (2002). Grouping of spindle activity during slow oscillations in human non-rapid eye movement sleep. *Journal of Neuroscience*, **22**, 10941–10947.

Muzio, J. W., Roffwarg, H. P., Anders, C. B., and **Muzio, L. G.** (1972). Retention of rote learned meaningful verbal material and alteration in the normal sleep EEG pattern. *Psychophysiology*, **9**, 108.

Newman, E. B. (1939). Forgetting of meaningful material during sleep and waking. *American Journal of Psychology*, **52**, 65–71.

Nofzinger, E. A., Mintun, M. A., Wiseman, M., Kupfer, D. J., and **Moore, R. Y.** (1997). Forebrain activation in REM sleep: an FDG PET study. *Brain Research*, **770**, 192–201.

Pavlides, C., Kimura, A., Magarinos, A. M., and **McEwen, B. S.** (1995*a*). Hippocampal homosynaptic long-term depression/depotentiation induced by adrenal steroids. *Neuroscience*, **68**, 379–385.

Pavlides, C., Watanabe, Y., Magarinos, A. M., and **McEwen, B. S.** (1995*b*). Opposing roles of type I and type II adrenal steroid receptors in hippocampal long-term potentiation. *Neuroscience*, **68**, 387–394.

Peigneux, P., Laureys, S., Delbeuck, X., and **Maquet, P.** (2001). Sleeping Brain, Learning Brain. The Role of Sleep and Memory Systems. *Neuroreport*, **12**, 111–124.

Plihal, W. and **Born, J.** (1997). Effects of early and late nocturnal sleep on declarative and procedural memory. *Journal of Cognitive Neuroscience*, **9**, 534–547.

Plihal, W. and Born, J. (1999*a*). Effects of early and late nocturnal sleep on priming and spatial memory. *Psychophysiology*, **36**, 571–582.

Plihal, W. and Born, J. (1999*b*). Memory consolidation in human sleep depends on inhibition of glucocorticoid release. *Neuroreport*, **10**, 2741–2747.

Plihal, W., Pietrowsky, R., and Born, J. (1999). Dexamethasone blocks sleep induced improvement of declarative memory. *Psychoneuroendocrinology*, **24**, 313–331.

Poldrack, R. A., Clark, J., Pare-Blagoev, E. J., Shohamy, D., Creso Moyano, J., Myers, C., and Gluck, M. A. (2001). Interactive memory systems in the human brain. *Nature*, **414**, 546–550.

Riedel, G., Micheau, J., Lam, A. G., Roloff, E., Martin, S. J., Bridge, H., Hoz, L., Poeschel, B., McCulloch, J., and Morris, R. G. (1999). Reversible neural inactivation reveals hippocampal participation in several memory processes. *Nature Neuroscience*, **2**, 898–905.

Sanes, J. N. and Donoghue, J. P. (2000). Plasticity and primary motor cortex. *Annual Review of Neuroscience*, **23**, 393–415.

Schacter, D. L. and Tulving, E. (1994). What are the memory systems of 1994? In *Memory systems* (eds D. L. Schacter and E. Tulving), pp. 1–38. MIT Press, Cambridge, MA.

Schoen, L. S. and Badia, P. (1984). Facilitated recall following REM and NREM naps. *Psychophysiology*, **21**, 299–306.

Sejnowski, T. J. and Destexhe, A. (2000). Why do we sleep? *Brain Research*, **886**, 208–223.

Shadmehr, R. and Brashers-Krug, T. (1997). Functional stages in the formation of human long-term motor memory. *Journal of Neuroscience*, **17**, 409–419.

Shadmehr, R. and Holcomb, H. H. (1997). Neural correlates of motor memory consolidation. *Science*, **227**, 821–825.

Smith, C. (1995). Sleep states and memory processes. *Behavioural Brain Research*, **69**, 137–145.

Smith, C. and Wong, P. T. (1991). Paradoxical sleep increases predict successful learning in a complex operant task. *Behavioral Neuroscience*, **105**, 282–288.

Spath-Schwalbe, E., Uthgenannt, D., Voget, G., Kern, W., Born, J., and Fehm, H. L. (1993). Corticotropin-releasing hormone-induced adrenocorticotropin and cortisol secretion depends on sleep and wakefulness. *Journal of Clinical Endocrinology and Metabolism*, **77**, 1170–1173.

Squire, L. R. (1992). Memory and the hippocampus: a synthesis from findings with rats, monkeys, and humans. *Psychological Review*, **99**, 195–231.

Squire, L. R. (1993). The hippocampus and spatial memory. *Trends in Neurosciences*, **16**, 56–57.

Squire, L. R., Ojemann, J. G., Miezin, F. M., Petersen, S. E., Videen, T. O., and Raichle, M. E. (1992). Activation of the hippocampus in normal humans: a functional anatomical study of memory. *Proceedings of the National Academy of Sciences, USA*, **89**, 1837–1841.

Squire, L. R. and Zola-Morgan, S. (1991). The medial temporal lobe memory system. *Science*, **253**, 1380–1386.

Steriade, M. (1999). Coherent oscillations and short-term plasticity in corticothalamic networks. *Trends in Neurosciences*, **22**, 337–345.

Steriade, M., Amzica, F., and **Contreras, D.** (1996). Synchronization of fast (30–40 Hz) spontaneous cortical rhythms during brain activation. *Journal of Neuroscience*, **16**, 392–417.

Stickgold, R., James, L., and **Hobson, J. A.** (2000*a*). Visual discrimination learning requires sleep after training. *Nature Neuroscience*, **3**, 1237–1238.

Stickgold, R., Whidbee, D., Schirmer, B., Patel, V., and **Hobson, J. A.** (2000*b*). Visual discrimination task improvement: a multi-step process occurring during sleep. *Journal of Cognitive Neuroscience*, **12**, 246–254.

Stones, M. J. (1973). The effect of prior sleep on rehearsal, recoding and memory. *British Journal of Psychology*, **64**, 537–543.

Stones, M. J. (1977). Memory performance after arousal from different sleep stages. *British Journal of Psychology*, **68**, 177–181.

Teng, E. and **Squire, L. R.** (1999). Memory for places learned long ago is intact after hippocampal damage. *Nature*, **400**, 675–677.

Tilley, A. J. and **Empson, J. A.** (1978). REM sleep and memory consolidation. *Biological Psychology*, **6**, 293–300.

Tilley, A. J. and **Empson, J. A.** (1981). Picture recall and recognition following total and selective sleep deprivation. In *Sleep '80* (ed. W. P. Koella), pp. 367–369. Karger, Basel.

Wagner, U., Fischer, S., and **Born, J.** (2002). Changes in emotional responses to aversive pictures across periods rich in slow wave sleep vs. rapid eye movement sleep. *Psychosomatic Medicine*, **64**, 627–634.

Wagner, U., Gais, S., and **Born, J.** (2001). Emotional memory formation is enhanced across sleep intervals with high amounts of rapid eye movement sleep. *Learning and Memory*, **8**, 112–119.

Winocur, G. (1990). Anterograde and retrograde amnesia in rats with dorsal hippocampal or dorsomedial thalamic lesions. *Behavioral Brain Sciences*, **38**, 145–154.

Yaroush, R., Sullivan, M. J., and **Ekstrand, B. R.** (1971). Effect of sleep on memory. II. Differential effect of the first and second half of the night. *Journal of Experimental Psychology*, **88**, 361–366.

CHAPTER 4

A ROLE FOR STAGE 2 SLEEP IN MEMORY PROCESSING

REBECCA NADER AND CARLYLE SMITH

Some basic characteristics of stage 2

Stage 2 sleep is the classification given to approximately 50 percent of the night of sleep in humans. It is recognized as having very salient features that distinguish it from other sleep stages. Traditionally, stage 2 sleep has been defined as having background EEG frequencies in the 5–8 Hz range, with intermittent 12–14 Hz spindle activity and K-complex slow wave activity (Rechtschaffen and Kales 1968). It occurs mainly in the last two-thirds of the night. Despite the presence of this stage in larger amounts than any other stage of sleep, the functions of stage 2 remain obscure.

A number of studies, driven by diverse hypotheses, have examined stage 2 in different contexts. Some unique characteristics have been identified. For example, stage 2 is not the first stage of sleep to recover after total sleep deprivation (TSD). Stage 3 and stage 4 sleep (SWS) appear to be the first priority, followed by REM sleep recovery and then stage 2 sleep recovery (Bonnet 2000). For this reason, stage 2 has often been considered less vital to the individual than the other two stages of sleep.

The average spectral power of stage 2 is relatively similar to that seen in REM sleep. The main difference, however, between the two stages is the 12–14 Hz (sigma) spindle activity of stage 2 that does not occur in REM sleep. Generation of this spindle activity is not evenly distributed throughout the brain and differs at central, parietal and frontal EEG recording sites (Tanguay *et al.* 1975; Sterman *et al.* 1978; Zeitlhofer *et al.* 1997).

The other distinctive wave form of stage 2 is the K-complex. This wave complex is composed of a well-delineated negative sharp wave immediately followed by a positive component. The duration of the K-complex is at least 0.5 s. K-complexes are observed to be largest when measured over the vertex area. K-complexes appear at the rate of 1–3 per min in young adults, with some individual variability. The K-complex appears spontaneously during stage 2 but can also be evoked by a variety of auditory stimuli (Carskadon and Rechtschaffen 1994).

Differences in stage 2 sleep architecture have been found to distinguish various pathological and drug groups. For example, Sterman *et al.* (1978) examined the sleep of normal, insomniac, and epileptic patients. He found that insomniacs and epileptics showed more activity in both the faster frequencies (beta) and slower frequencies (delta, theta, alpha) of stage 2 and lower amounts of spindle activity (12–14 Hz) than did the normal subjects in this stage.

Drugs can modulate stage 2 activity. Benzodiazepines have been observed to increase the amount of stage 2 as well as the density of sleep spindles (Hirshkowitz *et al.* 1982; Karacan *et al.* 1984; Carskadon and Rechtschaffen 1994). Phenobarbitol was also observed to increase the amount of stage 2, but the effect was much less pronounced than that of the benzodiazepines (Hirshkowitz *et al.* 1982).

Transition from stage 2 to waking involves an increase in faster frequency bands (alpha, beta) before there is a reduction in the slower frequencies (theta, delta) (Simons *et al.* 1990). Transition from stage 2 to REM sleep involves systematic changes of all of the frequencies, with delta, theta, and sigma decreasing while alpha increases (Hadjiyannakis *et al.* 1996).

Parasympathetic autonomic activities such as heart rate have been found to increase during stage 2 sleep while sympathetic activity is greater during REM sleep and the awake state (Bonnet and Arand 1996; Trinder *et al.* 2001).

Electrophysiology and neurophysiology of the sleep spindle

Rechtschaffen and Kales (1968) defined spindles as wave forms with frequencies between 12 and 14 Hz, with a minimum duration of 0.5 s. Since then, researchers have enlarged this original definition, particularly with respect to expanding the frequency range of sleep spindles (Jankel and Niedermeyer 1985).

With respect to duration and number of spindles occurring, in adults, sleep spindles last from 0.5 to 2 s and occur between 2 and 8 times a minute (Gaillard and Blois 1981; Carskadon and Rechtschaffen 1994). Sleep spindles are fusiform in shape, hence the name "spindle."

The topographic distribution of sleep spindles during stage 2 sleep was examined by Zeitlhofer *et al.* (1997). Spindle density was found to decrease from the beginning of the night to the end, and the topographic distribution of sleep spindles throughout the brain was observed to change over the course of the night, with maximal occurrences in the parietal, central, and left frontal regions at the beginning of the night and a more central distribution by the end of the night. However, despite the observed shift in the distribution of sleep spindles, Zeitlhofer *et al.* (1997) found that the maximum spindle density occurred in the centro-parietal region, regardless of time of night.

Evidence has also been found for two distinct types of sleep spindles, distinguished by both their frequency and the region of the brain in which they occur (Werth *et al.* 1997; Zeitlhofer *et al.* 1997; Zygierewicz *et al.* 1999). The slow spindle has a frequency of approximately 12 Hz (range of 11.5–14 Hz) and occurs predominantly in the frontal region of the brain, while the fast spindle has a frequency of approximately 14 Hz (14–16 Hz) and occurs primarily in the parietal region (Werth *et al.* 1997; Zeitlhofer *et al.* 1997). These results support the hypothesis that there are several spindle generators in the brain. Many researchers measure spindles only at the central location, and

Jobert *et al.* (1992) suggest that the activity that is thus being measured is actually an average of the activity occurring in the frontal and parietal regions.

The sleep spindle is a well-developed phenomenon in all mammalian species (Carskadon and Rechtschaffen 1994) and has now been physiologically described at the transmitter, cellular and neural network levels (Destexhe and Senjowski 2001). For example, Nunez *et al.* (1992) studied spindle activity in the cat. They concluded that spindles are waves of 11–16 Hz that are a result of oscillations between thalamocortical and corticothalamic cells. They further concluded that the spindle oscillations originate in the thalamus, generated by intrinsic properties of reticular thalamic neurons.

A suggested function of these sleep oscillations is synaptic plasticity (Steriade and Amzica 1998*a*; Steriade 1999; Destexhe and Sejnowski 2001; Steriade *et al.* 2001; see Chapter 13). One of the remarkable occurrences in the stage 2 sleep spindle is that during spindling, cortical pyramidal cells receive strong dendritic excitation from the thalamus. Simultaneously, these same cortical cells are inhibited from firing by inhibitory thalamic input to the cell bodies. The depolarization of these cortical cells coupled with inhibition to prevent the cells from firing results in a physiological state ideal for the influx of Ca^{++} ions, without excessive cell firing. It is suggested that this influx may serve to prime the synapses for permanent changes, since Ca^{++} mechanisms are clearly involved with synaptic plasticity (Ghosh and Greenburg 1995). This calcium influx may also be involved with the gene expression which occurs during synaptic plasticity (Abel *et al.* 1997; Li *et al.* 1998; see Chapters 15 and 16). Thus, the sleep spindle provides a physiological brain state which is theoretically ideal for synaptic plasticity.

Developmental aspects of the spindle

Tanguay *et al.* (1975) conducted a study that examined sleep spindles in young children. The participants ranged in age from 4 to 68 months. It was found that the number of spindles observed, their duration, and the percent of spindle activity reached a maximum between the ages of 4 and 6 months of age. After the age of 6 months, spindle activity was observed to decrease to a minimum at 27 months, to remain stable until approximately 54 months of age, and then to increase in the older subjects (i.e. up to 68 months). The mean frequency of the spindle activity however, appeared to decrease, as the child got older. The mean frequency was 13–14 Hz for children less than 40 months of age and for older children was 12–13 Hz. The researchers also found that the level of interhemispheric synchrony of spindle appearance was higher in the older children (>54 months) compared to the younger children (<22 months). It was suggested that due to the differences found between older and younger children, sleep spindles could be used as an indicator of neural maturation.

Frontal and parietal spindles appear to follow somewhat different developmental paths. The frequency of frontal spindles changes with age, with a frequency at 11–12 Hz prior to age 10 and then increasing to 12–14 Hz at approximately age 13, whereafter it appears to remain stable throughout adolescence and into adulthood. Frontal spindles appear to reach their peak power at approximately age 10 after which the power declines until early adulthood (age 13–14) when it stabilizes at a somewhat lower level (Shinomiya *et al.* 1999).

Parietal spindles also vary with the age of the individual (Shinomiya *et al.* 1999). During the first 10 years of life, children exhibit some low-frequency parietal spindles (i.e. <13 Hz), but the frequency of occurrence of these spindles declines until age 13 when the most common frequency of the parietal spindles is between 13.5 and 14.5 Hz. In contrast to the decline in power observed in frontal spindles, the power of the parietal spindles appears to be stable from childhood into young adulthood, suggesting that frontal and parietal spindles are following different developmental courses and may be serving different functions.

Researchers have consistently found that the rate of occurrence of sleep spindles can vary between 3 and 8 per minute in different individuals (Gaillard and Blois 1981). The peak frequency of those spindles has also been found to vary considerably between individuals (Werth *et al.* 1997). For example, Shinomiya *et al.* (1999) found that there was high stability for the peak frequency of spindles within individuals, although there were marked inter-individual differences. The stability of the number of spindles within an individual has been demonstrated in a number of laboratories (Gaillard and Blois 1981; Principe and Smith 1982; de Maertelaer *et al.* 1987; Nader and Smith 2001). Nader and Smith (2001) found that the number of spindles per minute correlated almost perfectly between night 1 and night 2 in a group of 10 normal young adults. The sigma power of the spindles was also very highly correlated between night 1 and night 2. These findings reinforce the idea that the native number of spindles, the power of those spindles and possibly the peak frequency, are all quite stable within an individual.

Perception and cognition during stage 2

Church and Johnson (1977) studied responses to auditory clicks in humans in order to determine whether or not sleep spindles inhibit sensory input. When spindle-synchronous auditory or spindle-asynchronous auditory clicks were presented during ascending stage 2, it was found that the number of K-complexes evoked by the clicks was greater for the spindle-synchronous condition. This result suggested that input was not suppressed by the sleep spindles. In the same study, when heart rate and finger pulse response magnitudes were examined, it was found that there were more evoked K-complexes and a larger heart rate response to the clicks presented during ascending stage 2 than to those presented during descending stage 2. Church and Johnson (1977) suggested that spindles are not inhibitory and might in fact occur during periods of increased central nervous system excitability.

A number of studies have focused on the possibility that learning could take place during stage 2. For example, Townsend *et al.* (1976) presented tone pulses during stage 2 and studied the subsequent auditory evoked potentials. They found that neither the amplitude nor the latencies of the evoked potentials changed over 30 days of stimulus exposure, suggesting that the participants were not habituating to the tones. They concluded that no memory trace was being formed during sleep.

Oltman *et al.* (1977) looked at perception and retention during stage 2 sleep. Single digit numbers were presented every 30 s and subjects were awakened during stage 2 either 1, 5, or 10 s after presentation and asked to recall the number presented. They concluded that while memory traces could be formed during stage 2, they decayed very quickly.

Tilley (1979) showed pictures to participants prior to sleep onset. For half of the pictures, equivalent words were presented either during subsequent stage 2 or REM sleep. Pictures connected with words presented during stage 2 were better remembered than those not connected with words. Pictures connected with words presented during REM sleep were not recalled any better than those not connected with words. The author concluded that repetition of information during stage 2 could enhance memory storage processes that were presumably already occurring.

Stage 2, learning, and memory

Smith and MacNeill (1992, 1994) examined the effects of imposing various kinds of sleep deprivation after simple motor task acquisition had occurred. Participants were trained on the pursuit rotor motor skills task on the evening after an acclimatization night in the lab. They were then split into groups that received either REM sleep deprivation (REMD), equivalent non-REM awakening (NREMD), total sleep deprivation for the last half of the night (LH-TSD), or total sleep deprivation for the entire night (TSD). There was also a non-deprived control group. Retesting on the task was done 1 week later. The LH-TSD group was used to deprive the subjects of a large amount of stage 2.

Results showed that the TSD and LH-TSD groups performed poorly compared to the REMD and Control groups. The NREMD group, that was not significantly different from any of the other groups, showed an intermediate level of performance. Since REM sleep and stage 2 are the two main stages of sleep during the last half of the night, the LH-TSD group was deprived of both stages. However, as the REMD group demonstrated, REM sleep was not important for this task. Thus, it was concluded that stage 2 sleep was the important stage of sleep for memory processing of this task. Further, the individual task scores were significantly correlated with the amount of stage 2 subjects from all groups got on the post-training night. Correlations of performance with the other sleep stages were not significant (Smith and MacNeill 1992, 1994; see Fig. 4.1).

Smith and Fazekas (1997) presented both a cognitive procedural (complex logic task) and a motor procedural (pursuit rotor) task to college students. Participants were allowed to sleep for the first half of the night and then were either exposed to REM sleep deprivation during the last half of the night or total sleep deprivation (TSD) during the last half of the night. A third group had an entire night of uninterrupted sleep in the lab (controls). The pursuit rotor task was poorly remembered by the group deprived of TSD in the last half of the night. This group also obtained the least amount of stage 2 sleep. The group deprived of REM sleep in the last half of the night managed to get a modest

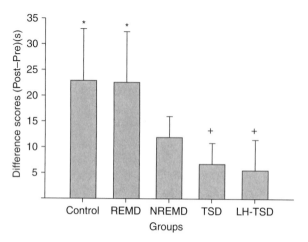

Figure 4.1 Shows the mean (+SEM) improvement in memory for the pursuit rotor task for groups exposed to either REM sleep deprivation (REMD), equivalent non-REMD (NREMD), total sleep deprivation for the entire night (TSD) or total sleep deprivation for the last half of the night only (LH-TSD). There was also a normally rested control group (Control). The REMD group performed as well as the Control group. The TSD and LH-TSD groups were significantly impaired compared to the REMD and Control groups ($p < 0.05$).

amount of stage 2 and had better scores on the pursuit rotor task than did the TSD group. The control group had the most stage 2 and also had the best pursuit rotor scores of all. The amount of REM sleep was not at all related to performance on the motor task, although as expected (Smith 1995, 2001), was very important for the logic task.

These results have important implications. First, post-training stage 2 would appear to be important for the efficient memory consolidation of procedural motor or skills tasks. On the other hand, memory for these skills tasks would appear to be completely unaffected by the amount of REM sleep that has occurred. The results may indicate two independent memory systems are at work here, one that requires REM sleep and the other that requires stage 2 (Smith 2001).

Walker *et al.* (2002) recently reported that memory for a simple finger tapping task was improved by 20 percent if subjects were allowed a night of sleep between training and retesting. Further, they observed that there was a very high correlation between post-sleep performance and the amount of stage 2 in the last quarter of the sleep night.

In another laboratory, Gais *et al.* (2002) have reported that spindle density increased following the learning of a paired associate task. The spindle density was most prominent at the first part of the night of sleep.

In an attempt to study the relationship between sleep and spatial memory, Meier-Koll *et al.* (1999) examined the effect of "walking" through a computer maze on sleep architecture. Participants traversed through either a complex or simple maze for a period of 8 h. They then slept over night in the sleep lab. Those that learned the simple maze spent significantly more time in stage 2 than those exploring the complex maze. While the count was not complete, and the spindles were not compared within subjects, the number of spindles in a 5-min period between groups was also higher for the group that learned the simple task compared to the complex test group and a control group. The results could mean that the number of spindles was increased following task acquisition.

These maze findings are similar to results from our own lab concerning increases in number of spindles following task acquisition (Fogel *et al.* 2001). In a preliminary study, subjects were asked to learn a number of procedural motor tasks. These skills tasks included the pursuit rotor, the ball and cup, a direct trace task and "Operation," a game where fine manual dexterity was required to remove toy body parts from the "patient." Subjects were exposed to an acclimatization and baseline night of sleep in the lab. On the evening prior to the third night of sleep, subjects were exposed to these tasks and then a third night of sleep was recorded. Task retesting was done 1 week later. It was hypothesized that there would be an increase in the number of spindles observed in the stage 2 of each experimental subject who acquired the task during the post-training night of sleep compared to their own baseline spindle levels. It was also predicted that subjects not exposed to the tasks would show the same number of spindles on both baseline and post-baseline nights. Results showed that there was a marked increase in the total number of spindles for the trained group. This increase averaged about 42 percent and there was a correlation between the increase in spindles and the scores on the skills tasks. Generally, the better the scores of the individual, the greater was the increase in number of post-training stage 2 spindles. Subjects that were not exposed to the tasks showed no changes in number of spindles and there were no initial differences in terms of number of baseline spindles between groups (Fogel *et al.* 2001; Fig. 4.2). Thus results support

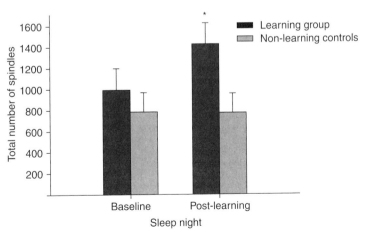

Figure 4.2 Shows the mean (+SEM) number of spindles for both the learning and non-learning groups. The number of spindles does not differ between groups on baseline night. The group exposed to the skills tasks showed a significant increase in number of spindles ($p < 0.01$) compared to baseline and non-learning controls.

the idea that spindle activity might reflect brain activity involved in memory processing of motor procedural material. The idea that synaptic plasticity is occurring during the oscillatory activity of the spindle has been suggested by others (Steriade and Amzica 1998; Steriade 1999; Destexhe and Sejnowski 2001).

Spindles and learning ability

Recently, some researchers have begun to investigate how sleep spindles might be related to learning ability. Briere *et al.* (2000) examined whether the number of native sleep spindles was related to implicit recall ability the next day. Participants spent 2 nights in the lab and the number of spindles was counted on the second night. The next day, participants were tested for explicit recall, implicit recall, and word span. These researchers found that the number of sleep spindles on the previous night was significantly positively correlated with implicit recall ability, but not with explicit recall or word span. These results suggest that some of our native cognitive abilities are related to number of stage 2 sleep spindles. Nader *et al.* (2001) proposed that spindle activity might be related to our potential to learn. These researchers had participants complete the Multidimensional Aptitude Battery II (MAB-II), which assesses the verbal and nonverbal intelligence of the individual. Subjects were then asked to spend the subsequent 2 nights (acclimatization and baseline) in the sleep lab. Sleep spindles (12–16 Hz and 0.5 s minimum duration) were counted from every page of the clean (i.e. no movement or other artifacts) baseline stage 2 sleep. Sigma power (12–14 Hz) was also assessed for the same pages in order to get an independent and objective measure of spindle activity.

Sigma power and spindle counts both provided the same pattern of results. Both correlated positively and significantly with Full Scale Intelligence Quotients (IQ) and with the Performance IQ subscale, respectively, but not with Verbal IQ subscale (see Fig. 4.3 for Full Scale IQ). The correlations of sigma power with Full Scale and Performance IQs were even stronger in the last third of the night, when a large proportion of sleep is stage 2. When the Performance and Verbal portions of the IQ test were broken down into their separate components, sigma power and spindle activity positively correlated with those subtests that require perceptual, analytical and reasoning skills. The correlations suggest that a higher level of spindle activity (as assessed by total number of spindles and sigma power) is related to a greater ability to perform tasks which require perceptual, analytical and reasoning abilities.

In a learning study, the number of spindles that a participant exhibited was significantly, positively correlated with the Performance IQ subscale of the MAB-II. A significant positive correlation was also found between sigma power (12–14 Hz) and Performance IQ (Fogel *et al.* 2001). These findings support those of Nader and Smith (2001) that higher scores on the Performance portion of the IQ test are related to higher amounts of "native" spindle activity. The results from these studies suggest that spindles are an indicator of current level of aptitude for learning certain types of material (Briere *et al.* 2000;

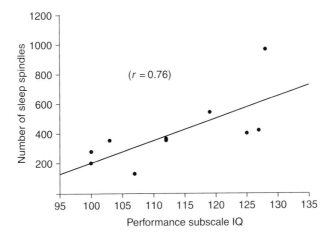

Figure 4.3 Shows the correlation between number of stage 2 spindles and Full Scale IQ score. Correlation is significant ($p < 0.01$).

Nader and Smith 2001). The spindle also increases in numbers following procedural motor learning and appears to be involved in memory consolidation of this material (Meier-Koll *et al.* 1999; Fogel *et al.* 2001).

Future directions

While stage 2 probably has a number of functions, there is evidence that this state of sleep is involved with the consolidation of procedural motor tasks. Although much remains to be done, minutes of stage 2 and number of spindles within stage 2 have both been related to memory for skills tasks.

From the developmental perspective, there is evidence to suggest that the native number of spindles exhibited by each individual is a biological marker for ability to learn certain kinds of tasks.

Many questions remain. The post-training time during which spindle activity remains elevated following skills task acquisition is unknown. Is the number of spindles determined at birth for an individual or can the number be enhanced by some kind of practice or enriched environment? What kinds of tasks are stage 2 sensitive?

The possibility that stage 2 sleep is important for motor learning (and perhaps other kinds of learning) has important practical implications for sleep quality, especially in the developing child. While emphasis is now being focused on the role of sleep and academic progress in school and while other stages of sleep are also important (Gozal 1998) these results reinforce the importance of further research to help realize the maximum motor skills potential of developing children.

References

Abel, T., Nguyen, P. V., Barad, M., Deuel, T. A. S., Kandel, E. R., and Bourtchouladze, R. (1997). Genetic demonstration of a role for PKA in the late phase of LTP and in hipppocampus—based long-term memory. *Cell*, **88**, 615–626.

Bonnet, M. H. (2000). Sleep deprivation. In *Principles and practice of sleep medicine* (eds M. Kryger, T. Roth, and W. Dement). Saunders, Philadelphia, pp. 53–71.

Bonnet, M. H., and Arand, D. L. (1996). Heart rate variability: sleep stage, time of night, and arousal effects. *Sleep Research*, **25**, 119.

Briere, M., Forest, G., Lussier, I., and Godbout, R. (2000). Implicit verbal recall correlates positively with EEG sleep spindle activity. *Sleep*, **23** (Suppl. 2), A219.

Carskadon, M. and Rechtschaffen, A. (1994). Monitoring and staging human sleep. In *Principles and practice of sleep medicine* (eds M. Kryger, T. Roth, and W. C. Dement), pp. 943–960. Saunders, Philadelphia.

Church, M. W. and Johnson, L. C. (1977). Human EEG and cardiovascular responses to spindle synchronous and spindle asynchronous clicks during stage 2 sleep. *Sleep Research*, **6**, 24.

de Maertelaer, V., Hoffmann, G., Lemaire, M., and Mendlewicz, J. (1987). Sleep spindle activity changes in patients with affective disorders. *Sleep*, **10**, 443–451.

Destexhe, A. and Sejnowski, T. J. (2001). Thalamocortical assemblies: how ion channels, single neurons and large—scale networks organize sleep oscillations. *Monographs of the Physiological Society 49*, Oxford University Press, Oxford.

Fogel, S., Jacob, J., and Smith, C. (2001). Increased sleep spindle activity following simple motor procedural learning in humans. *Actas de Fisiologia*, **7**, 123.

Gaillard, J.-M. and Blois, R. (1981). Spindle density in sleep of normal subjects. *Sleep*, **4**, 385–391.

Gais, S., Molle, M., Helms, K., and Born, J. (2002). Learning-dependent increases in sleep spindle density. *Journal of Neuroscience*, **22**, 6830–6834.

Ghosh, A. and Greenburg, M. E. (1995). Calcium signaling in neurons: molecular mechanisms and cellular consequences. *Science*, **268**, 239–247.

Gozal, D. (1998). Sleep-disordered breathing and school performance in children. *Pediatrics*, **102**, 616–620.

Hadjiyannakis, K., Ogilvie, R. D., Alloway, C. E. D., and Murphy, T. (1996). FFT analysis of the stage 2-REM sleep transitions in narcoleptics and controls. *Sleep Research*, **25**, 126.

Hirshkowitz, M., Thornby, J. I., and Karacan, I. (1982). Sleep spindles: pharmacological effects in humans. *Sleep*, **5**, 85–94.

Jankel, W. R. and Niedermeyer, E. (1985). Sleep spindles. *Journal of Clinical Neurophysiology*, **2**, 1–35.

Jobert, M., Poiseau, E., Jahnig, P., Schulz, H., and Kubicki, S. (1992). Topographical analysis of sleep spindle activity. *Neuropsychobiology*, **26**, 210–217.

Karacan, I., Orr, W., Kramer, M., Thornby, J. I., and Hirshkowitz, M. (1984). The effects of chronic flurazepam or phenobarbitol on stage 2 sleep in insomniacs. *Sleep Research*, **13**, 50.

Li, W., Llopis, J., Whitney, M., Zlokarnik, G., and **Tsien, R. Y.** (1998). Cell—permanent caged InsP3 ester shows that Ca^{++} spike frequency can optimize gene expression. *Nature*, **392**, 936–941.

Meier-Koll, A., Bussmann, B., Schmidt, C., and **Neuschwander, D.** (1999). Walking through a maze alters the architecture of sleep. *Perceptual and Motor Skills*, **88**, 1141–1159.

Nader, R. S. and **Smith, C. T.** (2001). The relationship between stage 2 sleep spindles and intelligence. *Sleep*, **24** (Suppl.), A160.

Nunez, A., Curo Dossi, R., Contreras, D., and **Steriade, M.** (1992). Intracellular evidence for incompatibility between spindle and delta oscillations in thalamocortical neurons of the cat. *Neuroscience*, **48**, 75–85.

Oltman, P. K., Goodenough, D. R., Koulack, D., Maclin, E., Schroeder, H. R., and **Flannagan, M. J.** (1977). Short-term memory during stage 2 sleep. *Psychophysiology*, **14**, 439–444.

Principe, J. C. and **Smith, J. R.** (1982). Spindle characteristics as a function of age. *Sleep*, **5**, 73–84.

Rechtschaffen, A. and **Kales, A.** (1968). *A manual of standardized terminology, techniques and scoring system for sleep scoring stages of human subjects.* US Department of Health, Education and Welfare, Public Health Services: Bethesda, MD.

Shinomiya, S., Nagata, K., Takahashi, K., and **Masumura, T.** (1999). Development of sleep spindles in young children and adolescents. *Clinical Electroencephalography*, **30**, 39–43.

Simons, I. A., Ogilvie, R. D., Segalowitz, S. J., and **Janicki, M. G.** (1990). EEG power spectrum changes during behaviorally indicated arousals from stage 2 sleep. *Sleep Research*, **19**, 131.

Smith, C. (1995). Sleep states and memory processes. *Behavioural Brain Research*, **69**, 137–145.

Smith, C. (2001). Sleep states and memory processes in humans: procedural vs declarative memory systems. *Sleep Medicine Reviews*, **5**, 491–506.

Smith, C. and **Fazekas, A.** (1997). Amounts of REM sleep and Stage 2 required for efficient learning. *Sleep Research*, **26**, 690.

Smith, C. and **MacNeill, C.** (1992). Memory for motor task is impaired by stage 2 sleep loss. *Sleep Research*, **21**, 139.

Smith, C. and **MacNeill, C.** (1994). Impaired motor memory for a pursuit rotor task following Stage 2 sleep loss in college students. *Journal of Sleep Research*, **3**, 206–213.

Steriade, M. (1999). Coherent oscillations and short term plasticity in corticothalamic networks. *Trends in Neurosciences*, **8**, 337–345.

Steriade, M. and **Amzica, F.** (1998). Coalescence of sleep rhythms and their chronology in corticothalamic networks. *Sleep Research Online*, **1**, 1–10.

Steriade, M., Timofeev, I., and **Grenier, F.** (2001). Natural waking and sleep states: a view from inside neocortical neurons. *Joural of Neurophysiology*, **85**, 1969–1985.

Sterman, M. B., Berntsen, I., and **Matsuno, D.** (1978). Quantitative comparison of stage 2 sleep EEG characteristics in normal, insomniac and epileptic subjects. *Sleep Research*, **7**, 52.

Tanguay, P. E., Ornitz, E. M., Kaplan, A., and **Bozzo, E. S.** (1975). Evolution of sleep spindles in childhood. *Electroencephalography and Clinical Neurophysiology*, **38**, 175–181.

Tilley, A. J. (1979). Sleep learning during stage 2 and REM sleep. *Biological Psychology*, **9**, 155–161.

Townsend, R. E., House, J. F., and Johnson, L. C. (1976). Auditory evoked potential in Stage 2 and REM sleepduring a 30 day exposure to tone pulses. *Psychophysiology*, **13**, 54–57.

Trinder, J., Kleiman, J., Carrington, M., Smith, S., Breen, S., Tan, N., and Kim, Y. (2001). Autonomic activity during human sleep as a function of time and sleep stage. *Journal of Sleep Research*, **10**, 253–264.

Walker, M., Brakefield, T., Morgan, A., Hobson, J., and Stickgold, R. (2002). Practice with sleep makes perfect: Sleep dependent motor skill learning. *Neuron*, **35**, 205–211.

Werth, E., Acherman, P., Dijk, D.-J., and Borbely, A. A. (1997). Spindle frequency activity in the sleep EEG: Individual differences and topographic distribution. *Electroencephalography and Clinical Neurophysiology*, **103**, 535–542.

Zeitlhofer, J., Gruber, G., Anderer, P., Asenbaum, S., Schimicek, P., and Saletu, B. (1997). Topographic distribution of sleep spindles in young healthy subjects. *Journal of Sleep Research*, **6**, 149–155.

Zygierewicz, J., Blinowska, K. J., Durka, P. J., Szelenberger, Q., Niemcwicz, S., and Androsiuk, Q. (1999). High resolution study of sleep spindles. *Clinical Electroencephalography*, **110**, 2136–2147.

ANIMAL BEHAVIOR

This section is composed of the animal behavioral and electrophysiological data that have accumulated over the last 35 years or so in support of the idea that there is a close relationship between memory processing or consolidation and sleep states. Some of the earliest intensive work on this problem was carried out in the laboratory of Dr Vincent Bloch at the University of Paris. The first chapter, by Dr Elizabeth Hennevin, describes the early EEG sleep recording and sleep-deprivation studies. Despite the short post-training examination period (usually 3–4 h), the results of these studies indicated that REM sleep increases were correlated with successful learning while non-learning animals did not show these increases. Conversely, selective REM sleep-deprivation impaired memory for the task. In later studies this lab showed that stimulation of the reticular formation could replace the post-learning REM sleep activity and reverse the REM sleep-deprivation effect. They also showed modulation of memory during REM sleep by presenting reminder stimuli to the sleeping rat. Further, they also showed that the pairing of internal neural stimuli resulted in learning if the pairing took place during REM sleep. This learning could be observed in the awake state as well but did not occur in SWS. They also showed that conditioning in the awake state could be observed again in the sleep state, particularly REM sleep and identified the neural structures most involved. These early studies were important in answering some very basic questions about sleep and memory consolidation which are ignored by critics today, yet the data are of high quality.

The second chapter is written by Carlyle Smith. The first work by this author was done in the laboratory of Dr Michel Jouvet at the Université Claude-Bernard in Lyon, France. The first study was also published in the early 1970s. This work continued at Trent University in Peterborough, Canada. In adding to the work of the Paris lab, the technique of EEG recording continuously over long periods of time revealed more complex timing relationships between sleep and memory while at the same time confirming earlier work that suggested a strong role for REM sleep in post-training memory processing. Studies from this lab resulted in the concept of the REM sleep window (RSW), which identified important post-training REM sleep times when memory was apparently being processed and when REM sleep loss was devastating for memory formation. More recent work focuses on the transmitter acetylcholine during these REM sleep windows as well as its activity in the lateral amygdala during the RSWs. A section in this chapter is also devoted to dealing with the long continuing argument that stress is the explanation for the REM sleep changes observed and the memory loss following platform REM sleep-deprivation. Recent and older data make this idea unlikely.

The fourth chapter is a contribution by Dr Antonio Giuditta, another early pioneer in the field of sleep and memory. Dr Giuditta's contribution is the emphasis he places on slow wave sleep (SWS) which was not focused upon in the earlier studies simply because it did not change in number of minutes after training. Further, other manipulations during SWS did not seem to be very fruitful. Dr Giuditta takes us through his early work and up to the present with an excellent examination of how SWS fits into the equation as well as REM sleep. With the more sophisticated methods of examining the wave characteristics of SWS, we are introduced to a state of sleep that appears to be a very important correlate of successful learning, the transitional sleep state. One of his most important contributions may well be the idea that the sequences of the different states of sleep are important to successful memory processing.

Meanwhile, the third chapter in this section has been contributed by Subimal Datta and Elissa Patterson at the Boston University School of Medicine. The work from this lab is consistent with the earlier work and extends those findings. The chapter provides an excellent description of the possible REM sleep mechanisms involved in the post-raining sleep memory processing in the rat. The chapter provides a detailed description of the physiological mechanisms and neural structures involved in the phenomenon we call REM sleep, including the ponto-geniculo-occipital (PGO) equivalent in the rat, the P wave. They argue that the P wave generator is capable and has all the properties necessary to induce physiological long-term potentiation (LTP). They provide both electrophysiological and behavioral data to support their ideas. Rats learned a two-way shuttle avoidance task and the subsequent sleep showed a 181 percent increase in the transitional stage between SWS and REM sleep and a 30 percent increase in REM sleep. They also observed a marked increase in the density of P waves at this time. There was a high correlation between P wave density and avoidance score improvement. It is interesting to note here that the transitional stage of sleep described by Giuditta and by Datta and Patterson is probably the same sleep state.

Finally, it is interesting to note the discrepancy between the models proposed by Datta and Patterson on the one hand and Buzsáki et al. (Chapter 13) on the other hand. The flows of information between the neocortex and the hippocampus during SWS and REM sleep go in completely opposite directions in the two models. Although the available data favor the Buzsáki's hypothesis, future research is probably needed to provide a definitive description the hippocampal–neocortical dialog during sleep.

CHAPTER 5

EXPRESSION AND MODULATION OF MEMORY TRACES DURING PARADOXICAL SLEEP

ELIZABETH HENNEVIN

The ups and downs of the research on sleep and memory

That sleep can aid in the memorization of waking experiences is an old idea, which found its first experimental support in the pioneering study of Jenkins and Dallenbach (1924). Awake subjects memorized lists of nonsense syllables, and after an interval spent either in sleep or in waking, they were asked to reproduce the lists. Retention performance was better after sleep than after an equivalent amount of wake time. This beneficial effect of sleep on memory was replicated many times and has given rise to three interpretations, each deriving from a theory about memory and forgetting: the decay theory (memory traces are subjected to a time-dependent decay process, and the decay rate would be slower during sleep than during wakefulness); the interference theory (forgetting results from interfering learning, and sleep would prevent activities that interfere with what has been learned); the consolidation theory (new memories consolidate over time, and sleep would facilitate the consolidation process). Note that the last two interpretations are not necessarily exclusive.

The discovery of a brain-activated state of sleep having dramatic physiological and oneiric properties, the rapid eye movement (REM) sleep, also called paradoxical sleep (PS), reactivated the hypothesis of memory consolidation during sleep. Indeed, among the various hypotheses proposed concerning the functional significance of PS, the view rapidly emerged within different disciplines that it might contribute to the stabilization, reinforcement, restructuring or adaptive integration of waking experiences (e.g. Newman and Evans 1965; Gaarder 1966; Feinberg and Evarts 1969; Dewan 1970; Greenberg 1970). At that time, this view primarily relied on the observations that (i) PS is associated with dreaming, (ii) it is a state of intense cerebral activity, (iii) its amount is greater during early life, a critical time for basic learning.

During the 1970s, the potential relationship between PS and memory was the subject of extensive experimental investigation in both humans and animals. Two main strategies were used: post-training PS deprivation and post-training sleep recording. The results obtained in particular by William Fishbein (review in Fishbein and Gutwein 1977), Ramon Greenberg, and Chester Pearlman (review in Pearlman 1979), as well as those collected in our laboratory (review in Bloch *et al.* 1979) provided concordant evidence for the involvement of PS in memory processing. However, negative or puzzling findings were also reported (review in McGrath and Cohen 1978). In parallel, using a quite different approach which compared retention rates following undisturbed periods of early or late nocturnal sleep, other authors pointed out the positive effect of slow wave sleep (SWS) on memory. They showed that the recall was better after early or late sleep than after waking. However, after early sleep, during which the stages 3 and 4 of SWS prevail, retention was better than after late sleep, during which PS predominates. Nonetheless, because the same authors found a detrimental effect of prior sleep on memory, which could account for the worse performance obtained for late sleep than for early sleep, they kept wise and rather dwelled on the beneficial effect of sleep taken as a whole on memory (review in Ekstrand *et al.* 1977).

Despite these significant advances, from the early 1980s the interest in sleep and memory waned, for various reasons. Some of them are easily understandable: inconsistencies had been observed across studies, and the use of sleep-deprivation in many experiments had raised (and continues to raise) important criticisms. Other reasons are more obscure: from the beginning, the view that active processes occurring during sleep (especially PS) could contribute to memory formation has not been easily accepted and is still controversial (Horne 2000; Vertes and Eastman 2000; Siegel 2001).

Two articles reinvigorated interest in the question of sleep and memory. One report demonstrated that overnight improvement of a perceptual skill in humans was dependent upon PS (Karni *et al.* 1994). The second showed that place cells in rat hippocampus which had fired together during spatial exploration exhibited an increased tendency to also fire together during the subsequent periods of quiet waking and SWS (Wilson and McNaughton 1994). Since then, a substantial number of studies have been carried out in humans and animals, from the cognitive to the molecular level. Some of them have enlightened us on discordances previously observed across studies, particularly in humans, and all of them have brought further support to the idea that sleep and memory are functionally related. These interactions are admittedly complex, but how could it be otherwise given the heterogeneity of sleep states and the diversity of memories?

Importance of post-learning paradoxical sleep

From the end of the 1960s, when Pierre Leconte and I were working in the department of Vincent Bloch, we embarked upon a set of studies in rats aimed at determining whether a functional link exists between learning and PS. The experiments relied on the rationale that, if learning and PS are functionally related, then they should covary. The experiments involved two complementary approaches: the analysis of the effects of post-training PS deprivation on subsequent learning performance and the analysis of the effects of learning on subsequent amount of PS. Across the experiments we have varied the nature (aversive or appetitive) and the type of training task (two-way avoidance conditioning, appetitive bar-press conditioning, complex maze learning), the number of training days (from one up to 18 days), and the number of trials per training session (from 70 trials to one single trial).

Convergent results were obtained, which clearly suggested that learning processes and post-training PS are closely related. On the one hand, when rats were PS-deprived during the 3 h following training (the longest deprivation period we used), retention performance tested 21 h later was impaired (Leconte and Hennevin 1973; Leconte *et al.* 1974; Hars and Hennevin 1983). On the other hand, when rats were allowed to sleep freely for 3–4 h after training, they spent increased time in PS (but not in SWS), compared both with their baseline levels and with control animals exposed to the same training conditions but without the possibility of effective learning (Hennevin *et al.* 1971, 1974; Leconte and Hennevin 1971, 1981).

These post-training PS elevations did result from learning and not from non-specific effects (such as stress or fatigue), because (i) they were not observed in trained but unsuccessful animals (Leconte *et al.* 1973), (ii) they were observed even when only one daily training trial was given (Bloch *et al.* 1977), and (iii) they were closely related to the degree of learning achieved. In the course of distributed training, the greatest PS increase did not occur after the first training trials (when the situation was yet the most stressful for the animals), but when the learning curve approached the asymptote; thereafter, when the performance was stabilized, PS returned to baseline level. But if the task to be learned was changed (e.g. if the maze was modified), then PS augmentations were manifested again (Hennevin *et al.* 1974; Hennevin and Leconte 1977; Bloch *et al.* 1981).

Admittedly, the functional significance of the post-learning PS elevations is unclear. We cannot preclude the possibility that they are merely a delayed consequence of what has occurred during learning in wakefulness: for example, in line with the suggestion proposed long ago by Moruzzi (1966), they might reflect a neural restorative process. However, two types of experimental data (in addition to those discussed by Carlyle Smith in Chapter 6) rather suggest that post-learning PS increase reflects an ongoing active process engaged in memory formation. First, we found a striking parallelism between the time course of post-training PS augmentation and the development of the reminiscence phenomenon, that is, a time-dependent improvement in performance which spontaneously develops in the hours following incomplete learning (Destrade *et al.* 1978). Note that this result is in accordance with the finding that PS deprivation in humans prevents overnight improvement of a perceptual skill (Karni *et al.* 1994). Second, we found an interdependence between the consolidation process taking place shortly after learning, during what was initially called "the consolidation period," and subsequent PS. It is known that a low level electrical stimulation of the mesencephalic reticular formation (MRF) administered soon after training enhances retention performance (discussion in Bloch and Laroche 1984). This post-training MRF stimulation reduced the normally deleterious effect of 3-h PS deprivation and also attenuated the normally occurring post-training PS increase (Bloch *et al.* 1977). Thus, these results reinforced the view that, like post-training MRF stimulation, some events taking place during post-learning PS actively contribute to facilitate memory consolidation. As we have repeatedly stressed, this does not imply that PS is an absolute requisite for memory to be formed, but rather that PS optimizes the formation of memory, or at least of some types of memories.

Modulation of memory during post-learning paradoxical sleep

At that point, we believed that the most crucial experiments using the PS deprivation and the post-training sleep recording methods had been exhausted. This led us to employ a new strategy to progress in the question of sleep and memory.

It has long been proposed (Lewis 1979) that a particular memory can be in two different states: a dynamic state (when the pattern of neural firing characteristic of that memory is active) and a dormant state (nonactive memory). As opposed to a nonactive memory, a memory in a presumed active state is labile and can be subjected to further processing (in the case of a newly acquired memory) or reprocessing (in the case of an old memory that has just been reactivated; for a recent review, see Sara 2000). This notion implies that whenever a memory is in an active state, it is accessible and susceptible to disruption by amnestic agents or enhancement by promnestic treatments. Within this framework, and on the basis of our previous data, Bernard Hars and I have postulated that a newly acquired memory would be in an active state during post-learning PS. To test this hypothesis, we applied experimental treatments during post-training PS and assessed their effects on subsequent retention performance. The choice of possible treatments was restricted, because each selected treatment had to meet three criteria: (i) to be precise and easy to present, so that it can be administered rapidly and with a great accuracy of intensity and duration during sleep; (ii) to never produce any awakening in sleeping animals; and (iii) to be effective in influencing memory processing in awake animals. We used two types of treatments that fulfill these requirements.

The first one was a cueing treatment. An extensive literature in humans and animals has demonstrated that exposing subjects, before the retention test, to cues associated with the original training enhances memory retrieval. A widely accepted interpretation of the efficacy of these "reminders" is that the cue stimulus facilitates access to the entire target memory and triggers its reactivation (Spear 1973). We used the rationale that, if memory consolidation occurs during post-learning PS, then it could be reinforced by reactivating neural circuits related to the original learning. Thus, we presented a reminder stimulus during PS (Hars *et al.* 1985). Rats were trained in an active avoidance task during which slight electrotactile stimulations (ETSs) applied to the pinna signaled footshock delivery. Some of them were given the same ETSs, at a non-awaking intensity, during PS episodes following training. When tested 24 h later, these animals exhibited better avoidance performance than control rats that had not received ETSs during PS. In a control experiment, ETSs were not used during conditioning (it was a tone that signaled footshock), but were applied during post-training PS; under these conditions, they had no effect on subsequent avoidance performance. Thus, ETSs did not act through nonspecific effects. To be effective, they had to have been associated with the learning. Opposite results were obtained during SWS: avoidance performance was impaired when learning-associated ETSs were given during post-learning SWS; it was unchanged when ETSs were not behaviorally significant (Hars and Hennevin 1987).

The other treatment we applied during sleep was a weak electrical stimulation of the MRF (Hennevin *et al.* 1989). As mentioned above, this stimulation improves retention when delivered within a short time after acquisition. It also facilitates retention when it is applied during wakefulness after a reactivation treatment (presentation of the conditioned stimulus, CS; DeVietti *et al.* 1977). Thus, application of MRF stimulation during PS appeared to be a potent tool for testing whether memory is in an active state during PS. Rats were trained to run in a maze for food reward with one trial per day. After each trial, some of them received non-awaking MRF stimulation during PS episodes. Compared with control, nonstimulated rats, they showed a marked improvement in performance, making fewer errors in the maze. This facilitatory effect was demonstrated in two independent experiments. In contrast, improved performance was not observed in rats that received MRF stimulation during SWS episodes. Thus, just as MRF stimulation applied in wakefulness is able to improve a newly acquired or a newly reactivated memory so is it effective in enhancing memory when it is applied during post-learning PS.

The results obtained in these two sets of experiments indicate that a newly acquired memory is accessible and can effectively be reprocessed during post-learning PS. Because such characteristics are typically those of a memory in an active state, and in accordance with the theoretical proposal suggested by Spear and Gordon (1981), for more than 15 years we have held the view that post-learning PS would constitute a special period for the reactivation of new memories (Hennevin and Hars 1985; Hennevin *et al.* 1995*a,b*). This reactivation would allow further processing or reinforcing of the neural circuits underlying the learning, that is, it would allow memory to undergo a further consolidation process in the same way that reactivation cues presented in wakefulness allow reconsolidation (see Sara 2000).

This hypothesis of memory reactivation during PS has long been ignored, probably because there was not direct evidence that the neural circuits involved in learning are spontaneously reactivated during PS. Of course, the lack of such evidence was a critical caveat, but I wish to stress the following point. Because memory is a psychological function, it can only be inferred from performance expressed at a behavioral level. Therefore, demonstrating that patterned neural activities expressed during waking are reexpressed during sleep is not sufficient to conclude that this replay is important for memory. To be conclusive, it must be accompanied by data showing that learned behavior does depend on this replay. However that may be, recent studies using functional imaging in humans (Maquet *et al.* 2000; Laureys *et al.* 2001) or electrophysiological recordings in animals (Poe *et al.* 2000; Louie and Wilson 2001) have now provided physiological support for the view that memory undergoes reactivation during PS, by showing that some brain areas or neuronal ensembles activated during waking behavior are again activated during subsequent PS. An obvious question that remains unanswered is—which type of event occurring during PS could trigger memory reactivation? We had suggested (Hennevin *et al.* 1995*a*) that the widespread neural activation which originates from the brainstem and characterizes PS might play this role, postulating that nonspecific factors (diffuse neural activation) might have specific functional effects (reactivation of relevant circuits). This is in agreement with the recent proposal that the phasic pontine waves (the homolog in rats of PGO waves in cats), which invade numerous forebrain structures and which increase in density after learning, could serve as reactivating agents of learning-related networks (Datta 2000, See Chapter 7).

Neuronal plasticity and expression of memory traces during paradoxical sleep

All of the results presented above argue in favor of the idea that newly acquired information is reprocessed during PS. Nonetheless, it seemed to us that to be fully credible, this hypothesis had to be supported by evidence that neural mechanisms involved in the processing of learned information are actually operational during PS. It is widely accepted that associative learning is underlain by changes in neuronal excitability and/or in synaptic transmission within the neural networks put into play during learning. Thus, our next studies were aimed at investigating whether the mechanisms underlying neuronal plasticity are functional in the PS state. These electrophysiological experiments were performed by Catherine Maho. Two types of issues were addressed. First, are neurons able to develop new associative plastic changes during PS? Second, are they able to express plastic changes previously induced by learning in wakefulness?

Cellular conditioning during PS

To test if new associations can be formed during sleep, Catherine Maho and Vincent Bloch (1992) designed a classical conditioning paradigm in which two non-awaking intracerebral stimulations were paired (instead of two external stimuli such as a tone and a footshock). An electrical stimulation of the auditory thalamus (medial geniculate body, MGB) was used as the CS. An electrical stimulation of the central gray, applied at CS offset, was used as the unconditioned stimulus (UCS); stimulation of this brain area has aversive effects in awake animals. Because neurons in the hippocampus are known to readily develop conditioned changes during learning in wakefulness, an increase in hippocampal multiunit activity was taken as the conditioned response. Three groups of rats were used: all three were first given a habituation session (presentation of the CS alone), then a daily session of 15 CS–UCS pairing trials for 14 days. Trials were exclusively given during episodes of wakefuness, PS, or SWS, according to the groups.

Before pairing, CS presentation did not affect hippocampal activity in any group. Pairing in wakefulness resulted in increased hippocampal discharges during CS presentation.

So it was for pairing in PS. By contrast, pairing in SWS was ineffective. In addition, after conditioning had been established during PS, the CS alone was presented during waking to rats of the PS group. Despite the change in state, the CS elicited the hippocampal conditioned response.

These results support two major conclusions. First, the mechanisms allowing the development of associative plasticity are operative during PS, at least in the hippocampus, whereas they do not seem to be during SWS. This is in line with other data showing that the induction of long-term potentiation is possible during PS, but not during SWS (Leonard *et al.* 1987; Bramham and Srebro 1989). Second, associative plastic changes induced during the PS state are maintained and can be expressed in the awake state. In the following experiments, we have examined whether the converse is also true.

Expression during PS of neuronal plasticity induced by fear conditioning

Everyone knows that external stimuli endowed with a strong emotional content, and in particular those associated with a potential danger, are the most able to be detected by the sleeping organism. The paradigm most often used to study emotional memory in animals is auditory fear conditioning, and the main neural circuitry underlying this form of learning is now well determined. Therefore, this paradigm was first used to assess whether neuronal plasticity induced by learning in wakefulness can be expressed during PS.

The experimental protocol was as follows. After a habituation session to a tone, awake rats underwent conditioning in three sessions of 10 trials each, during which the tone was used as the CS preceding a footshock (UCS); control rats received unpaired presentations of tone and footshock. Behavioral conditioned responses were measured by quantifying the changes in neck-muscle electromyographic (EMG) activity at tone presentation. After each daily session, 10 presentations of the tone alone were given during PS episodes. The tone intensity used never produced any awakening from PS, as attested by careful on-line examination of polygraphic recordings and by off-line analysis of neck-muscle EMG activity. At each tone presentation during waking and PS, multiunit activity was recorded in one or two selected brain structures. We focused exclusively on the discharges occurring in the first 60–100 ms of tone, to be sure that neuronal activity recorded in waking was not contaminated by conditioned motor responses which, in all cases, occurred more than 100 ms after tone onset.

Neuronal recordings were first performed in the hippocampus (Maho *et al.* 1991). Before conditioning, tone presentation did not affect hippocampal activity. As expected, pairing the tone with footshock in wakefulness rapidly resulted in increased hippocampal discharges to the tone. The new finding was that this conditioned hippocampal response was also expressed when the tone was presented during subsequent PS. Thus, hippocampal neurons continue to process the tone as a behaviorally relevant stimulus during PS.

The next step was to evaluate whether this enhanced tone responsiveness in PS is characteristic of neurons in integrative structures, such as the hippocampus, or if it is already manifested downstream, in the sensory pathway that conveys auditory information. An extensive literature has demonstrated that highly selective plastic changes occur in the thalamo-cortical auditory system during learning in wakefulness (review in Weinberger 1998). Neuronal recordings were collected from the auditory thalamus, in the medial subdivision of the MGB (Hennevin *et al.* 1993). Here again, after having been paired with footshock in wakefulness, tone presentation in PS evoked neuronal responses that were largely above preconditioning levels. This result is consonant with a recent study in humans suggesting that long-term learning-related neural changes are accessible during PS, as revealed by the mismatch negativity (a measure of the automatic change detection in the auditory cortex; Atienza and Cantero 2001).

In both experiments (as well as in all the following ones), the enhancement of tone responses in post-learning PS cannot be attributed to arousal from sleep, because no change in EEG and EMG activities was detected throughout the entire PS episodes during which the tones were presented. It was reliable, because it was manifested after each of the training sessions during which behavioral and neuronal conditioned responses were expressed. It was associative in nature, because it was not observed in pseudoconditioned rats. Thus, the increased tone responsiveness in PS does result from associative plasticity induced by learning in the awake state.

The implication of the amygdala in emotional experience and behavior is definitively established. There is extensive evidence from animal (and also human) studies indicating that the amygdala plays a pivotal role in the acquisition and expression of conditioned fear. Anatomical tracing, lesion, and electrophysiological experiments in rats have revealed that the lateral nucleus of the amygdala (LA) is the sensory gateway to amygdala circuits: in particular, auditory information from the MGB (and the auditory cortex as well) reaches first the LA, before being distributed to other amygdaloid nuclei which in turn mediate the expression of conditioned emotional responses. Finally, the monosynaptic pathway linking the MGB to the LA has been shown to be crucial for auditory fear conditioning (review in LeDoux 2000).

This led us to examine whether LA neurons also display plastic discharges to an emotionally significant tone presented during PS. The same protocol as that previously described was used, and neuronal activity was simultaneously recorded in the LA and the MGB (Hennevin *et al.* 1998). As a result of auditory fear conditioning, LA and MGB neurons rapidly developed discharge plasticity, both exhibiting increased tone responses within the first five conditioning trials. As shown in Fig. 5.1, both also expressed enhanced responses when the tone was presented in PS, and this enhancement was observed after each of the three conditioning sessions. In addition, for both structures, the changes in tone-evoked discharges occurring during PS were correlated with those occurring during the conditioning sessions (see Fig. 5.3(a)). From these data, it appears that neurons critically involved in learning, from the afferent side to the efferent side of the fear conditioning circuit, can express during PS plastic changes induced in wakefulness. Reinforcing this

Fear conditioning

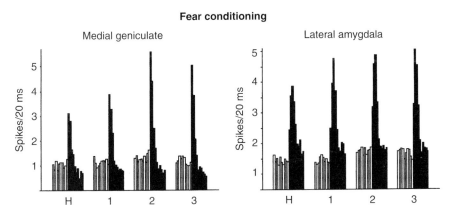

Figure 5.1 Expression of conditioned tone responses in the MGB and the LA during PS following fear conditioning. Averaged group histograms are from 14 recordings in the MGB and from 15 recordings in the LA. Each histogram represents the number of spikes per bin of 20 ms recorded during the 200 ms before (open bars) and the 200 ms after (solid bars) tone onset. H = PS after the habituation session; 1–3 = PS after each of the three conditioning sessions. During conditioning in wakefulness, like the conditioned behavioral responses, conditioned neuronal discharges were manifest in the MGB and the LA from the first to the third session. Note that during PS, the discharges evoked in the first 60 ms of tone were enhanced in both the MGB and the LA after each conditioning session.

view, we showed that an autonomic conditioned response can be evoked during PS. During fear conditioning in wakefulness, the tone CS elicited heart rate accelerations. Significant accelerative responses to the tone were also detected in PS following the conditioning sessions (Maho and Hennevin 1999). Thus, this set of results supports the conclusion that the memory traces formed during fear conditioning can be reactivated and expressed during PS.

Expression during PS of neuronal plasticity induced by appetitive conditioning

In all of the above described studies, the stimulus presented during PS had a negative emotional content: through its pairing with footshock in wakefulness, the tone had acquired fear-inducing properties. Is a stimulus endowed with a positive affect also able to evoke conditioned cellular responses during PS? We have recently addressed this question by using the same protocol as previously, except that slightly food-deprived rats were submitted to a classical conditioning procedure in which the tone signaled sucrose-pellet delivery. To allow comparison with the results obtained with an aversive CS, neuronal activity was simultaneously recorded in the MGB and the LA (Maho and Hennevin 2002). Note that numerous animal studies have demonstrated the involvement of the amygdala also in positively reinforced tasks (reviews in Gallagher and Schoenbaum 1999; Everitt *et al.* 2001).

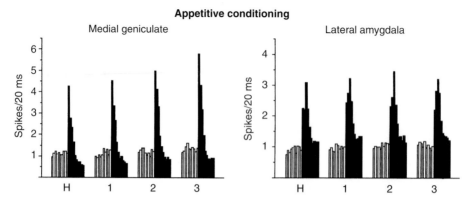

Figure 5.2 Expression of conditioned tone responses in the MGB but not in the LA during PS following appetitive conditioning. Averaged group histograms are from 14 recordings in each structure. Each histogram represents the number of spikes per bin of 20 ms recorded during the 200 ms before (open bars) and the 200 ms after (solid bars) tone onset. H = PS after the habituation session; 1–3 = PS after each of the three conditioning sessions. During conditioning in wakefulness, like the conditioned behavioral responses, conditioned neuronal discharges were manifest in both the MGB and the LA during the second and the third session. Note that during PS, the discharges evoked in the first 60 ms of tone were increased in the MGB after the second and third conditioning sessions, whereas they were not in the LA.

During waking, associative increases in tone-evoked discharges developed in the two structures from the beginning of the second conditioning session. During PS, as can be seen in Fig. 5.2, MGB neurons expressed conditioned tone responses after the second and third sessions, but LA neurons did not. As a consequence, the response changes observed in the MGB during waking and during PS were correlated, but those observed in the LA were not (see Fig 5.3(b)).

Combined with those obtained with fear conditioning, these results bring important clues into several fields of research. First of all, they further attest that the mechanisms underlying physiological plasticity are operative in the PS state. They also unambiguously demonstrate that some aspects of sensory processing are preserved during PS: environmental stimuli that are behaviorally relevant are recognized as such. That auditory processing is effective during PS is also supported by studies using other approaches: for example, a nonnegligible proportion of MGB neurons was shown to display basic functional properties in PS similar to those in wakefulness (Edeline *et al.* 2000).

Second, testing neuronal plasticity during PS allows the dissociation of thalamic and amygdalar plasticity, an issue that has been much debated in the recent years. The matter of controversy is which of the thalamus or the amygdala is the primary site of plasticity in emotional learning and determines the occurrence of plasticity in the other brain region. By showing that the plastic changes taking place in the MGB and the LA have different characteristics (they are or are not maintained during PS), the results obtained with

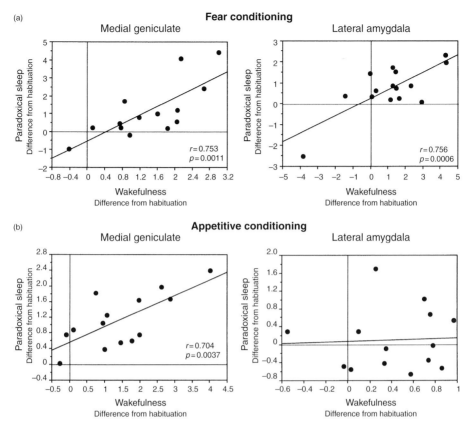

Figure 5.3 Relationship between the conditioned changes expressed during wakefulness and during PS. Data in (a) are from 14 recordings in the MGB and from 15 recordings in the LA. Data in (b) are from 14 recordings in each structure. For each recording, the tone-evoked response recorded during (i.e. in wakefulness) or after (i.e. in PS) the habituation session was subtracted from the response recorded during or after the third session of conditioning. For each structure, the values (expressed in spikes/20 ms) obtained during PS were plotted against those obtained during wakefulness, and the correlation coefficient was calculated. Note that both after fear conditioning and after appetitive conditioning, the response changes expressed by MGB neurons during PS were correlated with those expressed during conditioning in wakefulness. This was also the case for the responses of LA neurons after fear conditioning, but not after appetitive conditioning.

appetitive conditioning suggest that the plasticity developing in each region is specific and does not merely reflect the plasticity occurring in the other region.

Third, whereas MGB neurons behave similarly in PS after fear conditioning and appetitive conditioning, exhibiting increased responses to the acoustic CS regardless of its affective value, LA neurons behave differentially. The UCSs used in fear conditioning and in appetitive conditioning differ with regard to their aversive or appetitive nature, and also with regard to their relative emotional salience and arousal value: footshock is certainly more emotionally salient than are sucrose pellets for animals that are only slightly food deprived, as was the case in our experiment. Thus, the way amygdaloid neurons process the tone in PS appears to depend on the affective valence and/or emotional salience acquired by the tone in wakefulness. This is consonant with results obtained in awake human subjects showing a differential activation of the amygdala according to the emotional intensity and/or valence of stimuli (e.g. Morris *et al.* 1998; Whalen *et al.* 1998).

Is it necessary to stress the obvious adaptive function that has the maintenance of experience-dependent plasticity during PS? Through the expression of physiological plasticity that has developed during wakefulness in the sensory systems and the amygdala (and in functionally connected brain stuctures), the sleeping organism remains able to detect behaviorally meaningful stimuli and, further, to evaluate their biological importance. In other words, beyond its potential role in memory, the possibility for memory traces to be reactivated and expressed during PS has a basic survival function.

Looking back from more than 30 years ago, what is a good hypothesis? In my opinion, it is an hypothesis that can be experimentally tested, and that can be tested through various experimental approaches, because any approach has inherent limitations. Among all the hypotheses proposed for the function of PS, the PS-memory hypothesis is the one that has given rise to the most numerous and fierce criticisms. Why? Simply because it is the one that has been the most extensively tested. It is a good hypothesis. Does this hypothesis imply that PS is exclusively devoted to memory? That without PS there is no memory? No, it does not. In the field of behavioral neurosciences, to be simplistic can catch the attention but is never heuristic.

References

Atienza, M. and **Cantero, J. L.** (2001). Complex sound processing during human REM sleep by recovering information from long-term memory as revealed by the mismatch negativity (MMN). *Brain Research*, **901**, 151–160.

Bloch, V., Hennevin, E., and **Leconte, P.** (1977). Interaction between post-trial reticular stimulation and subsequent paradoxical sleep in memory consolidation processes. In *Neurobiology of sleep and memory* (eds R. Drucker-Colin and J. L. McGaugh), pp. 255–272. Academic Press, New York.

Bloch, V., Hennevin, E., and **Leconte, P.** (1979). Relationship between paradoxical sleep and memory processes. In *Brain mechanisms in memory and learning: from the single neuron to man* (ed. M. A. Brazier), pp. 329–343. Raven Press, New York.

Bloch, V., Hennevin, E., and **Leconte, P.** (1981). The phenomenon of paradoxical sleep augmentation after learning: experimental studies of its characteristics and significance. In *Sleep, dreams and memory* (ed. W. Fishbein), pp. 1–18. Spectrum Publications, New York.

Bloch, V. and **Laroche, S.** (1984). Facts and hypotheses related to the search for the engram. In *Neurobiology of learning and memory* (eds G. Lynch, J. L. McGaugh, and N. M. Weinberger), pp. 249–260. Guilford Press, New York.

Bramham, C. R. and **Srebro, B.** (1989). Synaptic plasticity in the hippocampus is modulated by behavioral state. *Brain Research*, **493**, 74–86.

Datta, S. (2000). Avoidance task training potentiates phasic pontine-wave density in the rat: a mechanism for sleep-dependent plasticity. *Journal of Neuroscience*, **20**, 8607–8613.

Destrade, C., Hennevin, E., Leconte, P., and **Soumireu-Mourat, B.** (1978). Relationships between paradoxical sleep and time-dependent improvement of performance in BALB/c mice. *Neuroscience Letters*, **7**, 239–244.

DeVietti, T. L., Conger, G. L., and **Kirkpatrick, B.** (1977). Comparison of the enhancement gradients of retention obtained with stimulation of the mesencephalic reticular formation after training or memory reactivation. *Physiology and Behavior*, **19**, 549–554.

Dewan, E. (1970). The programming "P" hypothesis for REM sleep. *International Psychiatric Clinics*, **7**, 295–307.

Edeline, J.-M., Manunta, Y., and **Hennevin, E.** (2000). Auditory thalamus neurons during sleep: changes in frequency selectivity, threshold, and receptive field size. *Journal of Neurophysiology*, **84**, 934–952.

Ekstrand, B. R., Barrett, T. R., West, J. N., and **Maier, W. G.** (1977). The effect of sleep on human long-term memory. In *Neurobiology of sleep and memory* (eds R. Drucker-Colín and J. L. McGaugh), pp. 419–438. Academic Press, New York.

Everitt, B. J., Cardinal, R. N., Hall, J., Parkinson, J. A., and **Robbins, T. W.** (2001). Differential involvement of amygdala subsystems in appetitive conditioning and drug addiction. In *The amygdala: a functional analysis* (ed. J. P. Aggleton), pp. 353–390. Oxford University Press, Oxford.

Feinberg, I. and **Evarts, E. V.** (1969). Changing concepts of the function of sleep: discovery of intense brain activity during sleep calls for revision of hypotheses as to its function. *Biological Psychiatry*, **1**, 331–348.

Fishbein, W. and **Gutwein, B. M.** (1977). Paradoxical sleep and memory storage processes. *Behavioral Biology*, **19**, 425–464.

Gaarder, K. (1966). A conceptual model of sleep. *Archives of General Psychiatry*, **14**, 253–260.

Gallagher, M. and **Schoenbaum, G.** (1999). Functions of the amygdala and related forebrain areas in attention and cognition. *Annals of the New York Academy of Sciences*, **877**, 397–411.

Greenberg, R. (1970). Dreaming and memory. In *Sleep and dreaming* (ed. E. Hartmann), pp. 258–267. Little-Brown, Boston.

Hars, B. and **Hennevin, E.** (1983). Reminder abolishes impairment of learning induced by paradoxical sleep retardation. *Physiology and Behavior*, **30**, 831–836.

Hars, B. and **Hennevin, E.** (1987). Impairment of learning by cueing during postlearning slow-wave sleep in rats. *Neuroscience Letters*, **79**, 290–294.

Hars, B., Hennevin, E., and **Pasques, P.** (1985). Improvement of learning by cueing during postlearning paradoxical sleep. *Behavioural Brain Research*, **18**, 241–250.

Hennevin, E. and **Hars, B.** (1985). Post-learning paradoxical sleep: a critical period when new memory is reactivated? In *Brain plasticity, learning and memory* (eds B. E. Will, P. Schmitt and J. C. Dalrymple-Alford), pp. 193–203. Plenum Press, New York.

Hennevin, E., Hars, B., and Bloch, V. (1989). Improvement of learning by mesencephalic reticular stimulation during postlearning paradoxical sleep. *Behavioral and Neural Biology*, **51**, 291–306.

Hennevin, E., Hars, B., and Maho, C. (1995*a*). Memory processing in paradoxical sleep. *Sleep Research Society Bulletin*, **1**, 44–50.

Hennevin, E., Hars, B., Maho, C., and Bloch, V. (1995*b*). Processing of learned information in paradoxical sleep: relevance for memory. *Behavioural Brain Research*, **69**, 125–135.

Hennevin, E. and Leconte, P. (1977). Etude des relations entre le sommeil paradoxal et les processus d'acquisition. *Physiology and Behavior*, **18**, 307–319.

Hennevin, E., Leconte, P., and Bloch, V. (1971). Effet du niveau d'acquisition sur l'augmentation de la durée du sommeil paradoxal consécutive à un conditionnement d'évitement chez le Rat. *Comptes Rendus de l'Académie des Sciences de Paris*, **273**, 2595–2598.

Hennevin, E., Leconte, P., and Bloch, V. (1974). Augmentation du sommeil paradoxal provoquée par l'acquisition, l'extinction et la réacquisition d'un apprentissage à renforcement positif. *Brain Research*, **70**, 43–54.

Hennevin, E., Maho, C., Hars, B., and Dutrieux, G. (1993). Learning-induced plasticity in the medial geniculate nucleus is expressed during paradoxical sleep. *Behavioral Neuroscience*, **107**, 1018–1030.

Hennevin, E., Maho, C., and Hars, B. (1998). Neuronal plasticity induced by fear conditioning is expressed during paradoxical sleep: evidence from simultaneous recordings in the lateral amygdala and the medial geniculate in rats. *Behavioral Neuroscience*, **112**, 839–862.

Horne, J. A. (2000). REM sleep—by default? *Neuroscience and Biobehavioral Reviews*, **24**, 777–797.

Jenkins, J. G. and Dallenbach, K. M. (1924). Obliviscence during sleep and waking. *American Journal of Psychology*, **35**, 605–612.

Karni, A., Tanne, D., Rubenstein, B. S., Askenasy, J. J. M., and Sagi, D. (1994). Dependence on REM sleep of overnight improvement of a perceptual skill. *Science*, **265**, 679–682.

Laureys, S., Peigneux, P., Phillips, C., *et al.* (2001). Experience-dependent changes in cerebral functional connectivity during human rapid eye movement sleep. *Neuroscience*, **105**, 521–525.

Leconte, P. and Hennevin, E. (1971). Augmentation de la durée de sommeil paradoxal consécutive à un apprentissage chez le Rat. *Comptes Rendus de l'Académie des Sciences de Paris*, **273**, 86–88.

Leconte, P. and Hennevin, E. (1973). Caractéristiques temporelles de l'augmentation de sommeil paradoxal consécutif à l'apprentissage chez le rat. *Physiology and Behavior*, **11**, 677–686.

Leconte, P. and Hennevin, E. (1981). Post-learning paradoxical sleep, reticular activation, and noradrenergic activity. *Physiology and Behavior*, **26**, 587–594.

Leconte, P., Hennevin, E., and Bloch, V. (1973). Analyse des effets d'un apprentissage et de son niveau d'acquisition sur le sommeil paradoxal consécutif. *Brain Research*, **49**, 367–379.

Leconte, P., Hennevin, E., and Bloch, V. (1974). Duration of paradoxical sleep necessary for the acquisition of conditioned avoidance in the rat. *Physiology and Behavior*, **13**, 675–681.

LeDoux, J. E. (2000). Emotion circuits in the brain. *Annual Review of Neuroscience*, **23**, 155–184.

Leonard, B. J., McNaughton, B. L., and Barnes, C. A. (1987). Suppression of hippocampal synaptic plasticity during slow-wave sleep. *Brain Research*, **425**, 174–177.

Lewis, D. J. (1979). Psychobiology of active and inactive memory. *Psychological Bulletin*, **86**, 1054–1083.

Louie, K. and **Wilson, M. A.** (2001). Temporally structured replay of awake hippocampal ensemble activity during rapid eye movement sleep. *Neuron*, **29**, 145–156.

Maho, C. and **Bloch, V.** (1992). Responses of hippocampal cells can be conditioned during paradoxical sleep. *Brain Research*, **581**, 115–122.

Maho, C. and **Hennevin, E.** (1999). Expression in paradoxical sleep of a conditioned heart rate response. *Neuroreport*, **10**, 3381–3385.

Maho, C. and **Hennevin, E.** (2002). Appetitive conditioning-induced plasticity is expressed during paradoxical sleep in the medial geniculate, but not in the lateral amygdala. *Behavioral Neuroscience*, **116**, 807–823.

Maho, C., Hennevin, E., Hars, B., and **Poincheval, S.** (1991). Evocation in paradoxical sleep of a hippocampal conditioned cellular response acquired during waking. *Psychobiology*, **19**, 193–205.

Maquet, P., Laureys, S., Peigneux, P., *et al.* (2000). Experience-dependent changes in cerebral activation during human REM sleep. *Nature Neuroscience*, **3**, 831–836.

McGrath, M. J. and **Cohen, D. B.** (1978). REM sleep facilitation of adaptive waking behavior: a review of the literature. *Psychological Bulletin*, **85**, 24–57.

Morris, J. S., Friston, K. J., Büchel, C., *et al.* (1998). A neuromodulatory role for the human amygdala in processing emotional facial expressions. *Brain*, **121**, 47–57.

Moruzzi, G. (1966). Functional significance of sleep for brain mechanisms. In *Brain and conscious experience* (ed. J. C. Eccles), pp. 345–388. Springer, Berlin.

Newman, E. A. and **Evans, C. R.** (1965). Human dream processes as analogous to computer programme clearance. *Nature*, **206**, 534.

Pearlman, C. A. (1979). REM sleep and information processing: evidence from animal studies. *Neuroscience and Biobehavioral Reviews*, **3**, 57–68.

Poe, G. R., Nitz, D. A., McNaughton, B. L., and **Barnes, C. A.** (2000). Experience-dependent phase-reversal of hippocampal neuron firing during REM sleep. *Brain Research*, **855**, 176–180.

Sara, S. J. (2000). Retrieval and reconsolidation: toward a neurobiology of remembering. *Learning and Memory*, **7**, 73–84.

Siegel, J. M. (2001). The REM sleep-memory consolidation hypothesis. *Science*, **294**, 1058–1063.

Spear, N. E. (1973). Retrieval of memory in animals. *Psychological Review*, **80**, 163–194.

Spear, N. E. and **Gordon, W. C.** (1981). Sleep, dreaming, and the retrieval of memories. In *Sleep, dreams and memory* (ed. W. Fishbein), pp. 183–203. Spectrum Publications, New York.

Vertes, R. P. and **Eastman, K. E.** (2000). The case against memory consolidation in REM sleep. *Behavioral Brain Sciences*, **23**, 867–876.

Weinberger, N. M. (1998). Physiological memory in primary auditory cortex: characteristics and mechanisms. *Neurobiology of Learning and Memory*, **70**, 226–251.

Whalen, P. J., Rauch, S. L., Etcoff, N. L., McInerney, S. C., Lee, M. B., and Jenike, M. A. (1998). Masked presentations of emotional facial expressions modulate amygdala activity without explicit knowledge. *Journal of Neuroscience*, **18**, 411–418.

Wilson, M. A. and McNaughton, B. L. (1994). Reactivation of hippocampal ensemble memories during sleep. *Science*, **265**, 676–679.

CHAPTER 6

THE REM SLEEP WINDOW AND MEMORY PROCESSING

CARLYLE SMITH

The REM sleep window

Background

Historically there have been two basic approaches to the study of the relationship of sleep states to memory processing. Using the first approach, animals were subjected to baseline electro-encephalographic (EEG) sleep recording. This procedure was followed by submitting the same animals to task acquisition. After the end of training, quantitative and qualitative post-learning changes in the sleep architecture were observed. The result most often found was an increase in the duration (number of minutes) of REM sleep with little change in the amount of slow wave sleep (SWS) in the animals that successfully learned the task. Thus, most researchers focused on REM sleep as the important sleep state for memory processing and the organisms most often studied were either rats or mice (Bloch 1970; Fishbein and Gutwein 1977; McGrath and Cohen 1978; Pearlman 1979; Smith 1985, 1996; Hennevin *et al.* 1995).

The second approach was to selectively prevent REM sleep (often termed paradoxical sleep or PS) following task acquisition, either by the "swimming pool" technique or by the injection of REM sleep-suppressing drugs. REM sleep deprivation (REMD) of the animal was followed by retesting at some later time. Many more experiments were done using the second approach compared to the first, and only a small number of labs used both approaches while keeping the same strain of animal, task and number of training trials (Bloch 1970; Smith *et al.* 1980; Smith and Lapp 1986; Hennevin *et al.* 1995). It was assumed in some of these earlier studies that the most important post-training time for memory consolidation was in the first few hours following the end of training. Thus, many sleep-recording studies did not monitor EEG for periods of time longer than 3–4 h after the end of the acquisition (Bloch 1970; McGrath and Cohen 1978; Pearlman 1979; Smith 1985; Hennevin *et al.* 1995). As we now know, consolidation or memory processing can take place many hours after the end of training. In retrospect, restricting EEG recording times or application of REMD to the first few hours following training resulted in some experiments not being able to observe any REM sleep increases or impaired memory (Bloch 1970; McGrath and Cohen 1978; Pearlman 1979; Smith 1985, 1996; Hennevin *et al.* 1995).

The concept of the REM sleep window (RSW), was first developed by doing continuous long term EEG recording and REMD experiments on the same strain of animal (Smith 1985). Following successful learning, the organism manifests an increase in amount of REM sleep (duration, min) or increased REM sleep intensity (number of REMs, REM density, etc.). These increases over the organism's own baseline REM sleep levels can persist for a period of hours or days. If selective REM sleep deprivation is applied to coincide with these expected post-training increases in REM sleep, memory is subsequently impaired. *The RSW is the relatively short period where REMD (3–4 h) can induce memory impairment.* It should be noted that the amount of applied REMD to impair memory need not be nearly as long as the observed REM sleep increases.

Some characteristics of the RSW

One of the characteristics of the RSW is its time of occurrence, which varies with respect to at least three variables: (i) strain and type of organism learning the task (Smith 1985, 1996), (ii) the type of task being trained (Smith 1985, 1996), and (iii) the number of training trials per session during training (Smith 1985, 1996). An example of the flexibility of the appearance and character of RSWs has been done in our own lab by varying the number of training trials per session. Over the years, we examined the sleep and memory of the male Sprague–Dawley rat, using the two-way shuttle shock avoidance task. Thus, male rats of the same strain were subjected to 100 trials in this avoidance task. The only difference between the various groups was the distribution of the training sessions.

Using the EEG sleep-recording approach, one study required the rats to learn the task in a single 1.5 h session (Smith *et al.* 1980). In another study, we required the rats to learn the task during two consecutive daily sessions of 50 trials per day (Smith and Lapp 1986). In yet another study, we required the rats to learn the task in 5 consecutive sessions of 20 trials per day (Smith *et al.* 1980). Thus, while all animals were ultimately exposed to 100 training trials in this task, the distribution of sessions was varied.

Since animals in all groups were continuously sleep recorded, we can compare the results of the various groups. It was clear from the EEG recording studies that 100 trials in a single session resulted in the most dramatic increases in REM sleep. These increases persisted in a cyclic manner for at least 6 days (see Fig. 6.1). (Rats that did not learn showed REM sleep similar to non-learning controls.) In the rats exposed to 50 trials per day for two consecutive days, the increases in REM sleep were again remarkably high. These increases persisted for about a week, but did not reach quite as high as did the REM sleep for the single session group (see Fig. 6.2). Those rats exposed to 20 trials per day in the avoidance task showed much more modest (although statistically significant) increases in REM sleep (see Fig. 6.3). Using this paradigm, rats exhibited their largest increase in REM sleep within the 24-h period prior to showing a maximum increase in correct performance (MIP). While recording after the end of the final training session did not extend for as long as for the other two groups, some interesting comparisons can be made. A kind of gradation of above normal REM sleep was observed, depending on the

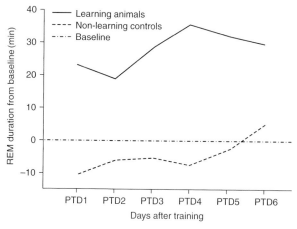

Figure 6.1 Mean number of minutes of REM sleep above or below normal baseline levels for the rats that learned the task in a single session of 100 trials and the combined values of non-trained animals and animals that were trained but did not learn the task.

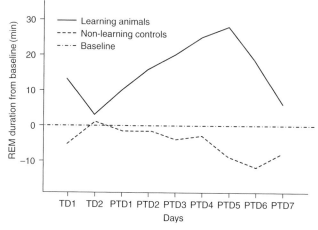

Figure 6.2 Mean number of minutes of REM sleep above or below normal baseline levels for the rats that learned the task in two consecutive daily training sessions of 50 trials each and the combined values of non-trained animals and animals that were trained but did not learn the task.

number of trials per session. Generally, the more training trials that were given at one session, the more subsequent REM sleep occurred in those animals that were successful in learning the avoidance task.

These same training paradigms were repeated using the second approach of REMD to establish RSWs for each of the groups of rats. The usual method for finding these RSWs was to impose post-training REMD for a 24-h period. If this initial treatment resulted in subsequent memory loss, smaller periods of REMD were then used. Various groups of animals, given the same training, were exposed to short, 4-h periods of REMD,

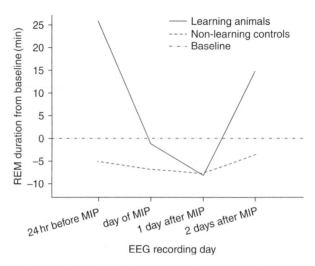

Figure 6.3 Mean number of minutes of REM sleep above or below normal baseline levels for rats that learned the task in five consecutive daily training sessions of 20 trials each. Because the rats learned at different rates, the REM sleep values were arranged to coincide with the MIP of each animal. It also shows the combined values of non-trained animals and animals that were trained but did not learn the task.

either immediately after the last training trial (1–4 h), 5–8 h, 9–12 h, 13–16 h, 17–20 h, or 21–24 h later. In this way, we were able to establish the exact time in the 24-h period when REM sleep was really vital for memory. For the 100 trials (single training session) rats, an RSW was established at between 1–4 h after the end of training. For the rats given two 50 trial sessions, there were two RSWs, one at 9–12 h after the end of training and the other 53–56 h after training. For the rats given 20 trials a day for 5 days, there were also two RSWs, 9–12 h and 17–20 h after the end of training. While there are probably more RSWs for the 100 trial single session group (later windows have not been thoroughly explored for this condition), the data are complete enough to show how responsive subsequent REM sleep is to the change in number of training trials per day in a task.

An overview of these data show that when the number of training trials per day was the only variable changed, the times at which the above normal post-training REM sleep appeared and its duration varied markedly. Further, when same strain rats were differentially deprived of REM sleep following identical training, the times at which short 4-h REMD exposures were effective in impairing memory coincided with the changes in appearance of above normal amounts of post-training REM sleep. Thus, RSWs are unique to the training history of the animal. The RSW has subsequently been found in a number of different tasks, including a complex operant appetitive task (Smith and Wong 1991), the Morris water maze (MWM) (Smith and Rose 1996, 1997), the 8-arm radial maze (Smith *et al.* 1998a), a conditioned cue preference (CCP) task (Vallance *et al.* 1999) as well as the two-way shuttle avoidance task (Smith *et al.* 1980; Smith and Lapp 1986). These RSWs appeared as early as the first 4 h after training and were delayed

Table 6.1 Values of RSWs established in the laboratory for different tasks

Description of task	Details of training	RSWs after last training trial (h)	Reference
Two-way shuttle shock avoidance	100 trials, single session	1–4	Smith *et al.* 1980
Two-way shuttle shock avoidance	50 trials, 2 days	9–12, 53–56	Smith and Lapp 1986
Two-way shuttle shock avoidance	20 trials, 5 days	9–12, 17–20	Smith *et al.* 1980
Morris water Maze spatial	4 trials/day for 3 days, 4 retest trials on day 4	5–8	Smith and Rose 1996
Morris water Maze spatial	12 trials/day, 4 retest trials	1–4	Smith and Rose 1997
Eight-arm radial maze spatial	1 trial/day, 10 days	1–4	Smith *et al.* 1988*a*
Conditioned cue preference (S–R)	1 trial/day, 8 days	9–12	Vallance *et al.* 1999
Complex operant appetitive	3 days bar press, 2 days FR-10, 3 days complex operant	1–4 (EEG estimate)	Smith and Wong 1991

as much as 53–56 h after the last training trial (Smith and Kelly 1988; Smith and MacNeill 1993). As with the shuttle avoidance task, the number of training trials per session in the MWM was varied in two separate studies. If the number of trials was 4 per day for 3 consecutive days, the RSW was found to be in the 5–8-h post-training time period. If rats were given 12 trials in a single training session, the RSW was found to be in the 1–4-h time period after the last training trial. Table 6.1 has a summary of the RSWs established in our lab to date for several tasks.

Stress as an explanation for memory loss

It could be argued that post-training REM sleep increases reflect stress and not memory processing. However, the idea that the stress resulting from the task induces above normal levels of REM sleep seems unlikely. The best evidence is provided by the non-learning control groups that have been exposed to the same appetitive tasks and the yoked control shock groups in the avoidance tasks. Animals unable to learn the tasks have never shown post-training REM sleep increases (Smith *et al.* 1974, 1980; Smith 1985; Smith and Lapp 1986; Smith and Wong 1991).

Memory loss following REMD has also been attributed to the stress of the deprivation situation (Vertes 2000; Siegal 2001). There is some merit in considering this option.

A much used method for REMD, often called the "swimming pool" or "platform" technique, consists of placing the animal on a platform that is surrounded by water. The animal, when placed on the platform, has enough room to relax and get SWS or NREM sleep, but not enough to lie in a position such that they can attain the complete muscle relaxation required for REM sleep to occur without falling into the water.

A number of studies have utilized the large platform control which allows the animal to attain REM sleep while at the same time being exposed to the equally stressful situation of being near water, confinement, etc. Rats placed on sufficiently large platforms are capable of almost normal (90% of baseline) REM sleep while those placed on small platforms are not (less than 10% of baseline; Smith and Gisquet-Verrier 1996). On the other hand, the stress induced by placing animals on platforms is very similar, since measures of corticosterone are found to be the same regardless of platform size (Coenen and Van Luijtelaar 1985; Coll-Andreu *et al.* 1989).

Results over the years have generally shown that animals placed on the small platforms exhibited post-training memory loss while the large platform animals behaved much like non-deprived cage controls. These studies can be found in several reviews (McGrath and Cohen 1978; Pearlman 1979; Smith 1985).

Many studies have used a REM sleep-suppressing drug as an alternative to this technique and have found comparable results to the platform REMD studies (Pearlman and Becker 1973, 1974*a,b*, 1975; Pearlman and Greenberg 1973; Kitahama *et al.* 1976; Smith *et al.* 1991). The stress involved in injecting a rat is not equal to the stress of sitting on a platform for several hours. Intraperitoneal (IP) injections take less than 5 s and if done properly, the rat has a minimum of discomfort. The animal is then placed back in its home cage as opposed to being in the more stressful platform situation for at least several hours.

Another argument against the stress hypothesis is the number of studies that have used short-lasting (2–4 h) platform REMDs, which impose minimal stress (McGrath and Cohen 1978; Bloch *et al.* 1979; Pearlman 1979; Smith 1985, 1996; Hennevin *et al.* 1995). The deprivations were applied to many groups of rats, all of equal length, but at various times following the end of training. The only groups to show memory deficits were those where the REMD coincided with the RSW. While it could still be argued theoretically that even this small amount of stress was the cause of the memory loss, the memory loss effects are very time-specific and the most obvious alternative explanation would be the existence of a "stress window." At this point there is not much evidence for such a window.

Another argument against the stress hypothesis is based on a study done in our lab (Smith and Butler 1982). The RSWs of the rats in the shuttle avoidance task were found to be at 9–12 h and 17–20 h after the end of training. At 20 trials per day, when rats were selectively deprived of REM sleep (platform) during either of these two time periods, they showed memory impairment. In a second experiment, we allowed animals to sleep only during these RSWs. This meant that they could have REM sleep during these two special times, but otherwise would be completely deprived of REM sleep. The REMD controls were exposed to the same amount of REM sleep loss but the REMD time always coincided with one of the two RSWs mentioned above. All of these REMD control groups showed deficits on the learning task. *The only rats that did as well as the non-deprived controls were the rats allowed REM sleep during the previously established, two short RSWs.* Thus, we had a situation where all rats but the non-deprived group were deprived of REM sleep approximately 17.5 h per day. Near the end of the 5 days, the deprived groups all showed obvious signs of stress. Despite this stressed behavior, the group that had the opportunity for REM sleep that coincided with the previously established RSWs—during the 3.5 h which corresponded to the 9–12 h window and the 3 h coinciding with the 17–20 h REMD window—did well on the task. Thus, there was equivalent stress on these rats that did not result in memory loss. It was concluded in this study that the timing of the REM sleep was the important variable and not the stress. The other equally stressed groups were not able to remember the task as well, because their REMD times included those times when the REM sleep window was previously found to be important (Smith and Butler 1982).

In summary, the stress of being in the learning situation does not adequately explain the above normal post-training REM sleep increases observed. Only animals that have learned the tasks show this phenomenon. Further, while the platform REMD technique might be somewhat stressful, it fails to adequately explain the memory losses. A better explanation is that REM sleep at specific post-training times is vital for efficient memory processing.

Mechanisms of action during the REM sleep window

It seems clear that REM sleep is very important for efficient memory at certain post-training times. There is some evidence for post-training biochemical windows relating to memory consolidation (Graves *et al.* 2001). However, there are not many studies that have reported post-training windows of important biochemical events which coincide with an RSW. In one preliminary study, mice were given fear conditioning and then hand deprived of sleep for either 0–5 h or 6–10 h after the end of training. They found a sleep window that coincided with the biochemical protein kinase A (PKA) window from hours 0–5, but not hours 6–10 (Graves *et al.* 2000).

Acetylcholine (ACh) is a transmitter that has long been linked with both memory processes (Corkin 1981; Coyle *et al.* 1983; Deutsch 1983; Hasselmo 1999) and REM sleep activity (Jouvet 1975; Sitaram *et al.* 1978; McGinty and Drucker-Colin 1982; Gillin and Sitaram 1984; Baghdoyan *et al.* 1987). It would seem to be a perfect candidate for a role in memory processing during REM sleep. A number of preliminary studies have been carried out in our lab which suggest that ACh does play a role in memory consolidation at these special time periods.

In an attempt to replicate our 9–12 h RSW using the two-way shuttle shock avoidance task and the "swimming pool" or platform REMD technique, we chose two drugs, anisomycin and scopolamine. In our first study, we injected the protein synthesis inhibitor anisomycin at post-training times that either preceded the RSW, coincided with the onset of the RSW, or took place after the end of the RSW. Each anisomycin group also had a saline control injection group that was injected at the same post-training time. The only group that showed memory deficits (30% drop in correct performance) on retest was the anisomycin group injected at 9-h after training to coincide with the beginning of the previously established RSW. These behavioral results were identical to those previously observed using the non-injection (swimming pool) technique (Smith *et al.* 1991).

The brains of these rats were removed after the injection of the drug and after the end of the retest session. They were analyzed for amount of ACh as well as acetylcholine esterase (AChE) activity. For AChE activity, as expected, the 9-h post-injection group had lower values than any of the other groups. Further, the increase in REM sleep levels normally seen in rats at the 12-h post-training time period was reflected in higher AChE activity at this time period compared to the 9- and 6-h periods. The levels of ACh in the whole brain provided the same profile of transmitter distribution as the AChE activity (Smith *et al.* 1991).

The results suggested that protein synthesis inhibition *during the RSW* was devastating to memory consolidation in these animals. However, anisomycin impairs the synthesis of many different proteins and it was decided to replicate this finding using a drug which specifically interferes with ACh transmission. The ACh antagonist scopolamine was chosen and it was injected at a dosage of 0.4 mg/kg IP in rats exposed to the same task as before. The timing of the injections was also as before, being either 6, 9, or 12-h after the end of the last training trial. Equivalent saline control groups were also trained. Behavioral results showed that the 9-h scopolamine injected animals were inferior on retest compared to all other saline and scopolamine groups. Thus, again, the result suggested that an ACh transmitter inhibitor active during the RSW impaired memory consolidation.

There were, of course, several possible mechanisms of action to explain these results. Both anisomycin (Rojas-Ramirez *et al.* 1977; Gutwein *et al.* 1980) and scopolamine (Domino *et al.* 1968; Jouvet 1975) have been reported to impair REM sleep. The behavioral results are very similar to the results observed using the mechanical or "swimming pool" technique (Smith *et al.* 1991). Thus REM sleep deprivation must be considered one possible memory impairing system. However, it is clear that these drugs have also impaired AChE activity and reduced the levels of ACh in rat whole brain. These results lead to the conclusion that mechanical REM sleep deprivation also induces a reduction in levels of the ACh transmitter. Few studies have examined the effect of ACh levels following mechanical sleep deprivation, although two reports indicate that the amount of ACh in rat telencephalon dropped after 96 h of REM sleep deprivation (Bowers *et al.* 1966; Tsuchiya *et al.* 1969). One author also reported an increase in rat whole brain ACh after 24 h of REMD (Tsuchiya *et al.* 1969). This result indicates that the level of transmitter can go either down or up. Although no study has applied mechanical REM sleep deprivation under the exact conditions of the studies mentioned above (Smith *et al.* 1991) and examined ACh changes directly, there is some support for the idea that REM sleep deprivation does induce reductions in whole brain ACh. This in turn strengthens the hypothesis that one of the transmitters involved in this sleep—memory system is ACh. The fact that ACh levels have been observed to decrease and increase after REMD (Bowers *et al.* 1966; Tsuchiya *et al.* 1969) also provides an explanation for those few studies that actually showed improved memory following REMD (Kitahama *et al.* 1976; Gisquet-Verrier and Smith 1989; Smith and Gisquet-Verrier 1996). ACh levels probably vary depending on strain of animal as well as hours of REMD.

Possible significance of the prolonged REM sleep elevations following learning

One of the results observed following task acquisition, such as the shuttle avoidance task has been the long-term increases in REM sleep which can persist for up to at least 6–7 days after the end of training. REM sleep deprivation at these times has not resulted in any marked reduction in subsequent performance except at discrete REM sleep windows (Smith *et al.* 1991). It seems likely from the levels of ACh and AChE activity observed in control rats at these post-training times, that there is a close relationship between amount of REM sleep and levels of the ACh transmitter. There has been no good explanation for why the RSWs are so small (4 h) compared to the total amount and extent of REM sleep increases following learning. It has been noted that the RSWs tend to coincide with a post-training time during which REM sleep is beginning to increase over normal levels. This suggests the start of an important memory process which is somewhat fragile and can be disrupted in its early stages. However, after it has been active for some hours, REM sleep deprivation is no longer able to interfere with the process. On the other hand, there is no obvious explanation for the very prolonged REM sleep increases following successful learning. However, one possible related group of studies are the enriched environment (EE) studies.

It is known that after rats are submitted to the informal learning situation of exposure to a variety of novel stimuli, they have thicker cortices which weigh more compared to controls of various kinds (Diamond *et al.* 1964; Diamond 1976). EE rats develop greater dendritic branching (Globus *et al.* 1973; Greenough and Volkmar 1973; Diamond *et al.* 1975) and there is greater cortical AChE activity (Rosensweig *et al.* 1962). Similar results of cortical weight increases, dendritic branching and brain chemistry have been found in formal training paradigms (Greenough 1976; Bennett *et al.* 1979; Chang and Greenough 1982). These changes take place over a period of weeks, but it has also been reported that these animals have more REM sleep than the impoverished controls (Tagney 1973; Gutwein and Fishbein 1980*a,b*; Kiyono *et al.* 1981; Mirmiram *et al.* 1982).

It has been proposed that permanent changes in ACh brain chemistry might occur following training in a formal learning task. Our lab decided to use the MWM to examine this possibility since we had established a clear RSW for this task at 1–4 h after the end of training when 12 massed trials were given in the hidden platform version (Smith and Rose 1997). The working hypothesis was that rats trained and allowed to rest for 1 week would show ACh levels above those of non-trained controls, or rats deprived of REM sleep during the 1–4 h RSW. As well they should have more ACh than those exposed to

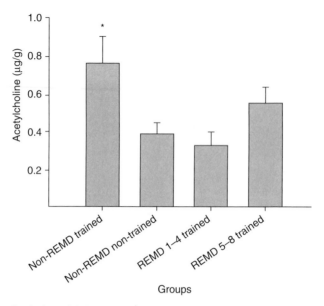

Figure 6.4 Mean level of acetylcholine (μg) in the whole brain of the various groups of rats (+ SEM). The trained non-REMD rats had significantly more ACh than either the non-trained or the REMD 1–4 groups, which did not differ significantly from each other. The REMD 5–8 group had slightly more ACh than the last mentioned groups but was not significantly different from any of the groups.

REM sleep deprivation 5–8 h after the end of training—a time just outside the previously established RSW. Our results showed that indeed, the trained animals that were allowed normal sleep had the largest amount of ACh in whole brain. The least amount of ACh was found in the rats deprived of REM sleep during the 1–4 h RSW. They did not differ from the non-trained cage controls that also had very low levels of ACh. The 5–8 h REM sleep deprived rats had less ACh than the rested animals but somewhat more than the cage control and 1–4 h RSW groups. It seems likely that there was some overlap in terms of a continuing high level of ACh which caught the "edge" of the RSW and caused some memory disruption (Smith *et al.* 1998*b*) (see Fig. 6.4). Overall, although the results are preliminary, they do suggest that "long term" changes in ACh related to learning can be impaired by relatively short periods of REM sleep deprivation which are strategically imposed following task acquisition. The results add support to the idea that the RSW is a time when special activities occur which are important for the final state of the brain at least 1 week later.

Specific neuroanatomical structures active during the RSW

As with knowledge of transmitter action during the RSWs, the understanding of which structures might be involved is also virtually nonexistent. One of the advantages of using the MWM task is that we know that the hippocampus is involved with this task (Morris *et al.* 1982) and that it must be active during REM sleep after acquisition (Smith and Rose 1997). It also must be the case that the brainstem REM sleep generating system is active, since REM sleep is involved (Datta 1995, 2000). Thus, the interaction of brainstem and hippocampal structures during the RSW are very likely part of the consolidation process following training in the MWM.

Another task in which the neuroanatomical structure involved has been identified is the CCP task (McDonald and White 1993). This task consists of two maze arms, one with a light cue near the food cup and the other arm (at 180° from the first) with no light cue near the food cup. Rats were required to run to the dark arm (no cue) for 4 consecutive trials, one per day. There was no food reward here. They were then required to run to the cued arm (light) of the maze for 4 trials, one per day. They received a food reward on each of these trials. All extra maze cues were eliminated. Damage to the lateral amygdala resulted in animals not being able to learn the CCP task (McDonald and White 1993). In our lab we ran the animals in this paradigm and using various 4-h REMD groups, we were able to establish a RSW at 9–12 h after the end of training (Vallance *et al.* 1999).

In further work, we decided to examine the possibility that the lateral amygdalae of these rats might be active during the 9–12 RSW and that one of the transmitters might be ACh. Rats were bilaterally implanted with cannulae in the lateral amygdalae. After recovery from the surgery, they were given 8 training trials (1 per day) in the CCP task. Groups were injected with the ACh antagonist scopolamine either immediately, at the beginning of the 9th hour after the end of training (to coincide with the RSW) or at the beginning of the 12th hour, to be present at a time just after the RSW was observed. As well, 3 saline control groups were run which were injected at the same times as each of the scopolamine groups. On day 9, all animals were tested in the maze and allowed to enter either arm of the maze. It was observed that while scopolamine had a marginal effect at the two times outside the RSW, it induced the greatest loss of memory for this simple task during the previously established RSW for the CCP task (Kenton and Smith 2001). Thus, we have preliminary data to specify that the lateral amygdala is most active during a RSW for the CCP task and that one of the transmitters is ACh (see Fig. 6.5).

Present status of the RSW

The presence of periods of time during REM sleep following successful task acquisition that are important for efficient memory processing seems reasonably well established in rats and mice. It has not been observed very often in humans. Stickgold (Stickgold *et al.* 2000*b*) has reported that following acquisition of a visual discrimination task, subjects that got REM sleep during the last two hours of an 8 h night of sleep were superior to subjects that did not. Thus, a RSW within a single night, from 6–8 h after sleep onset, would appear to have been identified for a simple visual discrimination task in humans. While precise REM sleep period deprivations have not yet been done, total sleep deprivation does markedly retard memory for this task (Stickgold *et al.* 2000*a*).

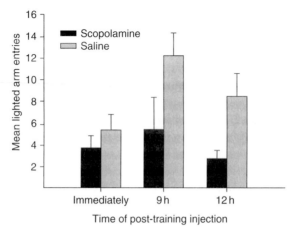

Figure 6.5 Mean number of lighted arm (reward) entries (+SEM) in the CCP task for the scopolamine and corresponding saline control groups for the three injection times. Only the 9 h post-training scopolamine and saline injection groups were significantly different.

While RSWs appear to exist within a sleep night for at least the visual discrimination task, it would also appear that REM sleep continues to be important for several nights after acquisition. In one study, subjects were trained to do a difficult logic task. Various groups were then exposed to total sleep deprivation (TSD) either the night of acquisition (day1), day 2 (24–48 h), day 3 (48–72 h), or day 4 (72–96 h) after acquisition. All groups were retested one week after initial acquisition. Participants deprived on the same night as acquisition were impaired on memory for this task. By contrast, participants deprived of TSD 24–48 h after acquisition were not impaired. However, participants deprived in a 48–72 h post-training "window" were also impaired on memory for the task. No effect was seen in memory of participants exposed to TSD 72–96 h after acquisition (Smith 1993). This effect was again seen when alcohol was used to impair normal REM sleep after acquisition of the same task. When alcohol was ingested after task acquisition, but just before bedtime on the same day as training (day 1), memory for the task was impaired on retest 1 week later. Ingestion of alcohol two nights after task acquisition (day 3; 48 h later) also resulted in memory impairment (Sandys-Wunsch and Smith 1991; Smith and Smith, submitted 2001). Thus, taken together, the results suggest that there are RSWs which occur on successive nights after acquisition as well as within a single night. It is not yet clear if all REM sleep periods are required on these nights.

Future directions

While the idea that the REM sleep window is an important time for memory processing appears to be well established in animals at the behavioral and EEG sleep levels, it is important that these special times be examined at the neurophysiological and biochemical levels as well. At least one group has pointed out that there are post-training biochemical windows in animals (Graves *et al.* 2001) and suggest the possibility of RSWs coinciding with these special times.

The RSW has only begun to be defined in humans (Sandys-Wunsch and Smith 1991; Smith 1993; Stickgold *et al.* 2000*a,b*). Presumably, as with rats and mice, there are RSWs that occur within a night of sleep as well as several days after learning, but only future research can support this hypothesis.

Acknowledgments

This research has been funded by the Natural Sciences and Engineering Research Council of Canada (NSERC).

References

Baghdoyan, H. A., Rodrigo-Angulo, M. L., Assens, F., McCarley, R. W., and **Hobson, J. A.** (1987). A neuroanatomical gradient in the pontine tegmentum for the cholinoceptive induction of desynchronized sleep signs. *Brain Research,* **414,** 245–261.

Bennett, E. L., Rosenzweig, M. R., and **Flood, J. F.** (1979). Role of neurotransmitters and protein synthesis in short- and long-term memory. In *Biological psychiatry today* (eds J. Obiols, C. Ballus, E. Gonzales Monclus, and J. Pujol), Elsevier/North Holland Biomedical Press, Amsterdam.

Bloch, V. (1970). Facts and hypotheses concerning memory consolidation processes. *Brain Research,* **24,** 561–575.

Bloch, V., Hennevin, E., and **Leconte, P.** (1979). Relationship between paradoxical sleep and memory processes. In *Brain mechanisms in memory and learning: from the single neuron to man* (ed. M. A. B. Brazier), pp. 329–343. Raven Press, New York.

Bowers, M. B., Hartmann, E. L., and **Freedman, D. X.** (1966). Sleep deprivation and acetylcholine. *Science,* **153,** 1416–1417.

Chang, F.-L. and **Greenough, W. T.** (1982). Lateralized effects of monocular training on dendritic branching in adult split brain rats. *Brain Research,* **232,** 283–292.

Coenen, A. M. and **Van Luijtelaar, E. N.** (1985). Stress induced by three procedures of deprivation of paradoxical sleep. *Physiology and Behavior,* **35,** 501–504.

Coll-Andreu, M., Ayora-Mascarell, L., Trullas-Oliva, R., and **Morgado-Bernal, I.** (1989). Behavioral evaluation of the stress induced by the platform method for short paradoxical sleep deprivation in rats. *Brain Research Bulletin,* **22,** 825–828.

Corkin, S. (1981). Acetylcholine, aging and Alzheimer's disease: implications for treatment. *Trends in Neurosciences,* **4,** 287–290.

Coyle, J., Price, D. L., and **DeLong, M.** (1983). Alzheimer's diease: a disorder of cortical cholinergic inervation. *Science,* **219,** 1184–1190.

Datta, S. (1995). Neuronal activity in the peribrachial area: relationship to behavioral state control. *Neuroscience and Biobehavioral Reviews,* **19,** 67–84.

Datta, S. (2000). Avoidance task training potentiates phasic pontine-wave density in the rat: a mechanism for sleep-dependent plasticity. *Journal of Neuroscience*, **20**, 8607–8613.

Deutsch, J. A. (1983). The cholinergic synapse and the site of memory. In *The physiological basis of memory* (ed. J. A. Deutsch), pp. 367–385. Academic Press, New York.

Diamond, M. C. (1976). Anatomical brain changes induced by environment. In *Knowing, thinking and believing* (eds L. Petrinovich and J. L. McGaugh), pp. 215–241. Plenum, New York.

Diamond, M. C., Krech, D., and **Rosenzweig, M. R.** (1964). The effects of an enriched environment on the histology of the rat cerebral cortex. *The Journal of Comparative Neurology*, **123**, 111–119.

Diamond, M. C., Lindner, B., Johnson, R., Bennett, E. L., and **Rosenzweig, M. R.** (1975). Differences in occipital cortical synapses from environmentally enriched, impoverished, and standard colony rats. *Journal of Neuroscience Research*, **1**, 109–119.

Domino, R. F., Yamamoto, K., and **Dren, T.** (1968). Role of cholinergic mechanisms in states of wakefulness and sleep. *Progress in Brain Research*, **28**, 113–133.

Fishbein, W. and **Gutwein, B. M.** (1977). Paradoxical sleep and memory storage processes. *Behavioral Biology*, **19**, 425–464.

Gillin, J. C. and **Sitaram, N.** (1984). Rapid eye movement (REM) sleep: cholinergic mechanisms. *Psychological Medicine*, **14**, 501–506.

Gisquet-Verrier, P. and **Smith, C.** (1989). Avoidance performance in rat enhanced by postlearning paradoxical sleep deprivation. *Behavioral and Neural Biology*, **53**, 152–169.

Globus, A., Rosenzweig, M. R., Bennett, E. L., and **Diamond, M. C.** (1973). Effect of differential experience on dendritic spine counts in rat cerebral cortex. *Journal of Comparative and Physiological Psychology*, **82**, 175–181.

Graves, L., Pack, A., and **Abel, T.** (2001). Sleep and memory: a molecular perspective. *Trends in Neurosciences*, **24**, 237–243.

Graves, L. A., Heller, E., Pack, A., and **Abel, T.** (2000). The role of sleep in hippocampus-dependent long-term memory. *Sleep*, **23**, A393.

Greenough, W. T. (1976). Enduring brain effects of differential experience and training. In *Neural mechanisms of learning and memory* (eds M. R. Rosenzweig and E. L. Bennett). MIT Press, Cambridge.

Greenough, W. T. and **Volkmar, F. R.** (1973). Pattern of dendritic branching in occipital cortex of rats reared in complex environments. *Experimental Neurology*, **40**, 491–504.

Gutwein, B. M. and **Fishbein, W.** (1980*a*). Paradoxical sleep and memory (i): selective alterations following enriched and impoverished environmental rearing. *Brain Research Bulletin*, **5**, 9–12.

Gutwein, B. M. and **Fishbein, W.** (1980*b*). Paradoxical sleep and memory (ii): sleep circadian rhythmicity following enriched and impoverished environmental rearing. *Brain Research Bulletin*, **5**, 105–109.

Gutwein, B. M., Shiromani, P. M., and **Fishbein, W.** (1980). Paradoxical sleep and memory: long term disruptive effects of anisomycin. *Pharmacology, Biochemistry and Behavior*, **12**, 377–384.

Hasselmo, M. E. (1999). Neuromodulation: acetylcholine and memory consolidation. *Trends in Cognitive Sciences*, **3**, 351–359.

Hennevin, E., Hars, B., Maho, C., and **Bloch, V.** (1995). Processing of learned information in paradoxical sleep: relevance for memory. *Behavioural Brain Research*, **69**, 125–135.

Jouvet, M. (1975). Cholinergic mechanisms and sleep. In *Cholinergic mechanisms* (ed. Waser, P.), pp. 455–476. Raven Press, New York.

Kenton, L. and **Smith, C.** (2001). Intra-amygdala scopolamine infusions during a paradoxical sleep window impairs conditioned cue preference acquisition. *Actas de Fisiologia*, **7**, 124.

Kitahama, K., Valatx, J.-L., and **Jouvet, M.** (1976). Apprentissage d'un labyrinthe en Y chez deux souches de souris. Effets de la privation instrumentale et pharmacologique du sommeil. *Brain Research*, **108**, 75–86.

Kiyono, S., Seo, M. L., and **Shibagaki, M.** (1981). Effects of rearing environments upon sleep waking parameters in rats. *Physiology and Behavior*, **26**, 391–394.

McDonald, R. J. and **White, N. M.** (1993). A triple dissociation of memory systems: hippocampus, amygdala and dorsal striatum. *Behavioral Neuroscience*, **107**, 3–22.

McGinty, D. J. and **Drucker-Colin, R. R.** (1982). Sleep mechanisms: biology and control of REM sleep. *International Review of Neurobiology*, **23**, 391–436.

McGrath, M. J. and **Cohen, D. B.** (1978). REM sleep facilitation of adaptive waking behavior: a review of the literature. *Psychological Bulletin*, **85**, 24–57.

Mirmiram, M., van den Dungen, H., and **Uylings, H. B. M.** (1982). Suppression of active sleep counteracts the environmental "enrichment" effect upon brain growth in rats. In *Experimental studies on the significance of active (c.q.REM sleep) sleep for maturation of brain and behavior in the rat* (ed. M. Mirmiram), pp. 79–85. Rhodopi, Amsterdam.

Morris, R. G. M., Garrud, P., Rawlins, J. N. P., and **O'Keefe, J.** (1982). Place navigation impaired in rats with hippocampal lesions. *Nature*, **297**, 681–683.

Pearlman, C. (1979). REM sleep and information processing: evidence from animal studies. *Neuroscience and Biobehavioral Reviews*, **3**, 57–68.

Pearlman, C. and **Becker, M.** (1975). Retroactive impairment of cooperative learning by imipramine and chlordiazepoxide. *Psychopharmacologia*, **42**, 63–66.

Pearlman, C. and **Becker, M.** (1974*a*). REM sleep deprivation impairs bar press acquisition in rats. *Physiology and Behavior*, **13**, 813–817.

Pearlman, C. A. and **Becker, M.** (1974*b*). REM sleep deprivation impairs serial reversal and probability maximizing in rats. *Physiological Psychology*, **2**, 509–512.

Pearlman, C. and **Becker, M.** (1973). Brief posttrial REM sleep deprivation impairs discrimination learning in rats. *Physiological Psychology*, **1**, 373–376.

Pearlman, C. A. and **Greenberg, R.** (1973). Posttrial REM sleep: a critical period for consolidation of shuttlebox avoidance. *Animal Learning and Behavior*, **1**, 49–51.

Rojas-Ramirez, J. A., Aguilar-Jiminez, E., Posadas-Andrews, A., Bernal-Pedraza, J. G., and **Drucker-Colin, R. R.** (1977). The effects of various protein synthesis inhibitors on the sleep–wake cycle of rats. *Psychopharmacology*, **53**, 147–150.

Rosensweig, M. R., Krech, D., Bennett, E. L., and **Diamond, M.** (1962). Effects of environmental complexity and training on brain chemistry and anatomy: a replication and extension. *Journal of Comparative and Physiological Psychology*, **55**, 429–437.

Sandys-Wunsch, H. and Smith, C. (1991). The effects of alcohol consumption on sleep and memory. *Sleep Research*, **20**, 419.

Siegal, J. M. (2001). The REM sleep-memory consolidation hypothesis. *Science*, **294**, 1058–1063.

Sitaram, N., Weingartner, H., and Gillin, J. C. (1978). Human serial learning: enhancement with arecholine and choline and impairment with scopolamine. *Science*, **201**, 274–276.

Smith, C. T. (1985). Sleep states and learning: a review of the animal literature. *Neuroscience and Biobehavioral Reviews*, **9**, 157–168.

Smith, C. (1993). REM sleep and learning: some recent findings. In *The Functions of Dreaming* (eds A. Moffitt, M. Kramer, and R. Hoffmann), pp. 341–361. SUNY Press, New York.

Smith, C. (1996). Sleep states, memory processes and synaptic plasticity. *Behavioural Brain Research*, **78**, 49–56.

Smith, C. and Butler, S. (1982). Paradoxical sleep at selective times following training is necessary for learning. *Physiology and Behavior*, **29**, 469–473.

Smith, C. and Gisquet-Verrier, P. (1996). Paradoxical sleep deprivation and sleep recording following training in a brightness discrimination avoidance task in Sprague-Dawley rats: paradoxical effects. *Neurobiology of Learning and Memory*, **66**, 283–294.

Smith, C. and Kelly, G. (1988). Paradoxical sleep deprivation applied two days after the end of training retards learning. *Physiology and Behavior*, **43**, 213–216.

Smith, C. and Lapp, L. (1986). Prolonged increases in both PS and number of REMS following a shuttle avoidance task. *Physiology and Behavior*, **36**, 1053–1057.

Smith, C. and MacNeill, C. (1993). A paradoxical sleep-dependent window for memory 53–56 h after the end of avoidance training. *Psychobiology*, **21**, 109–112.

Smith, C. and Rose, G. (1996). Evidence for a paradoxical sleep window for place learning in the Morris water maze. *Physiology and Behavior*, **59**, 93–97.

Smith, C. and Rose, G. (1997). Posttraining paradoxical sleep in rats is increased after spatial learning in the Morris water maze. *Behavioral Neuroscience*, **111**, 1197–1204.

Smith, C. and Smith, D. (2003). Ingestion of ethanol just prior to sleep onset impairs memory for procedural but not declarative tasks, *Sleep* **26** (in press).

Smith, C. and Wong, P. T. P. (1991). Paradoxical sleep increases predict successful learning in a complex operant task. *Behavioral Neuroscience*, **105**, 282–288.

Smith, C., Conway, J., and Rose, G. (1998a). Brief paradoxical sleep deprivation impairs reference, but not working memory in the radial maze task. *Neurobiology of Learning and Memory*, **69**, 211–217.

Smith, C., DeButte, M., and Annett, R. (1998b). Effects of paradoxical sleep deprivation on levels of acetylcholine and memory for a spatial task. *Sleep*, **21** (Suppl.), 7.

Smith, C., Tenn, C., and Annett, R. (1991). Some biochemical and behavioral aspects of the paradoxical sleep window. *Canadian Journal of Psychology*, **45**, 115–124.

Smith, C., Young, J., and Young, W. (1980). Prolonged increases in paradoxical sleep during and after avoidance task acquisition. *Sleep*, **3**, 67–81.

Smith, C. T., Kitahama, K., Valatx, J. L., and **Jouvet, M.** (1974). Increased paradoxical sleep in mice during acquisition of a shock avoidance task. *Brain Research*, **77**, 221–230.

Stickgold, R., LaTanya, J., and **Hobson, J. A.** (2000*a*). Visual discrimination learning requires sleep after training. *Nature Neuroscience*, **3**, 1237–1238.

Stickgold, R., Whidbee, D., Schirmer, B., Patel, V., and **Hobson, J. A.** (2000*b*). Visual discrimination task improvement: a multistep process occurring during sleep. *Journal of Cognitive Neuroscience*, **12**, 246–254.

Tagney, J. (1973). Sleep patterns related to rearing rats in enriched and impoverished environments. *Brain Research*, **53**, 353–361.

Tsuchiya, K., Toru, M., and **Kobashi, T.** (1969). Sleep deprivation: changes of monoamines and acetylcholine in rat brain. *Life Sciences*, **8**, 867–873.

Vallance, K., McDonald, R. J., and **Smith, C.** (1999). Effects of paradoxical sleep on the memory for a conditioned cue preference task in rats. *Sleep*, **22**, S243.

Vertes, R. (2000). The case against sleep and memory consolidation. *Behavioural and Brain Sciences*, **23**, 867.

CHAPTER 7

ACTIVATION OF PHASIC PONTINE WAVE (P-WAVE): A MECHANISM OF LEARNING AND MEMORY PROCESSING

SUBIMAL DATTA AND ELISSA H. PATTERSON

Introduction

Since the discovery of rapid eye movement (REM) sleep, many animal studies of sleep and learning have focused on the role of REM sleep in memory consolidation (Hennevin and Hars 1985; reviewed in Smith 1985, 1995; Hennevin *et al.* 1995). Using a variety of protocols and test paradigms, sleep and learning studies in animals have demonstrated the following results: (i) Training of rats on both appetitive and aversive tasks, including multiple-goal maze, operant bar press, shuttle avoidance, and classical conditioning tasks, leads to an increase in subsequent REM sleep (Lucero 1970; Fishbein *et al.* 1974; Hennevin *et al.* 1974; Smith and Young 1980; Smith *et al.* 1980; Portell-Cortes *et al.* 1989; Smith and Wong 1991; Bramham *et al.* 1994; Smith and Rose 1997; Datta 2000). These increases appear not to be due simply to the stress of the training protocol, but to active learning of new material (Hennevin *et al.* 1995; Datta 2000). (ii) The increased REM sleep often begins immediately after training and lasts for a limited period of time. (iii) REM sleep deprivation during critical periods of post-training REM sleep, called REM sleep windows (Smith 1985, 1995), but not during earlier or later periods, can partially or even totally block improved task performance on subsequent retesting (Fishbein 1971; Wolfowitz and Holdstock 1971; Pearlman 1973; Pearlman and Becker 1973; Smith and Butler 1982; Smith *et al.* 1998). Taken together, these animal studies suggest that memory consolidation following task training requires processes selectively active during REM sleep and that the organism homeostatically adjusts its REM sleep in response to memory consolidation demands.

Many human studies of sleep and learning have focused on REM sleep (reviewed in Smith 1995; Maquet 2001). Human studies have demonstrated that learning trials increase REM sleep in the subsequent sleep period (Verschoor and Holdstock 1984; DeKoninck *et al.* 1989; Mandai *et al.* 1989; Smith and Lapp 1991; Smith 1995). Some studies have looked at the effect of REM sleep deprivation on specific memory systems (Empson and Clarke 1970; McGrath and Cohen 1978; Lapp and Smith 1986; Smith and Whittaker 1987; Pirolli and Smith 1989; Smith and Pirolli 1989). In one study, REM sleep deprivation after training had no effect on declarative/explicit tasks such as word lists or paired-associates and word recognition tasks, but hindered subsequent performance of implicit/procedural tasks such as a word fragment completion task (Smith 1995). Another study using a visual discrimination task also reported that REM sleep deprivation prevents improvement on procedural memory (Karni *et al.* 1994). Complementary to these REM sleep-deprivation studies, one study compared the amount of learning on a declarative (paired-associates) learning task and a procedural (mirror writing) task following periods of wake or sleep (Plihal and Born 1997). It was found that slow wave sleep (SWS)-rich sleep (i.e. the first half of the night) enhanced subsequent performance on the declarative memory task—but not the procedural task—compared with an equivalent amount of either SWS-poor sleep (i.e. the second half of the night) or wake time. In contrast, REM sleep-rich periods (during the second half of the night) enhanced performance on the procedural but not the declarative task. These results suggest that REM sleep plays a larger role in the consolidation of procedural memories while SWS is more critical for declarative memory consolidation. More recently, another study using a procedural memory task (visual discrimination), demonstrated that overnight improvement was proportional to the amount of SWS during the first quarter of the night as well as to the amount of REM sleep in the last quarter (Stickgold 1998).

Taken together, the combined animal and human studies support the concept that REM sleep contributes importantly to the process of memory consolidation, especially of a procedural learning task. The goal of this chapter is to present arguments and supporting data for the hypothesis that the activation of phasic pontine-wave (P-wave) generating cells in the brainstem is critical for sleep-dependent learning and memory processing. Since the focus of this chapter is on the P-wave, and it is most frequent during REM sleep, the brainstem structures that are critical for REM sleep are briefly described in Box 7.1.

P-wave: description and functional significance

Activation of a group of neurons in the pontine tegmentum generates a prominent field potential just prior to the onset of and throughout REM sleep (Datta and Hobson 1994, 1995; Datta *et al.* 1998). This field potential has been recorded from the pons, lateral geniculate body, and occipital cortex. Since, in the cat, this potential originates in the pons (P) and propagates to the lateral geniculate body (G) and occipital cortex (O), it has been called the ponto-geniculo-occipital (PGO) wave (Brooks and Bizzi 1963; Jouvet *et al.* 1965). This field potential has also been recorded from many other parts of the brain which receive excitatory inputs from the PGO-wave generation site (Datta 1997; Datta *et al.* 1998). In addition to cats, the PGO wave has been documented and studied in other mammals including nonhuman primates, humans, and rodents (reviewed in Datta 1997). The P-wave in the rat is equivalent to the pontine component of the PGO wave in

Box 7.1 Brainstem structures trigger REM sleep signs

Sleep, especially REM sleep, provides an exceptional opportunity to study the brain based physical and physiological foundation of cognitive processes. As one proceeds from waking into NREM sleep and then REM sleep, a series of dramatic and well-defined changes occur in the neurophysiology and neurochemistry of the brain. REM sleep is characterized by a constellation of events including the following: (i) a desynchronized pattern of cortical activity; (ii) marked atonia of the postural muscles; (iii) REMs; (iv) a theta rhythm within the hippocampus; (v) field potentials in the pons (P-wave), lateral geniculate nucleus and occipital cortex (PGO) spikes; (vi) myoclonic twitches, most apparent in the facial and distal limb musculature; and (vii) pronounced cardiorespiratory fluctuations.

During the last decade, evidence from both rat and cat studies suggested that each of the events of REM sleep is executed by distinct cell groups in the brain stem (see Vertes 1984; Sakai 1985; Datta 1995, 1997, 1999 for reviews). These cell groups are discrete components of a widely distributed network rather than a single REM sleep "center" (Fig. 7.1). The cortical EEG desynchronization of REM sleep is executed by the ponto–mesencephalic reticular formation, muscle atonia by the locus coeruleus alpha, and REMs by the peri-abducens reticular formation. The PGO wave is executed by the caudolateral–peribrachial area (C-PBL) and nucleus subcoeruleus (SubC). Hippocampal theta rhythm is executed by the pontis oralis, and muscle twitches by the nucleus gigantocellularis especially the caudal part. Increased brain temperature and cardio-respiratory fluctuations are executed by the parabrachial nucleus. These REM sleep sign generating executive neurons are modulated and triggered by aminergic (in locus coeruleus and dorsal raphe nucleus) and cholinergic (in pedunculopontine tegmentum and laterodorsal tegmentum) cells of the brainstem to induce the behavioral state of REM sleep (Datta 1995). For the detailed mechanisms of REM sleep generation, readers are referred to recent reviews and a book elsewhere (Datta 1995; Mallick and Inoue 1999; Hobson *et al.* 2000).

the cat (Marks *et al.* 1980; Sanford *et al.* 1995; Datta *et al.* 1998, 1999). In the rat, this field potential is absent in the lateral geniculate body (LGB) due to the lack of afferent inputs from P-wave generating cells (Datta *et al.* 1998). Since this field potential is absent in the LGB of the rat (Stern *et al.* 1974), we call this field potential a P-wave rather than pontine PGO wave (Datta *et al.* 1999). The P-wave is 75–150 ms in duration and has amplitude of 100–150 μV (Fig. 7.2). This wave occurs as a singlet and as clusters containing a variable number of P-waves (3–5 waves/burst) at a frequency range of 30–60 spikes/min during REM sleep (Marks *et al.* 1980; Sanford *et al.* 1995; Datta *et al.* 1998, 2001). Detailed mechanisms for the generation of PGO/P-waves have been described in recent review articles (Datta 1997, 1999).

Since P-wave activity always precedes REM sleep, several investigators have proposed that P-wave mechanisms are causally linked to the cellular and molecular mechanisms that trigger and regulate the total amount of REM sleep (Duysan-Peyrethon *et al.* 1967; Dement *et al.* 1969; Malcolm *et al.* 1970; Foote 1973). In addition to REM sleep induction, it has been proposed that the P-wave is involved in several other important brain functions such as sensorimotor integration, learning, memory, cognition, dreaming, self-organization, development of the visual system, visual hallucination, and startle responses (Baust *et al.* 1972; Bowe-Anders *et al.* 1974; Morrison and Bowker 1975;

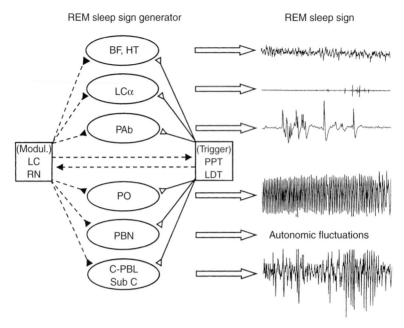

Figure 7.1 Structural and functional model for the generation of REM sleep. Each of the events of REM sleep (under the label "REM sleep sign") is executed by the activation of distinct cell groups (under the label "REM sleep sign generator") in the brainstem. These REM sleep sign generating executive neurons are excited by the activation of cholinergic cells in the pedunculopontine tegmentum (PPT) and laterodorsal tegmentum (LDT). Activation of aminergic cells in the locus coeruleus (LC) and dorsal raphe nucleus inhibits the REM sleep sign generating executive neurons. Abbreviations: LCα, locus coeruleus alpha; PAb, peri-abducence reticular formation; PO, pontis oralis; PBN, parabrachial nucleus; C-PBL, caudolateral peribrachial area; SubC, nucleus subcoeruleus; PMR, ponto-mesencephalic reticular formation (modified from Datta 1995).

Bowker and Morrison 1976, 1977; Orem and Barnes 1980; Crick and Mitchison 1983; Davenne and Adrien 1984; Sanford *et al.* 1992*a*,*b*, 1993; Kahn and Hobson 1993; Datta 1997, 1999; Shaffery *et al.* 1999). Although several functional roles for PGO and P-waves have been proposed, most of these ideas remain primarily speculative due to the lack of experimental evidence.

P-wave role in the memory consolidation process

Sites of consolidation process in the forebrain

Based on a number of neurophysiological studies, off-line reactivation of various neuronal structures involved in learning seems to be critical for the consolidation of memories. For example—when rats actively explore a new environment, pyramidal cells within the CA1 and CA3 regions of the hippocampus form a spatial map of the environment, wherein individual cells—referred to as place cells—become responsive

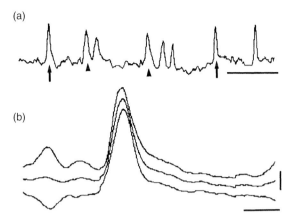

Figure 7.2 The waveform and amplitude of the P-wave in the rat. (a) shows a typical P-wave recorded from the P-wave generator. The arrow points to a single wave and arrowhead points to clustered waves. (b) Average (central trace) ± one unit of standard deviation (above and below the central trace) of 50 individual P-waves recorded in the P-wave generator. Time scale bars: in (a) = 1 s and in (b) = 100 ms. Amplitude scale bar in (b) = 25 μV (from Datta *et al.* 1998).

to specific locations within the environment. The development of these spatial maps is driven by the flow of sensory information from the neocortex into the hippocampus during active exploration. Following spatial exploration, when animals sleep, activity patterns of hippocampal place cells are reactivated. This reactivation is believed to be associated with memory formation and consolidation (Pavlides and Winson 1989; Wilson and McNaughton 1994; Skaggs and McNaughton 1996; Qin *et al.* 1997; Kudrimoti *et al.* 1999; Louie and Wilson 2001). Similarly, depending on the type of learning cues (e.g. auditory, visual, olfactory, tactile, etc.), this type of off-line reactivation may also occur in the amygdala, parahippocampal areas, neocortex, and many other brain structures involved in memory formation and consolidation (Maho *et al.* 1991; Hennevin *et al.* 1993, 1995). This reactivation hypothesis of memory consolidation is also supported by a number of hippocampal electrical stimulation studies (Stein and Chorover 1968; Erickson and Patel 1969; Destrade *et al.* 1973; Landfield *et al.* 1973; Destrade and Cardo 1974). These studies have shown that mice and rats receiving posttrial hippocampal stimulation showed better retention of learning than control animals. These studies also showed that when the hippocampus was reactivated by electrical stimulation, there was no need for sleep for the improvement of learning. In summary, reactivation of the hippocampus, amygdala, parahippocampal areas, and many other sites in the forebrain is critical for sleep-dependent memory processing.

Brainstem is the probable source of the triggering stimulus for consolidation

If reactivation of forebrain and cortical memory processing networks is critical for the consolidation of memory, then what is the physiological source of this reactivating stimulus during REM sleep? This reactivating stimulus is probably coming from the brainstem. This proposition is supported by the finding that in the rat, the electrical stimulation of the mesencephalic reticular formation (MRF) following training improves performance (Leconte *et al.* 1974; DeWeer 1976; Bloch *et al.* 1977; Devietti *et al.* 1977; Sara *et al.* 1980; Bloch and Laroche 1981; Hennevin *et al.* 1989). The improvement in learning performance by posttrial MRF stimulation was as effective as hippocampal stimulation. Posttrial MRF stimulation was shown to facilitate a classically conditioned association and also the development of associative changes in neuronal activity in the hippocampus as the conditioning proceeded (Bloch and Laroche 1981, 1984, 1985). Moreover, when this stimulation was administered after long-term potentiation (LTP) inducing stimulus, it enhanced the magnitude of LTP at the synapses of the perforant path on dentate granular cells and prolonged its duration by several days (Bloch and Laroche 1981, 1985). This MRF stimulation during the postacquisition period appeared to substitute the need for REM sleep by decreasing the post-training REM sleep elevation and by abolishing most of the learning impairment produced by posttrial REM sleep deprivation (Bloch *et al.* 1977). This evidence suggests that MRF stimulation has enhanced an ongoing physiological process which naturally occurs during post-learning REM sleep and which could be responsible, at least partially, for the beneficial effect of post-learning REM sleep on memorization. Based on the evidence above, it may be proposed that during REM sleep the MRF is the source of the reactivating stimulus for the memory processing network in the forebrain and cortical areas. However, these MRF electrical stimulation studies did not systematically localize a specific MRF site that is most effective at reactivating the memory processing network. Is the whole MRF or a specific nucleus the source of reactivation?

The MRF is an important part of the brainstem reticular formation, and it contains a number of specific cell groups involved in the generation of different signs of REM sleep (for review see Datta 1995 and Box 7.1 (Fig. 7.1)). During REM sleep, different parts of the brainstem reticular formation are activated for the generation of different phasic and tonic signs of REM sleep (for reviews see Vertes 1984; Datta 1995, 1997, 1999). It is likely that electrical stimulation of the MRF in these studies also stimulated other parts of the brainstem reticular formation involved in the generation of different phasic and tonic signs of REM sleep (Leconte *et al.* 1974; DeWeer 1976; Bloch *et al.* 1977; Devietti *et al.* 1977; Sara *et al.* 1980; Bloch and Laroche 1981; Hennevin *et al.* 1989). Which cell group(s) or structure(s) in the brainstem are responsible for the reactivation of the memory processing network in the forebrain and cortex? According to the general hypothesis of this chapter, the improvement of learning performance by posttrial MRF stimulation without REM sleep and after posttrial REM sleep without MRF stimulation is due to the activation of P-wave generating cells. The following evidence is presented in support of the idea that the activation of P-wave generating cells is responsible for the reactivation of the memory processing network in the forebrain and cortex.

Evidence that the brainstem P-wave generator is the triggering stimulus for consolidation processes in the forebrain

Physiological evidence

Long-term potentiation (LTP) of synaptic transmission is widely considered to be a model of activity-dependent synaptic plasticity that could be involved in certain forms of learning and memory (Lomo 1966; Bliss and Lomo 1973; McNaughton *et al.* 1986; Morris 1989; Morris *et al.* 1990; Bliss and Collingridge 1993). It has been shown that REM sleep increases following learning trials and that deprivation of REM sleep soon after learning trials causes a subsequent decrease in performance of a learned task (Smith 1985; Karni *et al.* 1994). Associated with these changes in REM sleep are changes in the efficacy of synaptic transmission in the brain, manifested as LTP (Ramirez and Carrer 1989; Silva *et al.* 1992; Bramham *et al.* 1994). Long-term potentiation is significant in that it is thought to be the physiological substrate of learning and memory at the level of the hippocampus and the amygdala (Bliss and Collingridge 1993). The standard protocols used by most researchers to induce LTP in the hippocampus, amygdala, neocortex, and many other areas of the brain are: (i) high-frequency stimulation in which several hundred pulses at frequencies of 250–400 Hz are given; and (ii) short high-frequency (>200 Hz) bursts of stimuli with an interburst interval of ~200 ms, called theta-patterned stimulation (Bliss and Gardner-Medwin 1973; Lee 1982; Racine *et al.* 1983; Rose and Dunwiddie 1986; Staubli and Lynch 1987; Diamond *et al.* 1988; Holscher *et al.* 1997). In an experimental situation, the high-frequency electrical stimulation of an afferent pathway is key for induction of LTP. However, during REM sleep, the physiological source of that presynaptic high-frequency stimulation is unclear. Therefore, the identification of the source of this presynaptic high-frequency stimulus for LTP during REM sleep would be a significant contribution to the current body of knowledge about the physiological substrates of learning and memory.

For REM sleep-dependent memory processing and learning, the source of the LTP inducing high-frequency stimulus must come from the REM sleep sign generating structures of the brainstem (brainstem structures that trigger REM sleep signs are described above). During the last 25 years, a number of laboratories have recorded the single cell activity patterns of the different REM sleep sign generating structures in the rat, cat, and nonhuman primate (for review see Steriade and McCarley 1990; Datta 1995, 1997). Depending on the specific REM sleep sign generating structure, neuronal activity patterns of those generating cells are classified as tonic single spike type, bursting type or both tonic and bursting type. The only type of cell within the REM sleep sign generating structures which fires as a high-frequency burst, similar to the high-frequency stimulus required for the generation of LTP, is located within the P-wave generator (Fig. 7.3 and Datta 1997). These P-wave generating neurons discharge

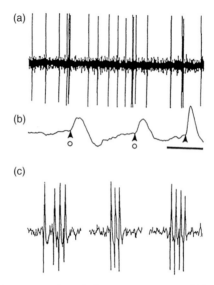

Figure 7.3 Single cell activity pattern of a typical P-wave generating cell during P-wave-related states of sleep (tS–R and REM sleep). (a) A train of action potentials from a P-wave generating neuron in the cat showing recurrent high-frequency bursts on a background of tonic action potentials. (b) Cluster PGO waves recorded simultaneously with A. (c) The three high-frequency bursts seen in (a) are displayed on an expanded time scale. The time scale in (a) and (b) is 100 ms; in (c), 10 ms (modified from Datta and Hobson 1994).

high-frequency (>500 Hz) spike bursts (3–5 spikes/burst) on the background of tonically increased firing rates (30–40 Hz) during the P-wave-related states of transition between SWS and REM sleep (tS–R) and REM sleep (Datta and Hobson 1994; Datta 1997). High-frequency bursting patterns of these P-wave generating cells support the idea that the P-wave generator may be the source of electrical stimulus for the induction of physiological LTP.

There is now experimental evidence that the activation of P-wave generating cells is capable of inducing LTP. Microinjection of the cholinergic agonist, carbachol, into the P-wave generator activates P-wave generating cells (Datta *et al.* 1991, 1998). The cholinergic activation of the P-wave generator in the cat markedly increases P-wave activity and REM sleep (Datta *et al.* 1991–1993). This cholinergic stimulation-induced potentiation of P-wave density and REM sleep lasts for about 7–10 days. This long-lasting increase in P-wave density and REM sleep is a physiological sign of synaptic as well as intracellular plasticity. Thus, the activation of P-wave generating cells is capable of inducing physiological LTP.

Anatomical evidence

If the P-wave generator is the presynaptic input for the induction of synaptic plasticity, a prerequisite for learning and memory processing, it is expected that the P-wave generating cells will send anatomical connections to the forebrain structures known to be involved in memory processing. To test this hypothesis, the anterograde tracer biotinylated dextran amine (BDA) was microinjected into the physiologically identified cholinoceptive pontine P-wave generating site of rats to identify brain structures receiving efferent projections from those P-wave generating sites (Datta et al. 1998). In all cases, small volume injections of BDA in the cholinoceptive P-wave generating sites resulted in anterograde labeling of fibers and terminals in many regions of the brain (Fig. 7.4). The most important output structures of those P-wave generating cells were the occipital cortex, entorhinal cortex, piriform cortex, amygdala, hippocampus, and many other thalamic, hypothalamic, and brainstem nuclei that participate in the generation of REM sleep (Datta 1995, 1997; Datta et al. 1998). All of these forebrain structures are already known to be involved in memory processing (Squire et al. 1990; LeDoux 1992; Silva et al. 1992; Izquierdo et al. 1995; Hatfield et al. 1996; Rampel-Clower et al. 1996; Poremba and Gabriel 1997; Young et al. 1997). These monosynaptic axonal connections between P-wave generating cells and forebrain structures provide anatomical evidence that P-wave generating cells have the necessary anatomical substrate to be the presynaptic input for the induction of synaptic plasticity, a required process for learning and memory processing.

Behavioral evidence

Several studies indicate that REMs may represent the element of REM sleep that is crucial for memory consolidation (Herman and Roffwarg 1983; Verschor and Holdstock 1984; Mandai et al. 1989; Smith and Weeden 1990; Smith and Lapp 1991). For example, when a background clicking noise was presented during acquisition of a learned skill, presentation of the same auditory stimulus during subsequent eye movements during REM sleep (cueing), was correlated with a 23 percent improvement on retest performance one week later. The same cueing applied during non-eye movement REM sleep episodes correlated with only an 8.8 percent retest improvement. It has been hypothesized, therefore, that the eye movements (or at least that segment of REM sleep in which they occur) are selectively important in REM sleep-dependent memory consolidation (Smith and Weeden 1990). Visual learning tests in human volunteers showed that in addition to increases in percentage of REM sleep, the percentage of eye bursts during post-training REM sleep increased (Verschoor and Holdstock 1984). These researchers hypothesize that these augmented eye bursts represent the scanning of visual stimuli encountered during the learning task, as part of the process of sorting, organizing, and consolidating daily input (Verschoor and Holdstock 1984). A study of Morse language learning in humans provides further evidence for an eye movement role in learning and memory processing during REM sleep. After a 90-min Morse language learning session immediately prior to bedtime, subjects who had the greatest success had the densest REMs (Mandai et al. 1989). It is well-established that the occurrence and direction of REMs during REM sleep depends exclusively on the excitation of P-wave generating cells (Datta and Hobson 1994). Therefore, the studies described above indirectly substantiate

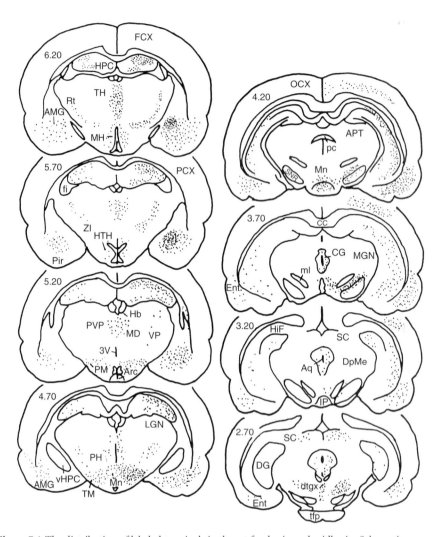

Figure 7.4 The distribution of labeled terminals in the rat forebrain and midbrain. Schematic representation of selected coronal forebrain and midbrain sections illustrating the distribution of labeled terminals (each dot = multiple labeled terminals) after a small injection of BDA into the cholinoceptive P-wave generation site in the subcoeruleus nucleus. The number on the upper left side of each section indicates the distance anterior to interaural line. Abbreviations: 3V, 3rd ventricle; AMG, amygdala; APT, anterior pretectal nucleus; Aq, aqueduct; Arc, arcuate hypothalamic nucleus; CC, splenium corpus callosum; CG, central gray; DG, dentate gyrus; DpMe, deep mesencephalic nucleus; dtgx, dorsal tegmental decussation; Ent, entorhinal cortex; FCX, frontal cortex; fi, fimbria hippocampus; Hb, habenular nucleus; HiF, hippocampal fissure; HPC, hippocampus; HTH, hypothalamus; IP, interpeduncular nucleus; LGN, lateral geniculate nucleus; MD, mediodorsal thalamic nucleus; MGN, medial geniculate nucleus; MH, medial hypothalamus; ml, medial lemniscus; Mn, medial mammillary nucleus; OCX, occipital cortex; pc, posterior commissure; PCX, parietal cortex; PH, posterior hypothalamic area; Pir, piriform cortex; PM, premammillary nucleus; PVP, paraventricular thalamic nucleus, posterior; Rt, reticular thalamic nucleus; SC, superior colliculus; SNR, substantia nigra, reticular; tfp, transverse fibers pons; TH, thalamus; TM, tuberomammillary nucleus; vHPC, ventral hippocampus; VP, ventral posterior thalamic nucleus; ZI, zona incerta (from Datta *et al.* 1998).

our hypothesis that the excitation of pontine P-wave generating cells is critical for REM sleep-dependent memory consolidation.

One recent study investigated the direct relationship between the P-wave and improvement of learning (Datta 2000). In this study, experiments were performed on adult male Sprague–Dawley rats. Rats were chronically implanted with a standard set of electrodes to objectively measure states of sleep and wakefulness. After 7–10 days of habituation, rats were placed in a shuttle box for the first session of active avoidance learning. All rats were subjected to 30 trials of conditioned stimulus (CS, 10 s light and sound) with an intertrial interval of 60 s. These rats were then randomly divided into two groups: group 1 (two-way active avoidance learning group) and group 2 (non-learning control group). Group 1 was subjected to 30 trials of CS paired with the unconditional stimulus (UCS, 5 s 0.3 mA FS, CS–UCS interval: 5 s) which they could avoid by moving to the other side of the shuttle box (training trials). Group 2 received 30 trials of CS and 10 trials of randomly delivered UCS (CS–UCS unpaired) which they could not avoid even by moving to the other side of the shuttle box. A PC using remote monitoring system software controlled experimental protocols and data collections. After these learning/non-learning experiments each rat was monitored for a 6-h free-moving polygraphic recording session between 10:00 h and 16:00 h. Immediately after the polygraphic recording session, the CS–UCS paired group (learning group) of rats was subjected to a second session (retrial session) of avoidance trials identical to the first session (training session). For the analysis, 30 avoidance trials were divided into six blocks (five trials per block). The level of learning was expressed as a percentage of avoidance. Six-hour polygraphic measures provided the following dependent variables that are quantified for each session: (i) percentage of recording time spent in wakefulness (W), SWS, transition between SWS and REM sleep (tS–R), and REM sleep, (ii) latencies to onset of the first episodes of tS–R and REM sleep after the onset of recordings, (iii) total number of tS–R and REM sleep episodes, (iv) mean duration of tS–R and REM sleep episodes, (v) P-wave density (waves/min) in REM sleep, (vi) theta wave frequency (waves/s) in REM sleep, and (vii) REM density (waves/min) in REM sleep.

In the initial learning session (training session), rats performed poorly in the first 10 trials and then learned to avoid UCS 50 percent of the time between trials 15 and 20. By 30 trials they learned to avoid 90 percent of UCS trials. During the second learning session (retrial session), rats avoided UCS trials 50 percent of the time from the beginning. By 15 trials they avoided almost 90 percent of UCS trials. These results indicate some changes in memory processing during the 6-h interval between the two learning sessions, causing improvement of learning by at least 50 percent. Six-hour polygraphic recordings show 181 percent increase of tS–R and 30 percent increase of REM sleep in the learning group relative to the non-learning control group. Because the P-wave is normally present only during the behavioral states of tS–R and REM sleep, we have referred to these as the P-wave states (PWS) (Datta *et al.* 1992; Datta and Hobson 2000). These results suggest a close association between the P-wave-related states and memory consolidation. Although no other learning study recorded the P-wave, based on only cortical electroencephalographic (EEG) pattern, the increase in transitional stage between SWS and REM sleep after learning trials was reported by another group of investigators using another learning task in the rat (Ambrosini *et al.* 1988; Giuditta *et al.* 1995, see Chapter 9).

Having documented a significant increase in the posttrial PWS percentage (combined percentage of tS–R and REM sleep) in the learning group compared to the control, we looked at P-wave density during the REM sleep episodes for 6 h of recordings after the shuttle box avoidance learning and control trials. The P-wave densities in the learning group of animals were significantly higher than those of the control group during REM sleep episodes from one to four (Fig. 7.5). This increase in P-wave density peaked in the third episode of REM sleep. Because there was a sharp rise of P-wave density between the first and third episodes of REM sleep after the training session, we expected to see a precise relationship between the increase in P-wave density

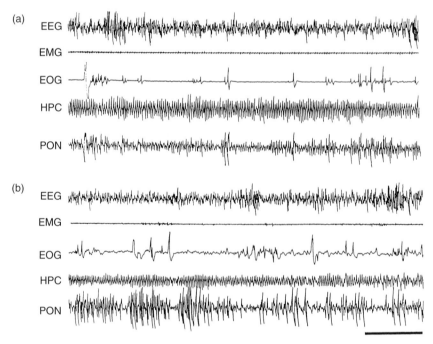

Figure 7.5 Sample polygraphic appearance of the third episode of REM sleep after the first session of control trials (a) and learning trials (b) Note qualitative similarity in both records showing characteristic electrographic signs of REM sleep: low-voltage, high-frequency or desynchronized waves recorded from the frontal cortex (EEG); muscle atonia (electromicrogram, EMG); rapid eye movements (electrooculogram, EOG); hippocampal theta waves in the hippocampal EEG (HPC); and P-waves (spiky waves) in the pontine EEG (PON). In spite of qualitative similarity, P-waves are more frequent in the learning trials than the control trials. Time scale = 5 s (from Datta 2000).

between the first and third REM sleep episodes and the improvement in performance. Indeed a strong correlation was observed. These results indicate that there is a significant relationship between the rate of change of P-wave generating cell activity and levels of memory retention. These findings provide behavioral evidence to support the hypotheses that the activation of P-wave generating cells is necessary for memory consolidation. As suggested by Carlyle Smith (1985, 1995), these findings also support that there is a "window of activation" (RSW) for the sleep-dependent consolidation process.

Conclusions

Based on all the evidence discussed in this chapter, it is clear that P-wave generating cells are capable of inducing physiological synaptic plasticity. It is also evident that the activation of P-wave generating cells is critical for the improvement of learning. If synaptic plasticity (LTP) is the physiological substrate for learning and memory, then P-wave generating cells are the presynaptic source for the high-frequency stimulus.

To account for sleep-dependent memory processing and learning, the following hypothesis has been suggested (Fig. 7.6). During wakefulness, external information is randomly input into the brain and temporarily stored in the neocortex. At the same time, this information is represented in a brief cataloged form in the amygdala, hippocampus, and parahippocampal areas. This process is called acquisition and temporary encoding of information. During subsequent SWS, the amygdala, hippocampus, and parahippocampal areas acquire the detailed information that was previously represented only by an abridged catalogue; the transmission of additional associative information from the neocortex helps to eliminate maladaptive and unnecessary information (Crick and Mitchison 1983; Buzsáki 1989, 1996). By eliminating maladaptive and unnecessary information, the system creates a high signal to noise ratio for the consolidation of important information. This is an important step in the consolidation process. During P-wave-related states (tS–R, REM sleep), P-wave generating cells are activated to stimulate the amygdala, hippocampus, and parahippocampal areas to organize and consolidate the random information acquired during wakefulness (Datta 2000). Almost at the same time, theta-frequency waves help to transfer and bind that consolidated information into the long-term memory storage in the neocortex and other storage areas. The evidence presented in this chapter is part of a continually growing, larger body of evidence that will be necessary to definitively detail the mechanisms involved in this schematic representation of a model for sleep-dependent learning and memory. The knowledge that P-wave generating cells are capable of inducing synaptic plasticity is an important building block upon which further investigation can be based in the quest to elucidate the mechanisms of sleep-dependent learning and memory.

Acquisition

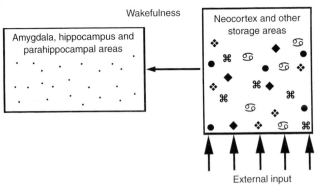

Pre-consolidation (Elimination of noise)

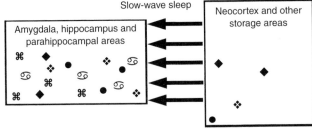

Consolidation and long-term storage

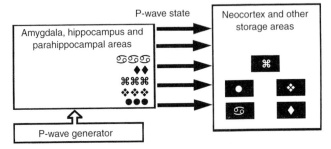

Figure 7.6 Model of sleep-dependent memory consolidation and long-term storage. During wakefulness, external information is randomly input into the brain and stored in the neocortex and other storage areas. This process is called acquisition of information. At the time of acquisition, a representational catalog of temporarily stored information is created in the amygdala, hippocampus, and parahippocampal areas. During slow wave sleep, the actual detailed information that had been temporarily stored in the neocortex and other storage areas is transferred to the amygdala, hippocampus, and parahippocampal areas. This is an important pre-consolidation phase. During this phase, some of the redundant information is eliminated to attenuate signal to noise ratio. During the P-wave-related sleep states (tS–R and REM sleep), activation of P-wave generating cells in the pons reactivates the amygdala, hippocampus, and parahippocampal areas to organize the random information acquired during wakefulness. This process is called consolidation of information. Once information is consolidated, it is ready to be stored in the permanent storage. Theta-frequency waves generated during REM sleep help to bind that consolidated information into the long-term memory storage in the neocortex and other storage areas. Symbols: five different types of external information (modified from Datta 1999).

Acknowledgments

This work was supported by National Institutes of Health (USA) Grants NS 34004 and MH 59839. The authors thank Soma M. Datta, Vijaya K. Mavanji, Donald F. Siwek, and Eric E. Spoley for their help.

References

Ambrosini, M. V., Sadile, A. G., Gironi-Carnevale, U. A., Mattiaccio, A., and Giuditta, A. (1988). The sequential hypothesis on sleep function. II. A correlative study between sleep variables and newly synthesized brain DNA. *Physiology and Behavior*, **43**, 339–350.

Baust, W., Holzbach, E., and Zechlin, O. (1972). Phasic changes in heart rate and respiration correlated with PGO-spike activity during REM sleep. *Pflugers Archiv*, **331**, 113–123.

Bliss, T. V. P. and Collingridge, G. L. (1993). A synaptic model of memory: long-term potentiation in the hippocampus. *Nature*, **361**, 31–39.

Bliss, T. V. P. and Gardner-Medwin, A. R. (1973). Long-lasting potentiation of synaptic transmission in the dentate area of the unanesthetized rabbit following stimulation of the perforant pathway. *Journal of Physiology (London)*, **232**, 357–374.

Bliss, T. V. P. and Lomo, T. (1973). Long-lasting potentiation of synaptic transmission in the dentate area of anaesthetized rabbit following stimulation of the perforant path. *Journal of Physiology (London)*, **232**, 331–356.

Bloch, V. and Laroche, S. (1981). Conditioning of hippocampal cells: It's acceleration and long-term facilitation by post-trial reticular stimulation. *Behavioral Brain Research*, **3**, 23–42.

Bloch, V. and Laroche, S. (1984). Facts and hypotheses related to the search for the engram. In *Neurobiology of learning and memory* (eds G. Lynch, J. L. McGaugh, and N. M. Weinberger), pp. 249–260. Guilford Press, New York.

Bloch, V. and Laroche, S. (1985). Enhancement of long-term potentiation in the rat dentate gyrus by post-trial stimulation of the reticular formation. *Journal of Physiology (London)*, **360**, 215–231.

Bloch, V., Hennevin, E., and Leconte, P. (1977). Interaction between post-trial reticular stimulation and subsequent paradoxical sleep in memory consolidation processes. In *Neurobiology of sleep and memory* (eds R. R. Drucker-Colin and J. L. McGaugh), pp. 255–272. Academic Press, New York.

Bowe-Anders, C., Adrien, J., and Roffwarg, H. P. (1974). Ontogenesis of ponto-geniculo-occipital activity in the lateral geniculate nucleus during deep sleep. *Experimental Neurology*, **43**, 242–260.

Bowker, R. M. and Morrison, A. R. (1976). The startle reflex and PGO spikes. *Brain Research*, **102**, 185–190.

Bowker, R. M. and Morrison, A. R. (1977). The PGO spikes: an indicator of hyper allertness. In *Sleep research* (eds W. P. Koella and P. Levin), pp. 23–77. Karger, Basel.

Bramham, C. R., Maho, C., and Laroche, S. (1994). Suppression of long-term potentiation induction during alert wakefulness but not during enhanced REM sleep after avoidance learning. *Neuroscience*, **59**, 501–509.

Brooks, D. C. and Bizzi, E. (1963). Brain stem electrical activity during deep sleep. *Archives Italiennes de Biologie*, **101**, 648–665.

Buzsáki, G. (1989). Two-stage model of memory trace formation: a role of "noisy" brain states. *Neuroscience*, **31**, 551–570.

Buzsáki, G. (1996). The hippocampo–neocortical dialogue. *Cerebral Cortex*, **6**, 81–92.

Crick, F. and Mitchison, G. (1983). The function of dream sleep. *Nature*, **304**, 111–114.

Datta, S. (1995). Neuronal activity in the peribrachial area: relationship to behavioral state control. *Neuroscience and Biobehavioral Reviews*, **19**, 67–84.

Datta, S. (1997). Cellular basis of pontine ponto-geniculo-occipital wave generation and modulation. *Cellular and Molecular Neurobiology*, **17**, 341–365.

Datta, S. (1999). PGO wave generation: mechanisms and functional significance. In *Rapid eye movement sleep* (eds B. N. Mallick and S. Inoue), pp. 91–106. Narosa Publishing House, New Delhi.

Datta, S. (2000). Avoidance task training potentiates phasic pontine-wave density in the rat: a mechanism for sleep-dependent plasticity. *Journal of Neuroscience*, **20**, 8607–8613.

Datta, S. and Hobson, J. A. (1994). Neuronal activity in the caudolateral peribrachial pons: relationship to PGO waves and rapid eye movements. *Journal of Neurophysiology*, **71**, 95–109.

Datta, S. and Hobson, J. A. (1995). Suppression of ponto-geniculo-occipital waves by neurotoxic lesions of pontine caudo-lateral peribrachial cells. *Neuroscience*, **67**, 703–712.

Datta, S. and Hobson, J. A. (2000). The rat as an experimental model for sleep neurophysiology. *Behavioral Neuroscience*, **114**, 1239–1244.

Datta, S., Calvo, J. M., Quattrochi, J. J., and Hobson, J. A. (1991). Long-term enhancement of REM sleep following cholinergic stimulation. *Neuroreport*, **2**, 619–622.

Datta, S., Calvo, J. M., Quattrochi, J. J., and Hobson, J. A. (1992). Cholinergic microstimulation of the peribrachial nucleus in the cat. I. Immediate and prolonged increases in ponto-geniculo-occipital waves. *Archives Italiennes de Biologie*, **130**, 263–284.

Datta, S., Patterson, E. H., and Siwek, D. F. (1999). Brainstem afferents of the cholinoceptive pontine wave generation sites in the rat. *Sleep Research Online*, **2**, 79–82.

Datta, S., Quattrochi, J. J., and Hobson, J. A. (1993). Effect of specific muscarinic M2 receptor antagonist on carbachol induced long-term REM sleep. *Sleep*, **16**, 8–14.

Datta, S., Siwek, D. F., Patterson, E. H., and Cipolloni, P. B. (1998). Localization of pontine PGO wave generation sites and their anatomical projections in the rat. *Synapse*, **30**, 409–423.

Datta, S., Spoley, E. E., and Patterson, E. H. (2001). Microinjection of glutamate into the pedunculopontine tegmentum induces REM sleep and wakefulness in the rat. *American Journal of Physiology*, **280**, R752–R759.

Davenne, D. and Adrien, J. (1984). Suppression of PGO waves in the kitten: anatomical effects on the lateral geniculate nucleus. *Neuroscience Letters*, **45**, 33–38.

DeKoninck, J., Lorrain, D., Christ, G., Proulx, G., and Coulombe, D. (1989). Intensive language learning and increases in REM sleep: evidence of a performance factor. *International Journal of Psychophysiology*, **8**, 43–47.

Dement, W., Ferguson, J., Cohen, H., and **Barchasa, J.** (1969). Nonchemical methods and data using a biochemical model: the REM quanta. In *Psychochemical research in man: Methods, strategy and theory* (eds A. J. Mandel and M. P. Mandel), pp. 275–325. Academic Press, New York.

Destrade, C. and **Cardo, B.** (1974). Effects of post-trial hippocampal stimulation on time-dependent improvement of performance in mice. *Brain Research*, **78**, 447–454.

Destrade, C., Soumireu-Mourat, B., and **Cardo, B.** (1973). Effects of post-trial hippocampal stimulation on acquisition of operant behavior in the mouse. *Behavioral Biology*, **8**, 713–724.

Devietti, T. L., Conger, G. L., and **Kirkpatrick, B. R.** (1977). Comparison of the enhancement gradients of retention obtained with stimulation of the mesencephalic reticular formation after training or memory reactivation. *Physiology and Behavior*, **19**, 549–554.

DeWeer, B. (1976). Selective facilitative effect of post-trial reticular stimulation in discriminative learning in the rat. *Behavioral Processes*, **1**, 243–257.

Diamond, D. M., Dunwiddie, T. V., and **Rose, G. M.** (1988). Characteristics of hippocampal primed burst potentiation *in vitro* and in the awake rat. *Journal of Neuroscience*, **8**, 4079–4088.

Duysan-Peyrethon, D., Peyrethon, J., and **Jouvet, M.** (1967). Etude quantitative des phenomenesphasiques du sommeil paradoxal pendent et apres sa deprivation instrumentale. *Comptes Rendus des Séances de la Société de Biologie et des Ses Filiales*, **161**, 2530–2533.

Empson, J. A. C. and **Clarke, P. R. F.** (1970). Rapid eye movements and remembering. *Nature*, **227**, 287–288.

Erickson, C. K. and **Patel, J. B.** (1969). Facilitation of avoidance learning by post-trial hippocampal electrical stimulation. *Journal of Comparative Physiology and Psychology*, **68**, 400–406.

Fishbein, W. (1971). Disruptive effects of rapid eye movement sleep deprivation on long-term memory. *Physiology and Behavior*, **6**, 279–282.

Fishbein, W., Kastaniotis, C., and **Chattman, D.** (1974). Paradoxical sleep: prolonged augmentation following learning. *Brain Research*, **79**, 61–75.

Foote, S. L. (1973). Compensatory changes in REM sleep time of cats during ad libitum sleep and following brief REM sleep deprivation. *Brain Research*, **54**, 261–276.

Giuditta, A., Ambrosini, M. V., Montagnese, P., Mandile, P., Cotugno, M., Grassi Zucconi, G., and **Vescia, S.** (1995). The sequential hypothesis of the function of sleep. *Behavioral Brain Research*, **69**, 157–166.

Hatfield, T., Han, J.-S., Conley, M., Gallagher, M., and **Holland, P.** (1996). Neurotoxic lesions of basolateral, but not central, amygdala interfere with pavlovian second-order conditioning and reinforcer devaluation effects. *Journal of Neuroscience*, **16**, 5256–5265.

Hennevin, E. and **Hars, B.** (1985). Post-learning paradoxical sleep: a critical period when new memory is reactivated. In *Brain plasticity, learning and memory* (eds B. E. Will and P. Schmitt, and J.-C. Dalrymple-Alford), *Advances in Behavioral Biology*, Vol. 28, pp. 193–203. Plenum Press, New York.

Hennevin, E., Hars, B., and **Bloch, V.** (1989). Improvement of learning by mesencephalic reticular stimulation during postlearning paradoxical sleep. *Behavior and Neural Biology*, **51**, 291–306.

Hennevin, E., Hars, B., Maho, C., and Bloch, V. (1995). Processing of learned information in paradoxical sleep: Relevance for memory. *Behavioral Brain Research*, **69**, 125–135.

Hennevin, E., Leconte, P., and Bloch, V. (1974). Augmentation du sommeil paradoxal provoquee par l'acquisition, l'extinction et la reacquisition d'un apprentissage a renforcement positif. *Brain Research*, **70**, 43–54.

Hennevin, E., Maho, C., Hars, B., and Dutrieux, G. (1993). Learning-induced plasticity in the medial geniculate nucleus is expressed during paradoxical sleep. *Behavioral Neuroscience*, **107**, 118–130.

Herman, J. H. and Roffwarg, H. P. (1983). Modifying oculomotor activity in awake subjects increases the amplitude of eye movements during REM sleep. *Science*, **220**, 1074–1076.

Hobson, J. A., Pace-Schott, E. F., and Stickgold, R. (2000). Dreaming and brain: toward a cognitive neuroscience of conscious states. *Behavioral and Brain Sciences*, **23**, 793–842.

Holscher, C., Anwyl, R., and Rowan, M. J. (1997). Stimulation on the positive phase of hippocampal theta rhythm induces long-term potentiation that can be depotentiated by stimulation on the negative phase in area CA1 *in vivo*. *Journal of Neuroscience*, **17**, 6470–6477.

Izquierdo, I., Fin, C., Schmitz, P. K., DaSilva, R. C., Jerusalinsky, D., Quillfeldt, J. A., Ferreira, M. B. G., Medina, J. H., and Bazan, N. G. (1995). Memory enhancement by intrahippocampal, intraamygdala, or intraentorhinal infusion of platelet-activating factor measured in an inhibitory avoidance task. *Proceedings of the National Academy of Sciences, USA*, **92**, 5047–5051.

Jouvet, M., Jeannerod, M., and Delorme, F. (1965). Organisation du systeme responsable de lactivite phasique au cours du sommeil paradoxal. *Comptes Rendus Séances de La Société de Biologie et de Ses Filiales*, **159**, 1599–1604.

Kahn, D. and Hobson, J. A. (1993). Self-organization theory of dreaming. *Dreaming*, **3**, 151–178.

Karni, A., Tanne, D., Rubenstein, B. S., Askenasy, J. J., and Sagi, D. (1994). Dependence on REM sleep of overnight improvement of a perceptual task. *Science*, **265**, 679–682.

Kudrimoti, H. S., Barnes, C. A., and McNaughton, B. L. (1999). Reactivation of hippocampal cell assemblies: effects of behavioral state, experience, and EEG dynamics. *Journal of Neuroscience*, **19**, 4090–4101.

Landfield, P. W., Tusa, R. J., and McGaugh, J. L. (1973). Effects of posttrial hippocampal stimulation memory storage and EEG activity. *Behavioral Biology*, **8**, 485–505.

Lapp, L. and Smith, C. (1986). The effects of one night's sleep loss on learning and memory in humans. *Sleep Research*, **15**, 73.

Leconte, P., Hennevin, E., and Bloch, V. (1974). Duration of paradoxical sleep necessary for the acquisition of conditioned avoidance in the rat. *Physiology and Behavior*, **13**, 675–681.

LeDoux, J. E. (1992). Emotion and the amygdala. In *The amygdala: Neurobiological aspects of emotion, memory, and mental dysfunction* (ed. J. Aggleton), pp. 339–351. Wiley-Liss, New York.

Lee, K. S. (1982). Sustained enhancement of evoked potentials following brief high-frequency electrical stimulation of the cerebral cortex *in vitro*. *Brain Research*, **239**, 617–623.

Lomo, T. (1966). Frequency potentiation of excitatory synaptic activity in the dentate area of the hippocampal formation. *Acta Physiologica Scandinavica*, **68** (Suppl. 277), 128.

Louie, K. and **Wilson, M. A.** (2001). Temporally structured replay of awake hippocampal ensemble activity during rapid eye movement sleep. *Neuron*, **29**, 145–156.

Lucero, M. (1970). Lengthening of REM sleep duration consecutive to learning in a rat. *Brain Research*, **20**, 319–322.

Maho, C., Hennevin, E., Hars, B., and **Poincheval, S.** (1991). Evocation in paradoxical sleep of a hippocampal conditioned cellular response acquired during waking. *Psychobiology*, **19**, 193–205.

Malcolm, L. J., Watson, J. A., and **Burke, W.** (1970). PGO waves as unitary events. *Brain Research*, **24**, 130–133.

Mallick, B. N. and **Inoue, S.** (1999). *Rapid eye movement sleep*. Narosa Publishing House, New Delhi.

Mandai, O., Guerrien, A., Sockeel, P., Dujardin, K., and **Leconte, P.** (1989). REM sleep modifications following a Morse code learning session in humans. *Physiology and Behavior*, **46**, 639–642.

Maquet, P. (2001). The role of sleep in learning and memory. *Science*, **294**, 1048–1052.

Marks, G. A., Farber, J., Rubinstein, M., and **Roffwarg, H. P.** (1980). Demonstration of ponto-geniculo-occipital waves in the albino rat. *Experimental Neurology*, **69**, 648–655.

McGrath, M. J. and **Cohen, D. B.** (1978). REM sleep facilitation of adaptive waking behavior: a review of the literature. *Psychological Bulletin*, **85**, 24–57.

McNaughton, B. L., Barnes, C. A., Baldwin, R. G., and **Rasmussen, M.** (1986). Long-term enhancement of hippocampal synaptic transmission and the acquisition of spatial information. *Journal of Neuroscience*, **6**, 563–571.

Morris, R. G. M. (1989). Synaptic plasticity and learning: selective impairment of learning in rats and blockade of long-term potentiation *in vivo* by the N-methyl-D-aspartate receptor agonist AP5. *Journal of Neuroscience*, **9**, 3040–3057.

Morris, R. G. M., Davis, S., and **Butcher, S. P.** (1990). Hippocampal synaptic plasticity and NMDA receptors: a role in information storage? *Philosophical Transactions of the Royal Society of London: Biological Sciences*, **329**, 187–204.

Morrison, A. R. and **Bowker, R. M.** (1975). The biological significance of PGO spikes in the sleeping cat. *Acta Neurobiologiae Experimentalis*, **35**, 821–840.

Orem, J. and **Barnes, C. D.** (1980). *Physiology in sleep*, Academic Press, New York.

Pavlides, C. and **Winson, J.** (1989). Influences of hippocampal place cell firing in the awake state on the activity of these cells during subsequent sleep episodes. *Journal of Neuroscience*, **9**, 2907–2918.

Pearlman, C. (1973). REM sleep deprivation impairs latent extinction in rats. *Physiology and Behavior*, **11**, 233–237.

Pearlman, C. and **Becker, M.** (1973). Brief Post-trial REM sleep deprivation impairs discrimination learning in rats. *Physiological Psychology*, **1**, 373–376.

Pirolli, A. and **Smith, C.** (1989). REM sleep deprivation in humans impairs learning of a complex task. *Sleep Research*, **18**, 375.

Plihal, W. and **Born, J.** (1997). Effects of early and late nocturnal sleep on declarative and procedural memory. *Journal of Cognitive Neuroscience*, **9**, 534–547.

Poremba, A. and **Gabriel, M.** (1997). Amygdalar lesions block discriminitive avoidance learning and cingulothalamic training-induced neuronal plasticity in rabbits. *Journal of Neuroscience*, **17**, 5237–5244.

Portell-Cortes, I., Marti-Nicolovius, M., Segura-Torres, P., and **Morgado-Bernal, I.** (1989). Correlation between paradoxical sleep and shuttlebox conditioning in rats. *Behavioral Neuroscience*, **103**, 984–990.

Qin, Y., McNaughton, B. L., Skaggs, W. E., and **Barnes, C. A.** (1997). Memory reprocessing in cortico-cortical and hippocampo-cortical neuronal ensembles. *Philosophical Transactions of the Royal Society of London: Biological Sciences*, **352**, 1525–1533.

Racine, R. J., Milgram, N. W., and **Hafner, S.** (1983). Long-term potentiation phenomena in rat limbic forebrain. *Brain Research*, **260**, 217–231.

Ramirez, O. A. and **Carrer, H. F.** (1989). Correlation between threshold to induce long-term potentiation in the hippocampus and performance in a shuttle box avoidance response in rats. *Neuroscience Letters*, **104**, 152–156.

Rempel-Clower, N. L., Zola, S. M., Squire, L. R., and **Amaral, D. G.** (1996). Three cases of enduring memory impairment after bilateral damage limited to the hippocampal formation. *Journal of Neuroscience*, **16**, 5233–5255.

Rose, G. M. and **Dunwiddie, T. V.** (1986). Induction of hippocampal long-term potentiation using physiologically patterned stimulation. *Neuroscience Letters*, **69**, 244–248.

Sakai, K. (1985). Anatomical and physiological basis of paradoxical sleep. In *Brain mechanisms of sleep* (eds D. McGinty, R. Drucker-Colin, A. Morrison, and L. Parmeggiani), pp. 111–137. Raven Press, New York.

Sanford, L. D., Ball, W. A., Morrison, A. R., and **Ross, R. J.** (1992*a*). Varying expression of alerting mechanisms in wakefulness and across sleep states. *Electroencephalography and Clinical Neurophysiology*, **83**, 458–468.

Sanford, L. D., Ball, W. A., Morrison, A. R., Ross, R. J., and **Mann, G. L.** (1992*b*). Peripheral and central components of alerting: habituation of acoustic startle, orienting responses and elicited waveforms. *Behavioral Neuroscience*, **106**, 112–120.

Sanford, L. D., Ball, W. A., Morrison, A. R., and **Ross, R. J.** (1993). The amplitude of elicited PGO waves: a correlate of orienting. *Electroencephalography and Clinical Neurophysiology*, **86**, 438–445.

Sanford, L. D., Tejani-Butt, S. M., Ross, R. J., and **Morrison, A. R.** (1995). Amygdaloid control of alerting and behavioral arousal in rats: involvement of serotonergic mechanisms. *Archives Italiennes de Biologie*, **134**, 81–99.

Sara, S. J., Deweer, B., and **Hars, B.** (1980). Reticular stimulation facilitates retrieval of a 'forgotten' maze habit. *Neuroscience Letters*, **18**, 211–217.

Shaffery, J. P., Roffwarg, H. P., Speciale, S. G., and **Marks, G. A.** (1999). Ponto-geniculo-occipital-wave suppression amplifies lateral geniculate nucleus cell-size changes in monocularly deprived kittens. *Developmental Brain Research*, **114**, 109–119.

Silva, A. J., Stevens, C. F., Tonegawa, S., and **Wang, Y.** (1992). Deficient hippocamal long-term potentiation in alpha-calcium-calmodulin kinase II mutant mice. *Science*, **257**, 201–206.

Skaggs, W. E. and **McNaughton, B. L.** (1996). Replay of neuronal firing sequences in rat hippocampus during sleep following spatial experience. *Science*, **271**, 1870–1873.

Smith, C. (1985). Sleep states and learning: a review of the animal literature. *Neuroscience and Biobehavioral Reviews*, **9**, 157–168.

Smith, C. (1995). Sleep states and memory processes. *Behavioral Brain Research*, **69**, 137–145.

Smith, C. and **Butler, S.** (1982). Paradoxical sleep at selective times following training is necessary for learning. *Physiology and Behavior*, **29**, 469–473.

Smith, C. and **Lapp, L.** (1991). Increases in number of REMS and REM sleep density in humans following an intensive learning period. *Sleep*, **14**, 325–330.

Smith, C. and **Pirolli, A.** (1989). Learning deficits following REM sleep deprivation of either the first two or the last two REM sleep periods of the night. *Sleep Research*, **18**, 377.

Smith, C. and **Rose, G. M.** (1997). Post-training paradoxical sleep in rats is increased after spatial learning in the Morris water maze. *Behavioral Neuroscience*, **111**, 1197–1204.

Smith, C. and **Weeden, K.** (1990). Post training REMs coincident auditory stimulation enhances memory in humans. *Psychiatric Journal of the University of Ottawa*, **15**, 85–90.

Smith, C. and **Whittaker, M.** (1987). Effects of total sleep deprivation in humans on the ability to solve a logic task. *Sleep Research*, **16**, 536.

Smith, C. and **Wong, P. T. P.** (1991). Paradoxical sleep increases predict successful learning in a complex operant task. *Behavioral Neuroscience*, **105**, 282–288.

Smith, C. and **Young, J.** (1980). Reversal of paradoxical sleep deprivation by amygdaloid stimulation during learning. *Physiology and Behavior*, **24**, 1035–1039.

Smith, C., Conway, J. M., and **Rose, G. M.** (1998). Brief paradoxical sleep deprivation impairs reference, but not working, memory in the Radial arm maze task. *Neurobiology of Learning and Memory*, **69**, 211–217.

Smith, C., Young, J., and **Young, W.** (1980). Prolonged increases in paradoxical sleep during and after avoidance task acquisition. *Sleep*, **3**, 67–81.

Squire, L. R., Amaral, D. G., and **Press, G. A.** (1990). Magnetic Resonance imaging of the hippocampal formation and mamillary nuclei distinguish medial temporal lobe diencephalic amnesia. *Journal of Neuroscience*, **10**, 3106–3117.

Staubli, U. and **Lynch, G.** (1987). Stable hippocampal long-term potentiation elicited by "theta" pattern stimulation. *Brain Research*, **435**, 227–234.

Stein, D. G. and **Chorover, S.** (1968). Effects of post-trial electrical stimulation of hippocampus and caudate nucleus on maze learning in the rat. *Physiology and Behavior*, **3**, 787–791.

Steriade, M. and **McCarley, R. W.** (1990). *Brainstem control of wakefulness and sleep.* Plenum Press, New York.

Stern, W. C., Forbes, W. B., and Morgane, P. J. (1974). Absence of ponto-geniculo-occipital (PGO) spikes in rats. *Physiology and Behavior*, **12**, 293–295.

Stickgold, R. (1998). Sleep: off-line memory reprocessing. *Trends in Cognitive Science*, **2**, 484–492.

Verschoor, G. J. and Holdstock, T. L. (1984). REM bursts and REM sleep following visual and auditory learning. *South African Journal of Psychology*, **14**, 69–74.

Vertes, R. P. (1984). Brainstem control of the events of REM sleep. *Progress in Neurobiology*, **22**, 241–288.

Wilson, M. A. and McNaughton, B. L. (1994). Reactivation of hippocampal ensemble memories during sleep. *Science*, **265**, 676–679.

Wolfowitz, B. E. and Holdstock, T. L. (1971). Paradoxical sleep deprivation and memory in rats. *Communications in Behavioral Biology*, **6**, 281–284.

Young, B., Otto, T., Fox, G. D., and Eichenbaum, H. (1997). Memory representation within the parahippocampal region. *Journal of Neuroscience*, **17**, 5183–5195.

CHAPTER 8

THE ROLE OF SLEEP IN MEMORY PROCESSING: THE SEQUENTIAL HYPOTHESIS

ANTONIO GIUDITTA, PAOLA MANDILE,
PAOLA MONTAGNESE, STEFANIA PISCOPO, AND
STEFANIA VESCIA

Introduction

It is common knowledge that slow wave sleep (SWS) was the first type of sleep to be described in human subjects by its high-amplitude, low-frequency electroencephalographic (EEG) waves, that sharply contrasted with the low-amplitude, high-frequency waves of active waking or wakefulness (W). Conversely, the later discovery of REM sleep was based on the occurrence of periodic episodes of rapid eye movements (REM) associated with a desynchronized EEG pattern resembling W. As this similarity envisaged an obvious paradox, REM sleep came to be also known as paradoxical sleep (PS). It is perhaps less well known that the discovery of PS elicited a remarkable wave of interest in its features that greatly contributed to highlight their relevance but, by contrast, outshadowed the role of SWS. The lesser attention paid to SWS is still reflected in its wide denomination as non-REM (NREM) sleep, underscoring REM sleep as the most important type of sleep.

Among the features of PS that contributed to its persisting popularity, one should include its heightened brain activity, the marked prevalence in the initial stages of brain development, and its alleged unique association with dreams (PS has also been called dream sleep) and with memory processing. Of the latter two features, the association with dreams is no longer deemed unique, as dreams have also been reported after SWS awakening (Cavallero *et al.* 1992; Nielsen 2000). Likewise, PS is not the only type of sleep involved in memory processing. As shown below and in other chapters of the book, SWS provides a primary contribution to this fundamental brain activity in laboratory animals (Giuditta 1977, 1985; Giuditta *et al.* 1995; Ambrosini and Giuditta 2001) and in human subjects (Ficca *et al.* 2000; Gais *et al.* 2000; Stickgold 2000*a*,*b*).

Almost a century ago, sleep was believed to promote memory retrieval by preventing the acquisition of additional inputs that would have impaired retention of previously acquired experiences (Jenkins and Dallenback 1924). More recently, such a "passive" hypothesis was replaced by the concept of an active involvement of sleep in memory events. The latter idea emerged approximately 30 years ago as a result of studies demonstrating a significant PS increment in learning rats (Lucero 1970; Leconte and Hennevin 1971). A large series of studies soon followed that confirmed and greatly extended the original data in laboratory animals (Greenberg and Pearlman 1974; Fishbein and Gutwein 1977; McGrath and Cohen 1978; Pearlman 1979; Smith 1985, 1995, 1996; Hennevin *et al.* 1995). The participation of PS in memory processing is now also well-established in humans (Gais *et al.* 2000; Maquet *et al.* 2000; Stickgold *et al.* 2000a,b; Smith 2001), except for a few dissenting opinions (Horne and McGrath 1984; Vertes and Eastman 2000). As data supporting the participation of PS in memory processing is discussed in separate chapters and have been repeatedly presented, the remaining body of the article will concern the evidence supporting the participation of SWS in memory processing, and the hypotheses concerning the roles of SWS and PS.

Theoretical considerations

In early years, when the selective involvement of PS in memory processing was proposed and actively investigated, we were impressed by several relevant features of sleep that included: (i) the strict interweaving of SWS and PS in the adult mammal, consistently requiring SWS to precede PS; (ii) the concomitant increment in SWS and PS in rats exposed to an enriched environment (reviewed in Smith 1985, 1996); (iii) the role of SWS in the retention deficit caused by PS deprivation (Rideout 1979); (iv) the higher energy flow in rat brain during a period of SWS that followed a period of active W, at variance with the decrease that followed a period of quiet W (Reich *et al.* 1972).

These considerations, and other thoughts, converged on the proposal that memory processing during sleep also involved the active and primary participation of SWS. Newly acquired memory traces were assumed to undergo a first processing step during SWS that allowed their further processing during PS. This proposal (the sequential hypothesis) was briefly mentioned in a review article by Giuditta *et al.* (1977) as "some of the initial steps in information processing occur during SWS and are required for the further processing that takes place during PS", and was more extensively presented later by Giuditta (1985). The evidence supporting the sequential hypothesis was recently reviewed (Giuditta *et al.* 1995; Ambrosini and Giuditta 2001).

But let us also mention the analogies that contributed to the formulation of the sequential hypothesis. One intriguing consideration regarded the essential roles played by food and information in allowing the organism's survival. In multicellular animals, food is sequentially processed in the intestinal tract and degraded to basic blocks eventually utilized for energy production and template-assisted syntheses; likewise, in the nervous system, experiential inputs are processed and reassembled into perceptions and knowledge.

Reasoning by analogy, it appeared reasonable that, as food undergoes sequential processing, experiential inputs might follow a comparable sequential course. We further reasoned that, as the role of the intestine may only be evaluated by providing food (gastric juice is not acidic during interprandial intervals), by analogy the role of sleep in brain information processing could only be evaluated by exposing the organism to novel experiences. Hence, in studies of the sleeping brain, due attention had to be paid to the previous waking experience, to compare the sleep effects of a familiar experience with those of novel, relevant experiences. This approach, already adopted in the study of PS, had to be extended to investigations of the whole structure of sleep.

An additional consideration concerned the dual capacity of homeostatic mechanisms to upregulate or downregulate biological variables, to oppose pressures otherwise displacing them beyond homeostatic boundaries. A suitable example was offered by the excretion of hypotonic or hypertonic urine by kidney, depending on the plasma osmotic pressure. Analogous to the operations performed by kidney on the massive inflow of glomerular filtrate, the massive inflow of experiences confronting the mammalian brain suggested that a dual capacity was at work to exert a homeostatic control on newly acquired memories. By discarding some while retaining others, the organism could adapt to changing circumstances.

As different mechanisms had to be responsible for memory clearance or retention, a number of reasons made us believe that SWS was better suited for clearing operations, while PS was more apt to implement retaining operations (see below). From a purely logical point of view, we were also convinced that it would be an advantage to have memory clearing occur first, before the retaining step. In turn, this logic offered independent support for the proposed role of SWS, in view of the systematic occurrence of SWS before PS starting from neonatal times, when waking experiences begin moulding brain circuitry (see below).

Two additional considerations supported our more specific proposal. One regarded the EEG features of SWS, PS, and active W. As it is well known, the latter two states are characterized by hippocampal theta waves, and neocortical higher frequency waves that reach towards the upper limit of the EEG frequency spectrum. On the other hand, during SWS and quiet W, sharp waves prevail in the hippocampus, and low-frequency waves invade the neocortex reaching the lower limit of the EEG frequency spectrum.

As memories are undoubtedly retained during active W, we reasoned that when a comparable need emerges during sleep, it would involve a state of sleep similar to active W, such as PS, rather than a state of sleep most different from active W, such as SWS. Conversely, as clearing operations are altogether different from those of memory retention, memory clearance was more likely to take place during SWS, as its features sharply contrasted with those of PS.

The second, perhaps more compelling consideration concerned the ontogenetic development of SWS, PS, and W (Giuditta 1977; Giuditta *et al.* 1984). As it is well known, active sleep is the ontogenetic precursor of PS that fills the day of the mature mammalian fetus, and markedly prevails during the first few months of postnatal life, to later undergo a progressive, substantial decrease in parallel with its differentiation into adult PS. On the other hand, at about the same postnatal times, SWS and W progressively gain longer shares of the day, become more differentiated, and SWS acquires its strategic position between W and PS. These substantial changes occur while the structuring of brain circuitry, initially modulated by innate instructions, becomes progressively more dependent on moulds generated by environmental experiences (see Chapter 10).

As innate instructions are clearly devoid of maladaptive contents to be cleared away, while memorized waking experiences include redundant, irrelevant, or erroneous contents that need clearing, active sleep presents itself as a physiological state favoring the retention of innate instructions into basic brain circuitry, while the strategic insertion of SWS between W and PS strongly suggests that the main role of SWS consists in clearing maladaptive contents from memorized waking inputs before the latter are allowed to mould brain circuits. It is of great interest that SWS was recently shown to mediate the down-regulation of synapses of the cat visual cortex following a period of monocular deprivation (Frank *et al.* 2001 and Chapter 10).

Experimental data

The sequential hypothesis has been largely tested using rats learning a two-way active avoidance task in a single session of massed training rather than in shorter sessions of daily training. The choice was prompted by our concurrent interest in the effect of sleep on brain DNA synthesized during training (Ambrosini *et al.* 1988*a,b*, 1992; Langella *et al.* 1992). This initial approach yielded supporting data, but later investigations were based on higher resolution methods of behavioral and EEG analysis.

In our early experiments, EEG records were analyzed with a time resolution that allowed the identification of SWS and PS, but was not sufficient to reveal the presence of transition sleep (TS), during which theta and alpha waves abruptly mixed with delta waves (see Box 8.1). In addition, trained rats were assigned to a fast learning (FL) group or to a non-learning (NL) group on the basis of a learning criterion attained in

Box 8.1 Transition sleep as compared to other sleep stages

During SWS, the rat keeps a typical posture, remaining immobile in a curled position, with eyelids closed, and head not fully relaxed. Breathing is calm and regular. Low-frequency, high-amplitude waves are prevalent in the EEG record, except for occasional periods of a few seconds during which spindlling occurs at higher frequency. Spectral density is maximal between 1 and 4 Hz and markedly declines at high frequencies.

Periods of TS generally follow SWS episodes. Behavioral features remain the same as during SWS but breathing becomes more frequent and irregular. The latter breathing pattern persists if TS is followed by PS, but quickly reverts to normal when TS is followed by W. The EEG trace shows the abrupt appearance of higher frequency waves (theta and alpha) that mix with the previously prevailing delta waves (see Fig. 8.1). The wave amplitude tends to decrease. The spectral density of TS episodes is high in a broad range (from delta to alpha), with a minor peak at 7 Hz.

Episodes of PS followed either SWS or TS. The sleep posture is maintained, but the head is fully relaxed and periodic twitches appear in the ears, vibrissae, and distal limbs. Breathing is frequent and irregular. The EEG trace displays homogeneous low-amplitude theta waves. Spectral analysis indicates the presence of a sharp peak at 7 Hz (from Mandile *et al.* 1996).

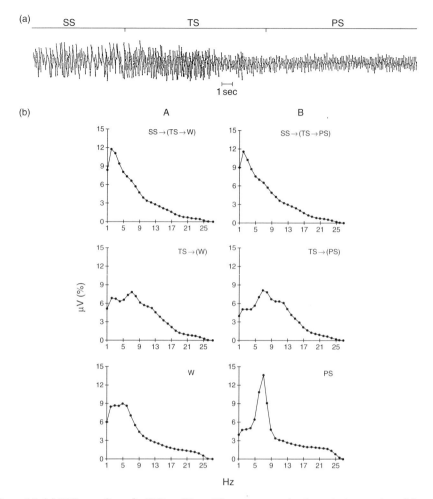

Figure 8.1 (a) EEG recording of a SWS → TS → PS sequence starting from the last portion of the initial SWS episode. (b) EEG power spectra of the components of SWS → TS → W and SWS → TS → PS sequences (left and right panels, respectively). SS or SWS, slow wave sleep (rearranged from Mandile *et al.* 1996).

the training session. On the other hand, in later experiments, TS was identified, and a consistent number of NL rats were found to attain the learning criterion in a retention session scheduled the day after training (slow learning or SL rats), while the remaining NL rats persisted in their failure to learn (persisting non-learning or NL* rats).

Recent data

Sleep sequences

To facilitate the presentation of our current views of memory processing during sleep, we will start with the more recent data and interpretations.

The identification of TS led to the identification of four sleep sequences that started with SWS and ended with W or PS, two of them including an intervening episode of TS. The sequences were labeled SWS → W, SWS → PS, SWS → TS → W, and SWS → TS → PS (Mandile *et al.* 1996 and Box 8.1). In our earlier experiments, we had identified only the former two sequences, each of which was still including the corresponding TS sequence.

Analysis of the sleep sequences occurring during a baseline session scheduled the day before training (Table 8.1(a)) indicated that the amount of SWS of the SWS → TS → W sequence and of SWS, TS, and PS of the SWS → TS → PS sequence were higher in FL rats than in SL and/or NL* rats. Conversely, the amounts of SWS of the SWS → W and SWS → PS sequences were essentially the same in all behavioral groups (Vescia *et al.* 1996). In addition, SWS and TS of the SWS → TS → W sequence correlated with the avoidances of the training session, while the components of the other sequences did not correlate (Table 8.1(b)). The correlative data were in good agreement with the intergroup differences concerning SWS → TS → W, SWS → W and SWS → PS sequences, but appeared at variance with regard to the components of the SWS → TS → PS sequence, as they did not correlate with avoidances despite their prevalence in FL rats (see later for an interpretation).

These results supported and clarified an earlier experiment in which the average duration of SWS episodes of baseline SWS → W sequences was found to be longer in FL rats than in NL rats, and to correlate with avoidances (Ambrosini *et al.* 1993). While these former observations indicated that the SWS component of the SWS → W sequences could be considered a reliable index of the capacity to learn, our later analyses allowed such a role to be more correctly attributed to the SWS component of the SWS → TS → W sequence.

Table 8.1 (a) Amounts of baseline SWS, TS, and PS in FL, SL, and NL* rats

Sleep sequence	Sleep component	FL	SL	NL*	
SWS → W	SWS	5047 ± 555	5721 ± 682	5233 ± 685	
SWS → PS	SWS	446 ± 129	456 ± 132	1021 ± 373	
SWS → TS → W	SWS	**3281 ± 375**	1630 ± 208	1788 ± 455	[§](SL),*(NL)
	TS	872 ± 81	783 ± 198	578 ± 130	
SWS → TS → PS	SWS	**1843 ± 238**	988 ± 238	1562 ± 454	*(SL)
	TS	**612 ± 121**	370 ± 106	333 ± 45	*(SL), [§](NL)
	PS	**2667 ± 179**	1958 ± 501	1967 ± 224	*(NL)

Results expressed in s (mean ± SEM). FL, SL, and NL*, fast learning, slow learning, and persisting non-learning rats. SWS, TS, and PS, slow wave, transition, and paradoxical sleep; W, waking. Significance of intergroup differences are shown in the last column with regard to the group in parenthesis and the group whose value appears in bold. Student *t* test for unpaired data.

Table 8.1 (b) Correlation coefficients between amounts of baseline SWS, TS, and PS and number of avoidances

Sleep sequence	Sleep component	Training period			
		1	2	3	4
SWS → W	SWS	0.216	0.001	−0.079	−0.157
SWS → PS	SWS	−0.118	−0.112	−0.078	−0.232
SWS → TS → W	SWS	&0.600	§0.740	§0.721	§0.713
	TS	*0.480	&0.581	0.421	0.412
SWS → TS → PS	SWS	0.264	0.435	0.382	0.345
	TS	0.094	0.464	0.316	0.329
	PS	0.106	0.404	0.286	0.279

Correlation coefficients calculated using the non-parametric Spearman's method.
*, $p < 0.05$; &, $p < 0.01$; §, $p < 0.005$. Rearranged from Vescia *et al.* 1996.

Analysis of the sleep sequences of the post-training rest period indicated that all components of the SWS → TS → PS sequence were markedly higher in FL rats than in SL rats, while the amounts of SWS episodes of the other sleep sequences did not differ among behavioral groups (Mandile *et al.* 2000). A longitudinal comparison of post-training sleep with baseline sleep showed that these differences were largely due to the training experience. In addition, avoidances inversely correlated with the amount of SWS of post-training SWS → W sequences, but did not correlate with the components of the SWS → TS → W or the SWS → TS → PS sequence.

Trains of sleep sequences

The selective association of TS sequences with the acquisition and processing of avoidance memories, confirmed in a recent experiment (Datta 2000), implied that TS, PS, or W did not follow SWS episodes at random, but presumably according to the outcome of processing operations they had performed. A similar consideration was accorded the W or PS state that followed TS episodes. This notion was actually implicit in the sequential hypothesis, in that memory processing was assumed to occur initially during SWS and subsequently during PS (Giuditta 1977, 1985).

Clearly, to account for the selective composition of sleep sequences, the putative forward influence of sleep episodes in selecting the appearance of the ensuing episodes could be envisaged to decay within minutes. By the same token, assuming that sleep sequences exerted a comparable forward influence, it was not unreasonable to envisage that the latter influence might last longer and progressively decay during W, thereby allowing long W periods to separate strings of sleep sequences (trains). To test this hypothesis, we plotted frequency histograms of durations of baseline W periods, and selected those of 1 min or longer as tentative delimiting units.

Using this criterion, several types of trains were identified in the baseline session and classified as homogeneous or mixed trains according to whether they included only one type of sleep sequence or more than one type (Piscopo *et al.* 2001a, see Box 8.2).

Box 8.2 The trains of sleep sequences

This box provides examples of trains of sleep sequences as well as quantitative data about the various trains and their constituent sequences and components. Figure 8.2 shows examples of trains of sleep sequences. The main properties of baseline trains are shown in Table 8.2.

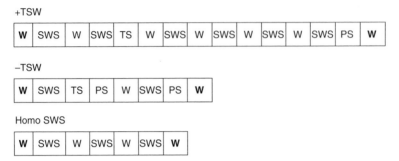

Figure 8.2 Examples of mixed +TSW trains, mixed −TSW trains, and homogeneous trains. +TSW, mixed train containing the SWS → TS → W sequence; −TSW, mixed train lacking the SWS → TS → W sequence; homo SWS, homogeneous train containing the SWS sequence. Mixed trains contain more than one type of sleep sequences, while homogeneous trains contain only one type of sleep sequence. W, waking epoch longer than 60 s; W, waking episode shorter than 60 s; SWS, slow wave sleep; TS, transition sleep; PS, paradoxical sleep (rearranged from Piscopo *et al.* 2001*a*).

Homogeneous trains turned out to be of four types, depending on the sleep sequence they included, while mixed trains were of two types differing from each other only in the presence or absence of the SWS → TS → W sequence (+TSW and −TSW trains, respectively). Homogeneous trains were relatively few and short, while +TSW trains were by far the most abundant, followed by −TSW trains.

Homogeneous and mixed trains were not homogeneously distributed among behavioral groups (Piscopo *et al.* 2001*b*). Notably, +TSW trains were most abundant in FL rats, but −TSW trains were most abundant in NL* rats (Table 8.3(a)). Furthermore, while in +TSW trains the amounts of TS sequences and of their SWS and PS components were higher in FL rats than in SL and/or NL* rats, in −TSW trains, the amounts of the SWS → TS → PS sequence and of its components were much more abundant in NL* rats. This led to the unexpected observation that the SWS → TS → PS sequence and its components were prevalent in FL rats when the sequence was included in +TSW trains, but were prevalent in NL* rats when it was included in −TSW trains. Conversely, in either mixed train, the amounts of SWS → W and SWS → PS sequences and of their components did not differ among behavioral groups.

These differences were in excellent agreement with the results of a correlative analysis between baseline train variables and number of avoidances of the training session (Table 8.2(b); Piscopo *et al.* 2001*b*). Indeed, the amounts of +TSW trains and of their TS sequences and components correlated with avoidances, while no correlations were

Table 8.2 Average values of baseline trains, and of their sleep sequences and components

Variable	Mixed trains		Homogeneous trains			
	+TSW	−TSW	SS(W)	SSTS(W)	SSTSPS	SSPS
Trains						
A	12881.7	1793.9	847.5	51.1	101.1	53.6
N	11.3	3.0	3.7	0.2	0.2	0.1
D	1271.5	462.0	256.0	51.1	101.1	53.6
Sleep sequences						
SS → (W)						
A	3777.5	637.8	668.6			
N	57.4	8.8	13.9			
D	70.0	61.5	56.6			
SS → TS → (W)						
A	2885.0			48.6		
N	28.6			0.3		
D	109.0			24.3		
SS → TS → PS						
A	3123.9	511.9			136.1	
N	17.9	2.6			0.4	
D	186.5	119.1			60.0	
SS → PS						
A	1016.9	387.5				51.1
N	8.9	2.6				0.2
D	155.8	101.9				25.6
Sleep components						
SS → (W)						
A	3777.5	637.8	668.6			
N	57.4	8.8	13.9			
D	70.0	61.4	56.5			
SS → (TS → W)						
A	2159.2			40.8		
N	25.5			0.3		
D	88.8			20.4		
SS → (TS → PS)						
A	1108.6	210.3			60.6	
N	16.6	2.6			0.4	
D	71.1	50.3			21.4	
SS → (PS)						
A	436.7	171.1				30.3
N	8.9	2.6				0.2
D	77.1	44.7				15.1

Table 8.2 *Continued*

Variable	Mixed trains		Homogeneous trains			
	+TSW	−TSW	SS(W)	SSTS(W)	SSTSPS	SSPS
(SS) → TS → (W)						
A	725.8			7.8		
N	28.6			0.3		
D	25.9			3.9		
(SS) → TS → (PS)						
A	304.4	50.3			7.8	
N	17.4	2.6			0.6	
D	17.5	12.2			2.9	
(SS → TS) → PS						
A	1710.8	250.8			67.8	
N	17.4	2.6			0.6	
D	100.1	56.5			27.9	
(SS) → PS						
A	579.7	216.4				20.8
N	8.9	2.6				0.2
D	78.4	56.7				10.4

+TSW and −TSW, mixed trains containing or lacking the SWS → TS → W sequence; SS(W), SSTS(W), SSTSPS, and SSPS, homogeneous trains only containing the SS → (W), SS → TS → (W), SS → TS → PS, and SS → PS sequence, respectively. Components identifying a sleep sequence but excluded from calculations are shown within brackets. *A*, total amount; *N*, number; and *D*, average duration of trains, sleep sequences, or components of sleep sequences SS or SWS, slow wave sleep.

In the baseline session the total amount of +TSW trains was significantly greater in FL rats than in NL rats, while the total amount of −TSW trains was significantly grater in NL rats than in SL rats. In addition, the SSTS(W) train was only present in FL rats, the SSTSPS train was only present in SL and NL rats, and the SSPS train was only present in NL rats. The SS(W) train was present in all groups (from Piscopo *et al.* 2001*b*).

present with −TSW trains and with the SWS → TS → PS sequence and components they included. Rather, all correlation coefficients were negative.

The average duration of +TSW trains markedly decreased in the post-training period of FL rats, but markedly increased in SL and NL* rats. In addition, the amount of SWS of the SWS → TS → PS sequence of +TSW trains selectively increased in FL rats, while the amount of SWS of the SWS → PS sequence selectively increased in NL* rats (Piscopo *et al.* unpublished).

Apparent discrepancies

On the whole, the sleep data suggested that SWS → TS → W and SWS → TS → PS sequences were processing memories of the novel avoidance response, respectively by implementing the initial processing step and the last processing step. On the other hand, SWS → W and SWS → PS sequences appeared involved in processing innate behavioral responses (escapes or freezings). Nonetheless, this tentative interpretation was not in

Table 8.3 (a) Amounts of mixed trains, and of their SWS → TS → PS sequences and components in the baseline session of FL, SL, and NL* rats

Train	Sleep sequence	Sleep component	FL	SL	NL*	
+TSW			**15238 ± 1211**	13116 ± 1326	10291 ± 1627	°(NL)
	SWS → TS → PS		**4438 ± 363**	2731 ± 690	2157 ± 284	°(SL), §(NL)
		SWS	**1693 ± 270**	813 ± 178	819 ± 142	*(SL, NL)
		PS	**2375 ± 201**	1618 ± 445	1139 ± 163	§(NL)
−TSW			1590 ± 787	825 ± 467	**3063 ± 628**	*(SL)
	SWS → TS → PS		359 ± 209	122 ± 91	**1052 ± 294**	&(SL)
		SWS	122 ± 76	49 ± 31	**459 ± 208**	*(SL)
		TS	42 ± 24	13 ± 9	**95 ± 20**	&(SL)
		PS	194 ± 128	60 ± 55	**498 ± 108**	&(SL)

Results expressed in s (mean ± SEM). FL, SL, and NL, fast learning, slow learning, and persistently non-learning rats. SWS, TS, and PS, slow wave, transition, and paradoxical sleep. Significance of intergroup differences are shown in the last column with regard to the group in parenthesis and the group whose value appears in bold. Student t test for unpaired data.

Table 8.3 (b) Correlation coefficients between baseline amounts of mixed trains and of their SWS → TS → PS sequences and components, and number of avoidances

Train	Sleep sequence	Sleep component	Training period			
			1	2	3	4
+TSW			*0.631	&0.723	°0.469	0.324
	SWS → TS → PS		0.302	§0.706	°0.547	*0.628
		SWS	0.003	&0.644	°0.547	*0.576
		TS	0.267	°0.555	0.024	0.297
		PS	0.238	&0.635	0.032	°0.551
−TSW			−0.332	−0.434	−0.356	°−0.534
	SWS → TS → PS		−0.349	−0.413	−0.246	−0.459
		SWS	−0.386	−0.391	−0.254	−0.438
		TS	−0.333	−0.378	−0.249	−0.434
		PS	−0.323	−0.389	−0.222	−0.436

Correlation coefficients calculated with the non-parametric Spearman's method. +TSW and −TSW, mixed trains with or without the SWS → TS → W sequence. °, $p < 0.1$; *, $p < 0.05$; &, $p < 0.01$; §, $p < 0.005$. Rearranged from Piscopo *et al.* 2001.

agreement with the following observations: (i) the lack of increment in the amount of SWS of the SWS → TS → W sequence in the post-training period of FL rats. Such an increment was expected, and its absence was all the more surprising when compared to the post-training increase in the amount of SWS of the SWS → TS → PS sequence; (ii) the lack of correlations between avoidances and components of the post-training

SWS → TS → W sequence; and (iii) the lack of correlations between avoidances and components of either the baseline or the post-training SWS → TS → PS sequence.

With regard to the first observation, the marked prevalence of SWS episodes in the baseline SWS → TS → W sequence of FL rats (Table 8.1(a); Vescia *et al.* 1996) suggested that the initial processing of avoidance memories could be implemented without further increment of this variable. While this possibility could not be excluded, it did not appear to account for the second observation (ii). Furthermore, an alternative, more intriguing explanation emerged from a comparison of the waking EEG power spectra of behaving rats with baseline waking spectra (Giuditta *et al.* 1995; Ambrosini and Giuditta 2001; Mandile *et al.* in press). In comparison with baseline, power spectra of FL rats recorded during training showed a selective increase in the delta region already in the first half of the first training period, when avoidances were still few, and a more conspicuous and significant increase in the second half of the same period, when avoidances markedly increased. Delta shift and increment in avoidances were completely lacking in SL and NL* rats. Hence, the improved performance of FL rats appeared to be causally related to the delta shift.

As the delta shift reflected an increase in amplitude/density of delta waves, it was considered the waking counterpart of an increment in the SWS component of the SWS → TS → W sequence, rather than of the SWS → W sequence, as only the former sequence was associated with the capacity to learn the avoidance task. Hence, we concluded that the post-training increment of this variable in FL rats had not occurred because a vicarious increment had already occurred during training. This explanation also accounted for the lack of correlations between avoidances and post-training SWS → TS → W sequences.

An altogether different explanation could be offered for the lack of correlations between avoidances and baseline or post-training SWS → TS → PS sequences. The main argument rested on the presence of this sequence in either mixed train, that is also in the −TSW train that did not include SWS → TS → W sequences (Piscopo *et al.* 2001*a*). As avoidance processing was assumed to start with the latter sequence, the SWS → TS → PS sequence of −TSW trains could not promote the subsequent processing step. Indeed, as mentioned above, variables of baseline SWS → TS → PS sequences prevailed in FL rats and correlated with avoidances when the SWS → TS → PS sequence was in +TSW trains, but prevailed in NL rats and did not show correlations when the same sequence was in −TSW trains (Piscopo *et al.* 2001*b*).

As correlative analyses between avoidances and SWS → TS → PS sequences (baseline or post-training) were performed irrespective of the sequence inclusion in +TSW or −TSW trains, the lack of correlations was likely to be due to the contrasting role played by the SWS → TS → PS sequence in +TSW and −TSW trains.

Earlier data

Before describing our earlier data, it might be of help to recall that, at that time, the only two sleep sequences we had identified (SWS → W and SWS → PS) were still including the corresponding TS sequences. Furthermore, the group of NL rats was still including SL rats.

What we initially found was that, in comparison with control rats, SWS episodes of the post-training SWS → W sequence were longer in FL and NL rats, but the effect prevailed in NL rats. On the other hand, the average duration and the amount of SWS episodes of the SWS → PS sequence displayed an early and persistent increase in FL rats, while the increase was delayed and shorter in NL rats. Increments in PS number and amount were only observed in FL rats (Ambrosini *et al.* 1988*a*, 1992). In addition, in comparison with baseline, the amount of SWS of the post-training SWS → W sequence increased in all rat groups, while the amount of SWS of the SWS → PS sequence only increased in FL rats (Ambrosini *et al.* 1992). Furthermore, in FL rats, avoidances inversely correlated with SWS episodes of the post-training SWS → W sequence, but directly correlated with SWS and PS of the SWS → PS sequence. Avoidances also correlated with the average duration of SWS episodes of the SWS → W sequence. Conversely, no correlations were present in NL rats (Langella *et al.* 1992).

On the whole, training appeared to have markedly modified post-training SWS (not only PS) in a selective way in the two rat groups (see Box 8.2). Processing of avoidance memories appeared responsible for most modifications of post-training SWS and PS in FL rats, while processing of memories of innate responses appeared responsible for most differences of post-training SWS in NL rats.

However, before this interpretation could be accepted, contingent effects such as sleep deprivation or stress, had to be excluded as possible factors of post-training sleep changes. This conclusion was reached on the basis of the following evidence: (i) the pattern of post-training sleep and the correlations with avoidances markedly differed between FL and NL rats, despite the fact that NL rats had experienced the same amount of sleep deprivation, and had received a higher number of footshocks eliciting more stress (Ambrosini 1988*a*, 1992); (ii) in a group of old rats exposed to the same training protocol but displaying only freezing responses, post-training SWS was not modified; yet, their sleep deprivation was the same as FL rats and their stress was markedly greater (Ambrosini *et al.* 1997); and (iii) in adult rats trained for a spatial habituation task in a training session lasting 10 min and not involving footshocks, the pattern of post-training SWS modifications was comparable to that of FL rats, despite the fact that their sleep deprivation and stress were minimal (Montagnese *et al.* 1993).

As a result, data were interpreted to indicate that SWS episodes were involved in processing, but that their processing operations were different in the two sleep sequences. As suggested in our paper (Langella *et al.* 1992): "adaptive behavioral responses favor the appearance of fewer SWS → W episodes of longer duration, and of more numerous SWS → PS and PS episodes of longer duration. Conversely, nonadaptive responses may favor the appearance of more numerous SWS → W episodes of somewhat longer duration." Hence, we proposed that "non adaptive memory traces may be destabilized during SWS → W episodes, and eventually cleared from the brain. On the other hand, adaptive memory traces may be destabilized during [the SWS segment of] SWS → PS episodes, to be stored again in more suitable form (better integrated with preexisting memory traces) during the ensuing PS episode" (Langella *et al.* 1992).

Newly synthesized brain DNA

In addition to behavior and sleep data, the above interpretation was in agreement with the results of a correlative analysis between post-training SWS and PS and radiolabeled brain DNA (DNA*). In this experiment, an intraventricular injection of [^{3}H]thymidine just before training allowed brain DNA* to be synthesized during training but not in the ensuing post-training period (Giuditta *et al.* 1985; Ambrosini *et al.* 1988a,b). This expectation was validated by the vanishing content of brain [^{3}H]thymidine triphosphate (the direct DNA precursor) at the end of the training session, at a time the content of brain DNA* was essentially the same in FL and NL rats (Scaroni *et al.* 1983; Giuditta *et al.* 1985).

Correlations between brain DNA* and post-training sleep were essentially lacking in control rats but were present in FL and NL rats, although with altogether different patterns (Table 8.4). In NL rats, correlations with SWS or PS of the SWS → PS sequence were numerous, rather robust, and of negative sign, while they were fewer and of positive sign with SWS of the SWS → W sequence. On the other hand, in FL rats, the few correlations with SWS of the SWS → PS sequence were of positive sign, and the correlations with SWS of the SWS → W sequence were of negative sign (Ambrosini *et al.* 1988b).

Furthermore, when FL and NL rats were separated in two subgroups using as a threshold the average amount of baseline PS, the content of brain DNA* was found to be essentially the same in the two FL subgroups, and in the NL subgroup showing less post-training PS than the average baseline value, but to be markedly lower (about one half) in the NL subgroup showing more post-training PS (Giuditta *et al.* 1985). As further synthesis of brain DNA* could not occur in the post-training period due to the lack of radiolabeled precursor, the data were interpreted to indicate that, in NL rats, a considerable amount of brain DNA* selectively disappeared during SWS → PS sequences.

Our interest in the fate of brain DNA* during sleep was elicited by evidence that its synthesis was modulated by training (Perrone Capano *et al.* 1982; Scaroni *et al.* 1983; Giuditta *et al.* 1986a; for reviews, see Giuditta 1983; Giuditta *et al.* 1986b). Upon the premise that synthesis of brain DNA was closely associated with the formation of memory traces, and would follow their fate, the destabilization/elimination of nonadaptive memories was assumed to also involve the loss of associated DNA* (Giuditta *et al.* 1985; Ambrosini *et al.* 1988b; Langella *et al.* 1992). Accordingly, the decrease of brain DNA* selectively occurring in NL rats in correlation with post-training SWS → PS sequences appeared in agreement with the proposed destabilizing role of SWS. The metabolic instability of brain DNA is further supported by additional independent data (Chun *et al.* 1991; Abeliovich *et al.* 1992). It is also in agreement with the observation that the expression of immediate early genes in brain is strongly activated during W, but drastically reduced during SWS (Grassi Zucconi *et al.* 1994; Cirelli and Tononi 2000a,b).

Table 8.4 Correlation coefficients between brain DNA* and amount of post-training SWS and PS

Rat group	Sleep sequence	Sleep component	Brain region	Post-training hours			
				1	2	3	1 → 3
FL	SWS → W	SWS	CC	−0.205	−0.064	* − 0.601	−0.191
			HP	−0.211	−0.055	−0.309	−0.145
			CB	−0.167	−0.059	* − 0.562	−0.161
			BS	−0.174	0.178	* − 0.574	−0.114
	SWS → PS	SWS	CC	0.033	0.361	§0.709	0.228
			HP	−0.112	0.416	0.391	0.109
			CB	0.063	0.311	**0.658	0.213
			BS	−0.012	0.001	0.442	−0.073
		PS	CC	−0.141	−0.128	−0.206	−0.174
			HP	−0.266	0.077	−0.362	0.018
			CB	−0.098	−0.151	−0.207	−0.225
			BS	−0.129	−0.321	−0.051	−0.341
NL	SWS → W	SWS	CC	0.167	0.182	−0.001	0.183
			HP	−0.043	0.156	0.111	0.162
			CB	*0.331	0.258	0.239	**0.391
			BS	*0.362	0.129	0.146	0.309
	SWS → PS	SWS	CC	−0.102	−0.273	−0.205	* − 0.348
			HP	−0.306	−0.127	& − 0.457	* − 0.381
			CB	* − 0.337	* − 0.339	§ − 0.542	§ − 0.614
			BS	* − 0.385	−0.205	§ − 0.537	§ − 0.554
		PS	CC	−0.121	& − 0.481	−0.181	** − 0.413
			HP	* − 0.353	** − 0.394	−0.298	& − 0.457
			CB	−0.327	§ − 0.603	** − 0.434	§ − 0.655
			BS	* − 0.365	§ − 0.578	§ − 0.511	§ − 0.682

Correlation coefficients calculated with the non-parametric Spearman method. DNA*, [^{3}H]DNA; FL, and NL rats, fast learning and non-learning rats. SWS and PS, slow wave and paradoxical sleep; W, waking, CC, cerebral cortex; HP, hippocampus; CB, cerebellum; BS, brainstem. *, $p < 0.05$; **, $p < 0.02$; &, $p < 0.01$; §, $p < 0.005$. Rearranged from Langella *et al.* 1992.

Reminiscent rats

We have already mentioned that, when NL rats were tested the day after training, one subgroup maintained a low level of avoidances (persistently non-learning, or NL* rats), while the remaining rats markedly improved their performance (SL rats; Ambrosini *et al.* 1995). This delayed, spontaneous improvement of performance, also called reminiscence, was known to be associated with a post-training increment in PS in the mouse BALB/c strain, and to be abolished by post-training PS deprivation (Destrade *et al.* 1978; Kitahama *et al.* 1981).

In our first experiment with NL* and SL rats, the reminiscence phenomenon was found to be also associated with modifications of post-training SWS (Ambrosini *et al.*

1995). In fact, in SL rats, SWS episodes of the SWS → W and SWS → PS sequences underwent a selective lengthening in the third hour of the post-training period, the amount of SWS increased in the fifth and sixth post-training hour, and the amount of PS increased in the sixth hour. These differences emerged from a comparison with home caged rats, and with the baseline values of SL rats.

As post-training sleep was not modified in NL* rats, despite their exposure to the same training session, the modifications of post-training sleep in SL rats were interpreted to reflect memory processing rather than training contingencies. Indeed, the variations displayed by SL rats reproduced the same pattern of sleep changes observed in FL rats, although they occurred with considerable delays, presumably due to the need to first dissipate their more intense stress. In addition, as the PS increment occurred with a greater delay than the SWS modifications, the SL sleep data confirmed that SWS was involved in memory processing before PS.

Additional data

In sleeping rats, hippocampal place cells active during a previous waking experience were shown to selectively resume their activity during SWS or PS (Pavlides and Winson 1989). These pioneering observations were confirmed and extended by analyses of hippocampal and entorhinal neurons using multiple neuronal recordings. In the latter studies, the spatio-temporal sequence of neuronal activation during waking was found to be replayed during posttrial SWS (Wilson and McNaughton 1994; Skaggs and McNaughton 1996; Kudrimoti et al. 1999; Nádasdy et al. 1999; Sutherland and McNaughton 2000; Hirase et al. 2001).

As better detailed in other chapters of this volume, memory processing in human subjects has been recently reported to require the dual involvement of SWS and PS, respectively occurring in the initial portion and in the last portion of the night (Gais et al. 2000; Stickgold et al. 2000a,b, 2001). These observations are in agreement with an additional study emphasizing the role of sleep cycles in human memory processing (Ficca et al. 2000).

On the whole, the above data add strong independent support to the participation of SWS in memory processing, and confirm the validity of the sequential hypothesis.

Alternative views

To provide a conceptual framework to what will be discussed in this section, it may not be irrelevant to recall that information flows from the neocortex to the hippocampus via the superficial layers of the entorhinal cortex, and flows back to the neocortex via the deep layers of the entorhinal cortex. This bidirectional traffic occurs in association with EEG waveforms of different vigilance states, that is, the hippocampal inflow with theta waves of active W or PS; the outflow with hippocampal sharp waves of quiet W or SWS. During the latter phase, synaptic connections are strengthened (Chrobak and Buzsáki 1994; Nádasdy et al. 1999; Chrobak et al. 2000), thus supporting the proposal that memories are potentiated during their hippocampal journey (Buzsáki 1989, 1998).

This suggestion is in apparent contrast with our view that SWS promotes synaptic down-regulation and memory clearing (Giuditta *et al.* 1995; Ambrosini and Giuditta 2001). However, memory consolidation during SWS may not occur outside the hippocampus (Buzsáki 1998; Steriade 2000; but see Sejnowski and Destexhe 2000 for a different view), in agreement with the observation that the expression of immediate early genes in brain is strongly activated during W, but drastically reduced during SWS (Grassi Zucconi *et al.* 1994; Cirelli and Tononi 2000*a,b*).

A plausible reconciliation of these two views might emerge from the assumption that synaptic strengthening during hippocampal sharp waves (Buzsáki 1998) only concerns the components of waking experiences to be retained. Such a selective potentiation might protect their neocortical representation from the presumably indiscriminate down-regulation exerted by delta waves on recently formed connections. As a result, non-protected features of the same experience or of competing memories would be selectively depressed, thereby increasing the relevance of the protected memory items. Interestingly, the neocortical expression of immediate early genes may not be completely abolished by SWS (Grassi Zucconi *et al.* 1994; Cirelli and Tononi 2000*a,b*). This suggested mechanism might start "on line" during active W, as in FL rats, and continue "off line" during sleep but with variable delays, as in SL rats.

An alternative view has also been expressed with regard to the role of PS, assumed to favor the elimination of non adaptive or irrelevant memories (Crick and Mitchison 1995). However, this hypothesis was proposed on the basis of theoretical considerations and analogies between brain and computer operations, and does not seem to have received experimental verification. Rather, it stands in sharp contrast with an extensive literature supporting the role of PS in memory formation and maintenance (Hennevin *et al.* 1995; Smith 1996, 2001). Nonetheless, the extensive remodeling of brain circuits that presumably allows the integration of novel memories with pre-existing memories during PS is likely to require the weakening of some synaptic connections, as also suggested by recent data (Poe *et al.* 2000), while largely promoting the potentiation/formation of additional connections (see below).

Conclusions

Studies with laboratory animals performed during the last 30 years have shown that memories are processed during sleep, presumably to enhance their relevant features and clear redundant or competing items, and to eventually integrate the resulting memories within existing brain circuits. These two main steps are presumed to occur initially during SWS and eventually during PS, in agreement with the sequential hypothesis (Giuditta 1977, 1985). Recent animal and human studies further support the validity of this hypothesis.

We have recently proposed (Ambrosini and Giuditta 2001) that synaptic connections involved in memory acquisition during W might be alternatively downregulated or upregulated during SWS or PS, irrespective of their substantially different roles. Thus, the prevailing capacity of SWS to depress recently formed connections related to irrelevant or nonadaptive aspects of waking experiences, while strengthening salient features, would reduce memories to their essential core, thereby increasing their signal to noise ratio. This view is in agreement with the ontogenetic pattern of SWS development.

Likewise, the integration of memory cores in the complex network of brain circuits, assumed to occur during PS, is also likely to require alternative weakening or strengthening of different sets of synaptic connections. We have proposed that this dual mechanism might be based on a down-regulation of newly formed connections, thereby allowing their renewed differential modulation by contingent influences (Hennevin *et al.* 1995). In view of the key role of brain noradrenergic and serotoninergic systems in waking consolidation, their substantial silence during PS might contribute to synaptic down-regulation. Interestingly, a process of memory labilization and subsequent reconsolidation has been recently reported for fear memories retrieved during W (Nader *et al.* 2000).

From a theoretical point of view, it is not surprising that the process of memory integration is fulfilled by PS, as integration allows waking stimuli to gain wider and easier access to memories, and PS resembles waking in most although not all features (Winson 1993). Support for this role of PS also derives from the observations that: (i) in human subjects, several brain regions active during a learning session undergo reactivation during PS (Maquet *et al.* 2000) and (ii) in rats exposed to an EE, brain immediate early genes are induced during PS (Ribeiro *et al.* 1999).

Clearly, the relevant role of sleep in memory processing does not imply that this activity only occurs during sleep. Besides our suggestion that EEG power spectra of behaving rats reflect on line processing of the acquired experience (Giuditta *et al.* 1995; Ambrosini *et al.* 2001; Mandile *et al.* in press), memory clearing and retention are widely accepted as normal occurrences during W. As a result, if these two complementing functions are assumed to be selectively associated with the different EEG waveforms of SWS or PS, how can we rationalize the notion that they simultaneously occur during W, PS, or SWS?

A plausible explanation is offered by an extension of the mosaic hypothesis of sleep to all vigilance states (Krueger *et al.* 1995; Nielsen 2000). Accordingly, states of SWS, PS, or W should not be viewed as including the entire set of neuronal circuits, but only a fraction of them, albeit sufficiently large to allow the correct classification of vigilance states. A well-known, extreme example regards the alternation of SWS in either brain hemisphere of dolphins, while the other hemisphere is kept awake. Hence, it may not be unreasonable that when we are awake, some brain circuits are asleep (either in SWS or PS), and conversely, that when we are asleep (either in SWS or PS), some brain circuits may be awake or in the other sleep state. In other words, local transgressions are possible and may actually be required to account for local processing needs.

References

Abeliovich, A., *et al.* (1992). On somatic recombination in the central nervous system of transgenic mice. *Science*, **257**, 404–410.

Ambrosini, M. V., *et al.* (1988*a*). The sequential hypothesis on sleep function. I. Evidence that the structure of sleep depends on the nature of previous waking experience. *Physiology and Behavior*, **43**, 325–337.

Ambrosini, M. V., *et al.* (1988*b*). The sequential hypothesis on sleep function. II. A correlative study between sleep variables and newly synthesized brain DNA. *Physiology and Behavior*, **43**, 339–350.

Ambrosini, M. V., *et al.* (1992). The sequential hypothesis of sleep function. III. The structure of postacquisition sleep in learning and non-learning rats. *Physiology and Behavior*, **51**, 217–226.

Ambrosini, M. V., *et al.* (1993). The structure of sleep is related to the learning ability of rats. *European Journal of Neuroscience*, **5**, 269–275.

Ambrosini, M. V., *et al.* (1995). The sequential hypothesis of sleep function. V. Lenghtening of post-trial SWS episodes in reminiscent rats. *Physiology and Behavior*, **58**, 1043–1049.

Ambrosini, M. V., *et al.* (1997). Post-trial sleep in old rats trained for a two-way active avoidance task. *Physiology and Behavior*, **62**, 773–778.

Ambrosini, M. V. and **Giuditta, A.** (2001). Learning and sleep: the sequential hypothesis. *Sleep Medicine Reviews*, **5**, 477–490.

Buzsáki, G. (1989). Two-stage model of memory trace formation: a role for "noisy" brain states. *Neuroscience*, **31**, 551–570.

Buzsáki, G. (1998). Memory consolidation during sleep: a neurophysiological perspective. *Journal of Sleep Research*, **7**, 17–23.

Cavallero, C., *et al.* (1992). Slow wave sleep dreaming. *Sleep* **15**, 562–566.

Chrobak, J. J. and **Buzsáki, G.** (1994). Selective activation of deep layer (V–VI) retrohippocampal cortical neurons during hippocampal sharp waves in the behaving rat. *Journal of Neuroscience*, **14**, 6160–6170.

Chrobak, J. J., *et al.* (2000). Physiological patterns in the hippocampo-entorhinal cortex system. *Hippocampus*, **10**, 457–465.

Chun, J. J., *et al.* (1991). The recombination activating gene-1 (RAG-1) transcript is present in the murine central nervous system. *Cell*, **64**, 189–200.

Cirelli, C. and **Tononi, G.** (2000*a*). On the functional significance of c-fos induction during the sleep–waking cycle. *Sleep*, **23**, 453–469.

Cirelli, C. and **Tononi, G.** (2000*b*). Differential expression of plasticity-related genes in waking and sleep and their regulation by the noradrenergic system. *Journal of Neuroscience*, **20**, 9187–9194.

Crick, F. and **Mitchison, G.** (1995). REM sleep and neural nets. *Behavioural Brain Research*, **69**, 147–155.

Datta, S. (2000). Avoidance task training potentiates phasic pontine-wave density in the rat: a mechanism for sleep-dependent plasticity. *Journal of Neuroscience*, **20**, 8607–8613.

Destrade, C., *et al.* (1978). Relationships between paradoxical sleep and time-dependent improvement of performance in BALB/c mice. *Neuroscience Letters*, **7**, 239–244.

Ficca, G., *et al.* (2000). Morning recall of verbal material depends on prior sleep organization. *Behavioural Brain Research*, **112**, 159–163.

Fishbein, W. and Gutwein, B. M. (1977). Paradoxical sleep and memory storage processes. *Behavioral Biology*, **19**, 425–464.

Frank, M. G., *et al.* (2001). Sleep enhances plasticity in the developing visual cortex. *Neuron*, **30**, 275–287.

Gais, S., *et al.* (2000). Early sleep triggers memory for early visual discrimination skills. *Nature Neuroscience*, **3**, 1335–1339.

Giuditta, A. (1977). The biochemistry of sleep. In *Biochemical correlates of brain structure and function* (ed. A. N. Davidson), pp. 293–337. Academic Press, New York.

Giuditta, A. (1983). Role of DNA in brain activity. In *Handbook of neurochemistry* (ed. A. Lajtha), pp. 251–276. Plenum Press, New York.

Giuditta, A. (1985). A sequential hypothesis for the function of sleep: In *Sleep '84* (eds W. P. Koella *et al.*), pp. 222–224. Fischer Verlag, Stuttgart.

Giuditta, A., *et al.* (1984). The neurochemical study of sleep: In *Handbook of neurochemistry* (ed. A. Lajtha), Vol. 8, 2nd edn, pp. 443–476. Plenum Press, New York.

Giuditta, A., *et al.* (1985). Effect of sleep on cerebral DNA synthesized during shuttle-box avoidance training. *Physiology and Behavior*, **34**, 769–778.

Giuditta, A., *et al.* (1986a). Synthesis of rat brain DNA during acquisition of an appetitive task. *Pharmacology, Biochemistry and Behavior*, **25**, 651–658.

Giuditta, A., *et al.* (1986b). *Role of RNA and DNA in brain function: A molecular biological approach*, p. 320. Martinus Nijhoff, Boston.

Giuditta, A., *et al.* (1995). The sequential hypothesis of the function of sleep. *Behavioural Brain Research*, **69**, 157–166.

Grassi Zucconi, G., *et al.* (1994). c-fos spontaneous expression during wakefulness is reversed during sleep in neuronal subsets of the rat cortex. *Journal of Physiology (Paris)*, **88**, 91–93.

Greenberg, R. and Pearlman, C. (1974). Cutting the REM sleep nerve: an approach to the adaptive function of REM sleep. *Perspectives in Biology and Medicine*, **17**, 513–521.

Hennevin, E., *et al.* (1995). Processing of learned information in paradoxical sleep: relevance for memory. *Behavioural Brain Research*, **69**, 125–135.

Hirase, H., *et al.* (2001). Firing rates of hippocampal neurons are preserved during subsequent sleep episodes and modified by novel awake experience. *Proceedings of the National Academy of Sciences, USA*, **98**, 9386–9390.

Horne, J. A. and McGrath, M. J. (1984). The consolidation hypothesis for REM sleep function: stress, SWS and other confounding factors—a review. *Biological Psychology*, **18**, 165–184.

Jenkins, J. and Dallenbach, K. (1924). Obliviscence during sleep and waking. *American Journal of Psychology*, **35**, 605–612.

Kitahama, K., *et al.* (1981). Paradoxical sleep deprivation and performance of an active avoidance task: impairment in C57BR mice and no effect in C57BL/6 mice. *Physiology and Behavior*, **27**, 41–50.

Kudrimoti, H. S., *et al.* (1999). Reactivation of hippocampal cell assemblies: effects of behavioral state, experience, and EEG dynamics. *Journal of Neuroscience*, **19**, 4090–4101.

Krueger, J. M., *et al.* (1995) Brain organization and sleep function. *Behavioural Brain Research*, **69**, 177–185.

Langella, M., *et al.* (1992). The sequential hypothesis of sleep function. IV. A correlative analysis among behavioral, biochemical and sleep variables in learning and non learning rats. *Physiology and Behavior*, **51**, 227–238.

Leconte, P. and **Hennevin, E.** (1971). Augmentation de la durée de sommeil paradoxal consécutif à un apprentissage chez le Rat. *Comptes Rendues de l' Académie de Sciences (Paris)*, **273**, 86–88.

Lucero, M. (1970). Lengthening of REM sleep duration consecutive to learning in the rat. *Brain Research*, **20**, 319–322.

Mandile, P., *et al.* (1996). Characterization of transition sleep episodes in baseline EEG recordings of adult rats. *Physiology and Behavior*, **60**, 1435–1439.

Mandile, P., *et al.* (2000). Post-trial sleep sequences including transition sleep are involved in avoidance learning of adult rats. *Behavioural Brain Research*, **112**, 23–31.

Maquet, P., *et al.* (2000). Experience-dependent changes in cerebral activation during human REM sleep. *Nature Neuroscience*, **3**, 831–836.

McGrath, M. J. and **Cohen, D. B.** (1978). REM sleep facilitation of adaptive waking behavior: a review of the literature. *Psychological Bulletin*, **85**, 24–57.

Montagnese, P., *et al.* (1993). Long-term habituation to spatial novelty modifies post-trial synchronized sleep followed by paradoxical sleep in rats. *Brain Research Bulletin*, **32**, 503–508.

Nádasdy, Z., *et al.* (1999). Replay and time compression of recurring spike sequences in the hippocampus. *Journal of Neuroscience*, **19**, 9497–9507.

Nader, K., *et al.* (2000). Fear memories require protein synthesis in the amygdala for reconsolidation after retrieval. *Nature*, **406**, 722–726.

Nielsen, T. A. (2000). A review of mentation in REM sleep and NREM sleep: "covert" REM sleep as a possible reconciliation of two opposing models. *Behavioral Brain Science*, **23**, 851–866.

Pavlides, C. and **Winson, J.** (1989). Influences of hippocampal place cell firing in the awake state on the activity of these cells during subsequent sleep episodes. *Journal of Neuroscience*, **9**, 2907–2918.

Pearlman, C. A. (1979). REM sleep and information processing: evidence from animal studies. *Neuroscience Biobehavioral Reviews*, **3**, 57–68.

Perrone Capano, C., *et al.* (1982). DNA turnover in rat cerebral cortex. *Journal of Neurochemistry*, **38**, 52–56.

Piscopo, S., *et al.* (2001*a*). Identification of trains of sleep sequences in adult rats. *Behavioural Brain Research*, **119**, 93–101.

Piscopo, S., *et al.* (2001*b*). Trains of sleep sequences are indices of learning capacity in rats. *Behavioural Brain Research*, **120**, 13–21.

Poe, G. R., *et al.* (2000). Experience-dependent phase-reversal of hippocampal neuron firing during REM sleep. *Brain Research*, **855**, 176–180.

Reich, P., *et al.* (1972). Metabolism of brain during sleep and wakefulness. *Journal of Neurochemistry*, **19**, 487–497.

Ribeiro, S., *et al.* (1999). Brain gene expression during REM sleep depends on prior waking experience. *Learning and Memory*, **6**, 500–508.

Rideout, B. E. (1979). Non-REM sleep as a source of learning deficits induced by REM sleep deprivation. *Physiology and Behavior*, **22**, 1043–1047.

Scaroni, R., *et al.* (1983) Synthesis of brain DNA during acquisition of an active avoidance task. *Physiology and Behavior*, **30**, 577–582.

Sejnowski, T. J. and Destexhe, A. (2000). Why do we sleep? *Brain Research*, **886**, 208–223.

Skaggs, W. E. and McNaughton, B. (1996). Replay of neuronal firing sequences in rat hippocampus during sleep following spatial experience. *Science*, **271**, 1870–1873.

Smith, C. (1985). Sleep states and learning: a review of the animal literature. *Neuroscience Biobehavioral Reviews*, **9**, 157–168.

Smith, C. (1995). Sleep states and memory processes. *Behavioural Brain Research*, **69**, 137–145.

Smith, C. (1996). Sleep states, memory processes and synaptic plasticity. *Behavioural Brain Research*, **78**, 49–56.

Smith, C. (2001). Sleep states and memory processes in humans: procedural versus declarative memory processes. *Sleep Medicine Reviews*, **5**, 491–506.

Steriade, M. (2000). Corticothalamic resonance, states of vigilance and mentation. *Neuroscience*, **101**, 243–276.

Stickgold, R., *et al.* (2000*a*). Visual discrimination learning requires sleep after training. *Nature Neuroscience*, **3**, 1237–1238.

Stickgold, R., *et al.* (2000*b*). Visual discrimination task improvement: a multi-step process occurring during sleep. *Journal of Cognitive Neuroscience*, **12**, 246–254.

Stickgold, R., *et al.* (2001). Sleep, learning, and dreams: off-line memory reprocessing. *Science*, **294**, 1052–1057.

Sutherland, G. R. and McNaughton, B. (2000). Memory trace reactivation in hippocampal and neocortical neuronal ensembles. *Current Opinions in Neurobiology*, **10**, 180–186.

Vertes, R. P. and Eastman, K. E. (2000). The case against memory consolidation in REM sleep. *Behavioral Brain Science*, **23**, 867–876.

Vescia, S., *et al.* (1996). Baseline transition sleep and associated sleep episodes are related to the learning ability of rats. *Physiology and Behavior*, **60**, 1513–1525.

Wilson, M. A. and McNaughton, B. (1994). Reactivation of hippocampal ensemble memories during sleep. *Science*, **265**, 676–679.

Winson, J. (1993). The biology and function of rapid eye movement sleep. *Current Opinions in Neurobiology*, **3**, 243–248.

SLEEP AND NEURAL DEVELOPMENT

The chapters of this section are concerned with the early neural development of the brain and its relationship to sleep states. It has long been noted that there are large amounts of sleep observed in the young. It has been speculated that sleep must be important for rapid brain growth and synaptic plasticity. Yet, proof for this idea has been elusive. While it might rank as extremely important, this research area has not involved a large number of scientists. Hopefully this book, and especially these chapters, will stimulate some new research activity. Majid Mirmiran has been studying in this area for many years at the Netherlands Institute for Brain Research. He and Ronald Ariagno (Stanford University) review the area and suggest useful approaches to studies in the very young. The existing data suggest that REM sleep deprivation (REMD) in infants may retard brain growth and synaptic plasticity. They review past findings and provide an interesting hypothesis about the possible role of REMD in the development of depression as well.

Marcos Frank and Michael Stryker (University of California at San Francisco) provide a developmental assessment of the role of sleep in the central visual pathways. They begin with a description of the visual system and the role of endogenous neural activity as well as that of external stimulation and experience. This is followed by an analysis of the role of sleep in the development and synaptic plasticity of central visual pathways. They evaluate the ontogenetic hypothesis that REM sleep alone provides an important source of endogenous neural activity for brain growth and synaptic plasticity. They conclude that both SWS and REM sleep probably play important, but probably different roles in the development of normal adult vision. They also have pointed out the pitfalls of some techniques and suggest fruitful directions for future research in this area.

CHAPTER 9

ROLE OF REM SLEEP IN BRAIN DEVELOPMENT AND PLASTICITY

MAJID MIRMIRAN AND RONALD L. ARIAGNO

Fetal and neonatal Rapid Eye Movement (REM) sleep

Rapid Eye Movement (REM) sleep occupies a large proportion of time during early brain development (Roffwarg *et al.* 1966). It serves a unique function in early life, namely to promote brain maturation. In an altricial mammal, such as the rat, the high amount of REM sleep declines to a low level during the first month of life. In the precocial mammal such as guinea pig, on the other hand, prenatally high levels of REM sleep are observed that decline to low (adult) values at birth. In both species as the rapid period of brain maturation is completed, the amount of REM sleep declines to a low adult level (Jouvet-Mounier *et al.* 1970). At birth, human newborns spend 16–18 h a day asleep, more than half of this is occupied by REM sleep (Anders *et al.* 1995). Both prenatal recording in the fetuses and postnatal studies in preterm infants showed a large proportion of time spent in REM sleep between 30 and 40 week postconceptional age (Mulder *et al.* 1987; Mirmiran 1995; Mirmiran *et al.* in press). The decline in REM sleep as a function of brain development is much slower in the human and does not reach low levels till preschool years period (Roffwarg *et al.* 1966; Anders *et al.* 1995). The time course of REM sleep development in human like other mammals corresponds well with the period of brain maturation.

   The high level of endogenous neuronal activation during REM sleep makes this state a good milieu for promoting brain development during a period in which environmental experiences are very limited (Roffwarg *et al.* 1966). It is not only the amount but also the intensity of phasic neuronal activity during REM sleep which is high in early development and diminishes as rapid brain maturation is completed (Mirmiran and Corner 1982; Mirmiran 1995). Eye movements during REM sleep are good indicator of phasic neuronal activity in the brain. We have studied the development of eye movements during REM sleep in rats from 10–25 days of age. At approximately 15–18 days there is a peak in the mean frequency of eye movements, burst density, burst duration and the mean number of eye movements within the burst. Since rat pups reared in constant dark showed similar increase in eye movements, this change seems to be part of an endogenous developmental timetable of REM sleep which is necessary for brain maturation rather than an association with an increase in visual stimuli (Van Someren *et al.* 1990). Similar developmental changes in eye movement density during REM sleep are also found *in utero* in the human between 30 and 40 week postconceptional age (Birnholz 1981; Inoue *et al.* 1986).

REM sleep and brain development

Although correlation studies indicating a relationship between REM sleep and the degree of brain maturation are interesting in their own right, the most straightforward experimental approach to study the function of REM sleep in brain development is to deprive as selectively as possible the rapidly developing mammal of its normal quota of REM sleep. Accordingly, the consequences of this deprivation on later brain function in adulthood can be elucidated. Since long-term instrumental deprivation or lesion studies are not feasible, we and other investigators have used a pharmacological approach (Mirmiran *et al.* 1981, 1983; Hilakivi 1987; Hilakivi *et al.* 1987; Vogel *et al.* 1990*a,b,c*). We have suppressed REM sleep during the second and third weeks of postnatal development in rats using an antidepressant drug such as clomipramine or an antihypertensive drug like clonidine. In adulthood, the neonatally REM sleep-deprived animals showed increased anxiety, reduced sexual activity and disturbed sleep (Mirmiran *et al.* 1981, 1983; Mirmiran 1986; De Boer *et al.* 1989). Other investigators found similar results which included despair behavior, reduced pleasure seeking and increased alcohol preference using clomipramine or other antidepressants in rats (Hilakivi *et al.* 1984; Hilakivi 1987; Hilakivi and Hilakivi 1987; Neill *et al.* 1990; Vogel *et al.* 2000). Subsequent regional brain measurements showed a significant reduction in the size of the cerebral cortex and brainstem in adult rats who were REM sleep-deprived during neonatal development. In addition, a proportional reduction of tissue protein was found in the affected brain areas (Mirmiran *et al.* 1983). We have pursued these structural changes at the functional level and found changes in the neurotransmitter circuitry of neonatally REM sleep-deprived animals. In the cerebral cortex the magnitude of the gamma-amino-butyric-acidergic (GABAergic) depression of the glutamate-induced single cortical neurons responses was greater in the neonatally REM sleep-deprived rats (Mirmiran *et al.* 1988, 1990). In the hippocampus there was a supersensitivity of the pyramidal cells to noradrenaline (Gorter *et al.* 1990). Based on these results we hypothesized that during the homeostatic adaptation of receptor sensitivity to a persistent change in the intensity of incoming neuronal stimulation, individual neurons have established "set-points," which were determined by the amount of synaptic activation in early development, most probably during REM sleep (Mirmiran *et al.* 1988).

REM sleep and brain plasticity

Environmental enrichment in rats has been shown to increase the size of the cerebral cortex, the number and efficacy of synapses and the problem-solving ability of the animal (Will *et al.* 1977; Juraska *et al.* 1980). When our neonatally REM sleep-deprived rats were subjected to an standard or an enriched environment (EE) after weaning, no significant plasticity effect was found (Mirmiran *et al.* 1983). The kindling phenomenon in rats has been used to assess hippocampal plasticity. In this model kindling causes a prolonged decrease in latency and an increase in sensitivity for epileptogenesis by electrical stimulation in the hippocampus. Neonatal REM sleep deprivation induced an increase in latency from the end of the kindling stimulation to the initiation of the epileptic activity (i.e. after discharge latency). Additionally, there was a reduced excitability ratio in these neonatally REM sleep-deprived kindled rats compared with the kindled controls (Gorter *et al.* 1991).

Ponto-geniculo-occipital (PGO) waves are endogenous phasic activity in the visual system characteristics of REM sleep. Monocular deprivation reduces the size of the lateral geniculate nucleus (LGN) contralateral to the deprived eye only during a critical period of brain development. Bilateral lesion of the brainstem generator of PGO waves in kittens has been shown to amplify the brain plasticity induced by monocular deprivation (Davenne and Adrien 1987; Marks *et al.* 1995; Shaffery *et al.* 1999). Selective suppression of REM sleep by manually keeping the kittens awake during the critical period of development induced similar results (Oksenberg *et al.* 1996). Amplification of plasticity induced by monocular deprivation with concomitant sleep deprivation has recently been demonstrated at the single cell level (Frank *et al.* 2001). Taken together, these results indicate that neonatal REM sleep deprivation not only impairs brain development but it also prevents further plasticity of the brain in adulthood.

REM sleep and depression

Neonatal suppression of REM sleep induced several long-lasting behavioral changes reviewed above. Vogel hypothesized that these behavioral changes can be interpreted as symptoms of endogenous depression (Vogel *et al.* 1990*a*). He and his group carried out a number of studies to support this hypothesis (Neill *et al.* 1990; Vogel *et al.* 1990*b*, 2000). First of all they found reduced shock-induced aggression and enhanced defensive responses in adult rats neonatally treated with clomipramine. Second, sexual activity in these neonatally REM sleep-deprived males showed fewer mountings, intromissions, ejaculations, and longer mount latencies and postejaculatory pauses. Third, in an open-field activity test these rats showed increased activity mainly in the outer part of the chamber, indicating a motor restlessness associated with the fear or stress of an open, exposed environment. Fourth, in an experimental pleasure-seeking behavior paradigm (hypothalamic self-stimulation), neonatally REM sleep-deprived rats showed reduced pleasure seeking. Fifth, these rats also showed increased voluntary alcohol consumption and despair behavior (Hilakivi *et al.* 1984; Hilakivi 1987; Hilakivi and Hilakivi 1987). Sixth, sleep studies showed reduced REM sleep latency, frequent sleep onset REM sleep and an abnormal temporal course of REM sleep rebound after REM sleep deprivation in adult rats neonatally treated with an antidepressant drug. Last, administration of antidepressant drugs to these animals in adulthood ameliorate several of these behavioral consequences of neonatal REM sleep deprivation. These findings suggest that neonatal REM sleep deprivation induces adult depression.

Concluding remarks

Although one may still argue that more selective methods for REM sleep deprivation during early development must be developed before a firm conclusion could be made of its function, the experimental evidence so far suggests that neonatal REM sleep plays an important role in brain growth, connectivity, and synaptic plasticity. For the sake of space and lack of experimental data, we have limited this chapter to the role of REM sleep. However, we do not want to exclude any role sleep as a whole may play in brain development/plasticity. Given the new data concerning the role of sleep in memory formation (Maquet 2000; Maquet *et al.* 2000; Smith 1995; Shaggs and McNaughton 1996; Stickgold *et al.* 2000; Wilson and McNaughton 1994), it would be very interesting to examine learning and memory processes in fetal/neonatally REM sleep-deprived animals. If the results show similar findings as above, this may have important public health implications. For example, depressed mothers continue to use antidepressants during pregnancy and lactation. Antihypertensive drugs such as clonidine are used during pregnancy. These drugs can suppress fetal and neonatal REM sleep. Furthermore, infants born prematurely suffer from sleep disturbances during a long stay in the Neonatal Intensive Care Unit (NICU). Many behavioral and physiological consequences in adulthood in these individuals may simply be explained by suppression of REM sleep in early life. We can only hope that the importance of these findings for clinical practice will be recognized and that appropriate clinical intervention will be developed, thereby the neurobehavioral outcome of human preterm newborn infants may be improved in the future.

References

Anders, T., Sadeh, A., and Appareddy, V. (1995). Normal sleep in neonates and children. In *Principles and practice of sleep medicine in the child* (eds R. Ferber and M. H. Kryger), pp. 7–18. Saunders, Philadelphia.

Birnholz, J. C. (1981). The development of human fetal eye movement patterns. *Science*, **213**, 679–681.

Davenne, D. and Adrien, J. (1987). Lesion of the ponto-geniculo-occipital pathways in kittens. I. Effects on sleep and on unitary discharge of the lateral geniculate nucleus. *Brain Research*, **409**, 1–9.

De Boer, S., Mirmiran, M., Van Haaren, F., Louwerse, A., and van de Poll, N. E. (1989). Neurobehavioral teratogenic effects of clomipramine and alpha-methyldopa. *Neurotoxicology and Teratology*, **11**, 77–84.

Frank, M. G., Issa, N. P., and Stryker, M. P. (2001). Sleep enhances plasticity in the developing visual cortex. *Neuron*, **30**, 275–287.

Gorter, J. A., Kamphuis, W., Huisman, E., Bos, N. P., and Mirmiran, M. (1990). Neonatal clonidine treatment results in long-lasting changes in noradrenaline sensitivity and kindling epileptogenesis. *Brain Research*, **535**, 62–66.

Gorter, J. A., Veerman, M., Mirmiran, M., Bos, N. P., and Corner, M. A. (1991). Spectral analysis of the electroencephalogram in neonatal rats chronically treated with the NMDA antagonist MK-801. *Brain Research, Developmental Brain Research*, **64**, 37–41.

Hilakivi, L. (1987). Adult alcohol consumption after pharmacological intervention in neonatal sleep. *Acta Physiologica Scandanavica Supplementum*, **562**, 1–58.

Hilakivi, L. A. and Hilakivi, I. (1987). Increased adult behavioral "despair" in rats neonatally exposed to desipramine or zimeldine: an animal model of depression? *Pharmacology Biochemistry and Behavior*, **28**, 367–369.

Hilakivi, L. A., Hilakivi, I., and Kiianmaa, K. (1987). Neonatal antidepressant administration suppresses concurrent active (REM sleep) sleep and increases adult alcohol consumption in rats. *Alcohol*, (Suppl.1), 339–343.

Hilakivi, L. A., Sinclair, J. D., and Hilakivi, I. T. (1984). Effects of neonatal treatment with clomipramine on adult ethanol related behavior in the rat. *Brain Research*, **317**, 129–132.

Inoue, M., Koyanagi, T., Nakahara, H., Hara, K., Hori, E., and Nakano, H. (1986). Functional development of human eye movement in utero assessed quantitatively with real-time ultrasound. *American Journal of Obstetrics and Gynecology*, **155**, 170–174.

Jouvet-Mounier, D., Astic, L., and Lacote, D. (1970). Ontogenesis of the states of sleep in rat, cat, and guinea pig during the first postnatal month. *Developmental Psychobiology*, **2**, 216–239.

Juraska, J. M., Greenough, W. T., Elliott, C., Mack, K. J., and Berkowitz, R. (1980). Plasticity in adult rat visual cortex: an examination of several cell populations after differential rearing. *Behavioral Neural Biology*, **29**, 157–167.

Maquet, P. (2000). Functional neuroimaging of normal human sleep by positron emission tomography. *Journal of Sleep Research*, **9**, 207–231.

Maquet, P., Laureys, S., Peigneux, P., Fuchs, S., Petiau, C., Phillips, C., Aerts, J., Del Fiore, G., Degueldre, C., Meulemans, T., Luxen, A., Franck, G., Van Der Linden, M., Smith, C., and Cleeremans, A. (2000). Experience-dependent changes in cerebral activation during human REM sleep. *Nature Neuroscience*, **3**, 831–836.

Marks, G. A., Shaffery, J. P., Oksenberg, A., Speciale, S. G., and Roffwarg, H. P. (1995). A functional role for REM sleep in brain maturation. *Behavioral Brain Research*, **69**, 1–11.

Mirmiran, M. (1986). The importance of fetal/neonatal REM sleep. *European Journal of Obstetrics Gynecology and Reproductive Biology*, **21**, 283–291.

Mirmiran, M. (1995). The function of fetal/neonatal rapid eye movement sleep. *Behavioural Brain Research*, **69**, 13–22.

Mirmiran, M. and Corner, M. (1982). Neuronal discharge patterns in the occipital cortex of developing rats during active and quiet sleep. *Brain Research*, **255**, 37–48.

Mirmiran, M., Dijcks, F. A., Bos, N. P., Gorter, J. A., and Van der Werf, D. (1990). Cortical neuron sensitivity to neurotransmitters following neonatal noradrenaline depletion. *International Journal of Developmental Neuroscience*, **8**, 217–221.

Mirmiran, M., Feenstra, M. G., Dijcks, F. A., Bos, N. P., and Van Haaren, F. (1988). Functional deprivation of noradrenaline neurotransmission: effects of clonidine on brain development. *Progress in Brain Research*, **73**, 159–172.

Mirmiran, M., Maas, Y., and Ariagno, R. Development of fetal and neonatal sleep and circadian rhythms. *Sleep Medicine Reviews*, in press.

Mirmiran, M., Scholtens, J., van de Poll, N. E., Uylings, H. B., van der Gugten, J., and Boer, G. J. (1983). Effects of experimental suppression of active (REM sleep) sleep during early development upon adult brain and behavior in the rat. *Brain Research*, **283**, 277–286.

Mirmiran, M., van de Poll, N. E., Corner, M. A., van Oyen, H. G., and Bour, H. L. (1981). Suppression of active sleep by chronic treatment with chlorimipramine during early postnatal development: effects upon adult sleep and behavior in the rat. *Brain Research*, **204**, 129–146.

Mulder, E. J., Visser, G. H., Bekedam, D. J., and Prechtl, H. F. (1987). Emergence of behavioural states in fetuses of type-1-diabetic women. *Early Human Development*, **15**, 231–251.

Neill, D., Vogel, G., Hagler, M., Kors, D., and Hennessey, A. (1990). Diminished sexual activity in a new animal model of endogenous depression. *Neuroscience and Biobehavioral Reviews*, **14**, 73–76.

Oksenberg, A., Shaffery, J. P., Marks, G. A., Speciale, S. G., Mihailoff, G., and Roffwarg, H. P. (1996). Rapid eye movement sleep deprivation in kittens amplifies LGN cell-size disparity induced by monocular deprivation. *Brain Research, Developmental Brain Research*, **97**, 51–61.

Roffwarg, H. P., Muzio, J. N., and Dement, W. C. (1966). Ontogenetic development of the human sleep–dream cycle. *Science*, **152**, 604–619.

Shaffery, J. P., Roffwarg, H. P., Speciale, S. G., and Marks, G. A. (1999). Ponto-geniculo-occipital-wave suppression amplifies lateral geniculate nucleus cell-size changes in monocularly deprived kittens. *Brain Research, Developmental Brain Research*, **114**, 109–119.

Skaggs, W. E. and McNaughton, B. L. (1996). Replay of neuronal firing sequences in rat hippocampus during sleep following spatial experience. *Science*, **271**, 1870–1873.

Smith, C. (1995). Sleep states and memory processes. *Behavioural Brain Research*, **69**, 137–145.

Stickgold, R., James, L., and Hobson, J. A. (2000). Visual discrimination learning requires sleep after training. *Nature Neuroscience*, **3**, 1237–1238.

Van Someren, E. J., Mirmiran, M., Bos, N. P., Lamur, A., Kumar, A., and Molenaar, P. C. (1990). Quantitative analysis of eye movements during REM sleep–sleep in developing rats. *Developmental Psychobiology*, **23**, 55–61.

Vogel, G., Neill, D., Hagler, M., and Kors, D. (1990*a*). A new animal model of endogenous depression: a summary of present findings. *Neuroscience and Biobehavioral Reviews*, **14**, 85–91.

Vogel, G., Neill, D., Hagler, M., Kors, D., and Hartley, P. (1990*b*). Decreased intracranial self-stimulation in a new animal model of endogenous depression. *Neuroscience and Biobehavioral Reviews*, **14**, 65–68.

Vogel, G., Neill, D., Kors, D., and Hagler, M. (1990*c*). REM sleep abnormalities in a new animal model of endogenous depression. *Neuroscience and Biobehavioral Reviews*, **14**, 77–83.

Vogel, G. W., Feng, P., and Kinney, G. G. (2000). Ontogeny of REM sleep in rats: possible implications for endogenous depression. *Physiology and Behavior*, **68**, 453–461.

Will, B. E., Rosenzweig, M. R., Bennett, E. L., Hebert, M., and **Morimoto, H.** (1977). Relatively brief environmental enrichment aids recovery of learning capacity and alters brain measures after postweaning brain lesions in rats. *Journal of Comparative Physiology and Psychology*, **91**, 33–50.

Wilson, M. A. and **McNaughton, B. L.** (1994). Reactivation of hippocampal ensemble memories during sleep. *Science*, **265**, 676–679.

CHAPTER 10

THE ROLE OF SLEEP IN THE DEVELOPMENT OF CENTRAL VISUAL PATHWAYS

MARCOS G. FRANK AND MICHAEL P. STRYKER

Introduction

In a variety of mammalian species, sleep amounts are much greater during periods of rapid brain development and plasticity than at any other time of life (Roffwarg *et al.* 1966; Jouvet-Mounier *et al.* 1970; Frank and Heller 1997). The abundance of sleep in infancy, and the fact that adult sleep is associated with complex patterns of brain activation (Wilson and McNaughton 1994; Skaggs and McNaughton 1996; Qin *et al.* 1997; Maquet 2001) and the release of neuromodulators that influence neural development (Lauder 1983; Jones 1994; Hobson 1999; Lauder and Schambra 1999), suggests that sleep may play an important role in brain maturation. In this chapter, we review the evidence in support of this general hypothesis. We focus primarily on the developing visual system since this system has provided a model for much of our understanding of the mechanisms of neural development (Hubel 1982, 1988; Wiesel 1982; Shatz 1996; Schmidt *et al.* 1999; Berardi *et al.* 2000; Sur and Leamey 2001). We begin by briefly reviewing the role of endogenous neural activity and experience in the development of central visual pathways. This is followed by a discussion of current findings that support a role for sleep in visual system development. We conclude with a discussion of several theories regarding the functions of sleep in developing animals; specifically, we review the "Ontogenetic Hypothesis" that posits REM sleep as an important source of endogenous activity in the developing brain (Roffwarg *et al.* 1966) and a second view which states that NREM sleep promotes the consolidation of waking experience; a process which begins at certain stages of development, but is retained throughout the lifespan.

The roles of endogenous activity and experience in visual system development

The development of precise neuronal connections in the mammalian brain requires both endogenous and exogenous sources of neuronal activity. In the developing visual system, endogenous activity in the retina and in thalamocortical circuits helps establish initial

Box 10.1 A brief overview of central visual pathways: LGN and primary visual cortex (V1)

The LGN receives bilateral retinal input via the optic tracts, where it is segregated into eye-specific lamina. The LGN also receives inputs from ascending brainstem centers, as well as from primary cortex, which modulate LGN response properties (Hubel 1982, 1988; Wandell 1995; Derrington 2001). Visual information is then relayed to V1, and further segregated into several functional domains arrayed in radial columns spanning the cortical plate (Hubel 1982, 1988; Wandell 1995). In animals with binocular vision, two basic functional domains are the ocular dominance and orientation columns. The ocular dominance columns are alternating regions of V1 that receive visual inputs representing one or the other eye (Hubel 1982, 1988; Wiesel 1982). While most normal cortical neurons respond to stimuli seen by either eye, neurons within a specific ocular dominance column respond more strongly to visual inputs that innervate that column. Neurons in V1 are also sensitive to the orientation of edges of the stimulus within their receptive fields. Cortical neurons preferentially activated by a specific stimulus orientation are arranged radially in columns. Tangentially, the preferred orientation of cortical columns changes gradually and progressively across the cortex, except at occasional discontinuities (Hubel 1982, 1988; Grinvald *et al.* 1986; Ferster and Miller 2000). Visual inputs relayed through the LGN terminate within these alternating cortical regions where they activate specific columns of neurons. In addition to these thalamic inputs, neurons in V1 receive numerous intracortical projections from neighboring ocular dominance and orientation domains and from extra-striate visual areas, which together determine their response properties (Singer 1982; Gilbert and Wiesel 1983; Sengpiel *et al.* 1998; Ferster and Miller 2000).

patterns of synaptic circuitry that are elaborated and sculpted by experience during subsequent critical periods of postnatal development (Shatz 1996; Sengpiel *et al.* 1998; Penn and Shatz 1999; Wong 1999; Sur and Leamey 2001). The interplay of these two sources of neural activity has been well documented in two visual structures, the lateral geniculate nucleus (LGN) of the thalamus and primary visual cortex (V1). A brief overview of central visual pathways is available in Box 10.1.

The role of endogenous neural activity in visual system development

LGN

The initial maturation of the LGN does not require visual experience, but is dependent upon endogenous neural activity. In fetal cats and newborn ferrets, the retinal projections to the LGN are initially diffuse and become progressively restricted to their eye-appropriate lamina during subsequent development (Shatz 1996; Penn and Shatz 1999; Wong 1999). This segregation of retinal afferents in the LGN occurs well before eye opening and appears to require spontaneous waves of retinal activity (Galli and Maffei 1988; Shatz and Stryker 1988). Spontaneous waves of retinal activity appear before eye opening, are transmitted to LGN, and coincide with the morphological and functional maturation of the LGN (Wong 1999). Pharmacological blockade of this retinal activity disrupts the normal segregation of retinal afferents into their proper laminar positions in the LGN (Sretavan *et al.* 1988) and prevents the normal maturational changes in NMDA current kinetics in LGN cells (Ramoa and Prusky 1997; Wong 1999).

V1

A similar stage of development is reported in V1. The segregation of LGN afferents into ocular dominance columns begins well before the onset of visual experience (Rakic 1977; Horton and Hocking 1996; Crair *et al.* 1998, 2001; Crowley and Katz 2000), and in the cat eye-preference is observed in cortical neurons shortly after the time of eye opening and is not delayed if the eyes are kept closed (Crair *et al.* 1998). Spatially distributed patterns of spontaneous activity in the LGN and visual cortex measured in unanesthetized developing animals are found to be consistent with the hypothesized activity needed to form cortical columns based on mathematical models (Miller *et al.* 1989; Weliky and Katz 1999; Chiu and Weliky 2001). Orientation selectivity of cortical neurons is also detected before the onset of visual experience and develops normally in the absence of patterned visual stimuli (Chapman and Stryker 1993; Crair *et al.* 1998; White *et al.* 2001). This early development of orientation selectivity in cortical neurons is paralleled by the formation of crude long-range, horizontal connections between cortical cells that in adult animals connect columns of similar orientation preference (Gilbert and Wiesel 1983; Ruthazer and Stryker 1996).

As is true for the LGN, alterations in endogenous neural activity lead to profound anatomical and physiological changes in the development of ocular dominance and orientation selectivity in cortical neurons. Complete blockade of retinal activity with tetrodotoxin (TTX) prevents the normal segregation of LGN afferents into ocular dominance columns (Stryker and Harris 1986), and TTX infusions in V1 prevent the normal extension of LGN afferents into their normal target regions (Catalano and Shatz 1998). TTX infusions in the developing visual cortex also prevent the initial development of orientation selectivity (Chapman and Stryker 1993) and inhibit the formation of rudimentary horizontal connections that link common functional domains (Ruthazer and Stryker 1996). Since these early processes in cortical development are disrupted by silencing cortical cells with TTX but not by altering visual experience, or even by the removal of the eyes, they are thought to depend on endogenous neuronal activity in the cortex. Recent recordings of such endogenous activity are consistent with this view (Weliky and Katz 1999; Chiu and Weliky 2001).

The role of experience in visual system development

The maintenance and further refinement of rudimentary circuits and response properties in central visual pathways is highly dependent on visual experience during critical developmental periods (Chapman *et al.* 1999; Berardi *et al.* 2000; Sur and Leamey 2001). For example, while rudimentary orientation selectivity can develop in the absence of patterned visual experience, this response property rapidly deteriorates if visual experience is prevented during a critical period that begins about 2 weeks after eye opening (Crair *et al.* 1998; White *et al.* 2001). Alterations in visual experience during the critical period also profoundly influence the subsequent refinement of ocular dominance and orientation selectivity in primary visual cortex (Wiesel and Hubel 1965; Hubel and Wiesel 1970).

If one eye is allowed to see normally while the vision of the other eye is occluded (monocular deprivation: MD) during a critical period of development, most of the cortical cells, even those in the deprived eye's columns, lose their ability to respond to the deprived eye and become much less selective for stimulus orientation (Wiesel and Hubel 1965; Hubel and Wiesel 1970; Shatz and Stryker 1978; Singer 1979; Crair et al. 1997). This physiological loss of response is followed in less than a week by a dramatic retraction of the branches of deprived geniculocortical arbors and is followed much later by a compensatory expansion of the arbors of the open eye (LeVay et al. 1980; Antonini and Stryker 1993). These physiological and anatomical changes in neurons are collectively known as ocular dominance plasticity. Related morphological changes occur in the LGN. The LGN cells receiving afferent input from the deprived eye shrink in size concurrent with an expansion of cell sizes in lamina innervated by the non-deprived eye (Guillery and Stelzner 1970; Hubel and Wiesel 1970; Tieman 1985). These processes depend on a competitive interaction between patterns of neural activity in the two visual pathways, and do not take place when the vision of both eyes is occluded (Wiesel and Hubel 1965; Guillery and Stelzner 1970; Guillery 1972).

In summary, the early development of both the LGN and visual cortex depends upon endogenous or spontaneous neural activity, which when blocked, results in profound malformation of these brain regions. Visual experience is not required for this initial developmental phase, but is required at later critical periods for the maintenance and refinement of selective and strong visual responses and precise columnar structure in the cortex. Disruption of normal binocular vision during the critical period can cause rapid and profound changes in subcortical and cortical anatomy and physiology.

Sleep and visual system development

The initial development of the central visual pathways and their subsequent sculpting by experience occur at ages when sleep amounts are very high, or during landmark changes in sleep expression (Jouvet-Mounier et al. 1970; Davis et al. 1999). Both REM sleep and NREM sleep could contribute to these developmental processes. REM sleep is accompanied by tonic excitation of thalamic and cortical neurons and phasic activations in visual structures (pontine-geniculate-occipital (PGO) waves) (Jones 1991; Siegel 1994). REM sleep is also associated with increased release of acetylcholine (Jones 1991), a neurotransmitter that influences neuronal development (Lauder and Schambra 1999) and synaptic remodeling (Rasmusson 2000). NREM sleep is also characterized by events conducive to synaptic plasticity and neural development, such as synchronized bursting in thalamocortical circuits, transient elevations of intracellular calcium, and in some mammals, the release of somatotropins (Steriade and Amzica 1998; Cauter and Spiegel 1999; Steriade 2000). Both REM sleep and NREM sleep also appear to promote processes dependent on synaptic remodeling, such as learning and memory (Smith 1995;

Maquet 2001; Stickgold *et al.* 2001), and therefore might influence periods of heightened synaptic plasticity and development in the maturing brain.

Sleep and subcortical development in central visual pathways

A role for REM sleep in brain development has been tested by studying the effects of REM sleep deprivation (REMD), or the elimination of REM sleep PGO waves (REMPD), on subsequent visual system development (additional tests of this hypothesis are discussed elsewhere in this volume).

Davenne and Adrien conducted the first of such studies, by examining changes in neuronal morphology in the LGN in kittens following brainstem lesions that eliminated PGO waves (Davenne and Adrien 1984). Bilateral electrolytic lesions of the X area, a nucleus close to the locus coeruleus, and regions near the rostral pontine tegmentum abolished PGO waves in the neonatal cat, resulting in smaller LGN volumes (22% reduction compared to sham or unilaterally lesioned control cats) and reduced LGN soma sizes (binocular segment: 20% reduction compared to sham or unilaterally lesioned cats). These findings were replicated and extended in a second study (Davenne *et al.* 1989), which showed that PGO wave elimination in developing cats produced much slower LGN responses to stimulation of the optic chiasm (compared to sham or unilaterally lesioned control cats), and also more LGN cells with "mixed" on–off responses (as opposed to pure "on" or "off" responses to an annulus of light centered in the receptive field), fewer X cell responses (relative to on–off responses). These morphological and functional changes in LGN cells are consistent with a delayed maturation of the LGN (Daniels *et al.* 1978; Williams and Jeffery 2001) and suggest that REM sleep neuronal activity may provide a source of endogenous neuronal activity necessary for normal LGN development.

Several findings in developing cats also suggest a possible role for sleep during later occurring, critical periods for visual development. Pompeiano *et al.* (1995) reported that total sleep deprivation (NREM sleep + REM sleep) combined with MD enhanced the effects of MD on LGN cell morphology. The results of this study, however, are difficult to interpret since the amount of visual experience was not equal across sleeping and sleep-deprived cats, and very little quantitative data on sleep architecture were presented. More persuasive evidence for a role for sleep in subcortical development is provided by studies using various forms of selective REMD, or REMPD combined with MD. Using the "flower pot" technique of REMD, Oksenberg *et al.* (1996) demonstrated that 1 week of REMD in kittens enhanced the effects of MD on cell morphology in the binocular segment of the LGN. LGN cells receiving input from the occluded eye were smaller when REMD was combined with MD compared to MD alone resulting in a greater difference in the size of LGN cells activated by the open and deprived eyes. A similar increase in LGN cell size disparity is reported when MD is combined with brainstem lesions that remove PGO waves, and in this case, LGN cells receiving input from the open eye appeared to increase in size (Shaffery *et al.* 1999). The REMD combined with MD also reduces cell sizes in the monocular segment of the LGN, which is normally little affected by competitive interactions between the two eyes (Shaffery *et al.* 1998). In addition, REMD for 1 week reduces immunoreactivity for the calcium binding protein parvalbumin in gamma-amino-butyric-acid-ergic (GABAergic) interneurons in the developing LGN (Hogan *et al.* 2001). These latter findings are particularly interesting since parvalbumin in neurons influences certain forms of synaptic plasticity (Caillard *et al.* 2000). Together these results suggest that REMD or REMPD can influence certain developmental events in the LGN during critical periods of visual system development.

Sleep and developmentally regulated cortical plasticity

A role for REM sleep has also been reported in a developmentally regulated form of long-term potentiation (LTP) elicited during the critical period for visual system development (Kirkwood *et al.* 1995). In this type of LTP, high-frequency white-matter stimulation in cortical slices obtained from juvenile rats [postnatal (P) day 28–30] produces synaptic potentiation in upper cortical layers, an effect that wanes with age (P35+), and is rarely observed in cortical slices from adult rat brains. Using a modified, less stressful version of the "flower-pot" technique of REMD ("multiple small-platform"), Shaffery *et al.* (2001) examined the effects of 1 week of REMD on this form of LTP in rat visual cortex.

The study reported that 1 week of REMD extended the critical period for this developmentally regulated form of LTP which was readily evoked from slices of visual cortex from REMD rats at ages when this type of LTP is not normally observed (P34–P40). A similar extension of the critical period was not observed in cortical slices from control rats that were left in their nests, or from rats placed on slightly larger platforms (large-platform control) that presumably permitted REM sleep. Conversely, a nondevelopmentally regulated form of LTP evoked by layer IV stimulation was not affected by REMD. The latter effects of REMD were similar to effects produced by dark rearing, which also prolongs the period of susceptibility to this form of LTP (Shaffery *et al.* 2001). These findings are consistent with a maturational delay, and are in general agreement with previous findings from the same group that show that REMD impairs or retards normal brain maturation.

A role for sleep in developmental cortical plasticity has also been demonstrated *in vivo*. In addition to its anatomical effects in the LGN, MD during the critical period for visual development induces rapid changes in cortical responses to the two eyes. Frank *et al.* (2001) investigated the role of sleep in this process by combining MD with periods of *ad lib* sleep or sleep deprivation. Cats at the peak of the critical period were divided into 4 experimental groups, all of which had one eye sutured shut and were kept awake in a lighted environment for 6 h. This MD period provided a standard stimulus for the induction of plasticity in all groups. The 4 groups differed in their experience thereafter. Cats in the first group (MD6) were immediately anesthetized for physiological measurement of ocular dominance in primary visual cortex using optical imaging of intrinsic cortical signals and extracellular unit recording. Cats in a second group (MDS) were allowed to sleep for an additional 6 h in complete darkness before making optical and unit recordings. Cats in the third group (MDSD) were treated identically to those in the

MDS group except that they were kept awake, rather than allowed to sleep, during the 6 h in complete darkness before the recordings. Cats in the fourth group (MD12) were also kept awake for 6 additional hours but remained in a lighted environment, effectively giving them 6 additional hours of monocular deprivation before the recordings.

These experiments determined, first, whether the effects of MD were enhanced by sleep immediately thereafter (MD6 compared to MDS); second, whether the enhancement of plasticity observed in group MDS was due to sleep or merely to the passage of time following the inducing stimulus (MDS compared to MDSD); third, whether the procedure used to sleep deprive the cats itself directly impeded ocular dominance plasticity (MD12 compared to MDSD).

Both optical imaging of intrinsic cortical signals and extracellular unit recording showed that sleep nearly doubled the effects of a preceding period of monocular deprivation on visual cortical responses, but wakefulness in complete darkness did not do so. Moreover, no brain state other than sleep is known have such enhancing effects on ocular dominance plasticity since anesthetic states and cortical inactivation suppress further ocular dominance plasticity (Freeman 1979; Reiter *et al.* 1986; Rauschecker and Hahn 1987; Imamura and Kasamatsu 1991). The enhancement of plasticity by sleep was at least as great as that produced by an equal amount of additional deprivation. While it was not possible to determine the precise contribution of REM and NREM sleep to this process, the enhancement of cortical plasticity was highly correlated with NREM sleep time and intensity, suggesting an important role for NREM sleep in the rapid cortical synaptic remodeling elicited by MD (Frank *et al.* 2001).

Some further considerations

Although the findings discussed above support a role for sleep in visual system development, a number of considerations should be kept in mind. First, one should consider the possible secondary effects of the experimental manipulation used in a study. For example, sleep deprivation has multiple behavioral and neurochemical effects that may in turn influence the results of an experiment (Vertes and Eastman 2000; Siegel 2001). In particular, the manipulations performed in one sleep state may also influence neural processing in other vigilance states as well, making it difficult to ascertain which vigilance state is responsible for the observed effects.

Secondary effects

In all of the experiments reviewed above, some manipulation of sleep structure, or lesions that damage parts of the brain active in sleep are used to test the putative role of sleep in visual system development. Some of these manipulations are likely to have complex effects on neural development and behavior outside of their impact on sleep. In the case of studies using brainstem lesions, it is not clear if the reported deficits are due to PGO suppression, or the removal of ascending innervation to target LGN neurons. The LGN is massively innervated by ascending cholinergic and monoaminergic brainstem projections (Steriade 1996; Derrington 2001). In addition to providing tonic excitatory input, these afferents may also promote neural growth and maturation since both cholinergic and monoaminergic neurotransmission have neurotrophic effects in developing animals (Lauder 1983; Lauder and Schambra 1999). Thus, the bilateral removal of this input, rather than the elimination of REM sleep PGO waves, may contribute to the results reported in the Davenne studies (though they are probably not a major factor in the Shaffery study since cell sizes increased following PGO elimination).

The effects of stress should also be considered in studies using sleep deprivation; REMD using the "flower-pot" or small-platform technique is stressful because the animal periodically falls into a pool of water, and often is unable to properly groom itself. Prolonged exposure to stress hormones can influence neuronal degeneration (Sapolsky 1996; Abraham *et al.* 2000; Yusim *et al.* 2000), and processes dependent upon synaptic plasticity (De Kloet *et al.* 1999). Thus, while the enhancement of the anatomical effects of MD in the LGN by REMD is consistent with a maturational delay induced by REMD, it may also reflect the influence of stress hormones on degenerative processes triggered by sensory deprivation. This seems an especially important consideration given that the anatomical effects of REMD are found in the monocular segment of the LGN, an area that normally does not remodel during developmental critical periods.

Stress, however, does not appear to be a factor in studies using sleep deprivation combined with *in situ* LTP, immunohistochemical assays of calcium binding proteins (parvalbumin) or cortical plasticity *in vivo*. In the case of the study by Shaffery *et al.* the chronic stress hormone release induced by long-term REMD might be expected to impair, not prolong, susceptibility to LTP (De Kloet *et al.* 1999; Shaffery *et al.* 2001). Nor is there evidence to suggest that stress associated with REMD down-regulates parvalbumin in the LGN. Elevated stress hormones have no effect on parvalbumin concentrations in the hippocampus—a brain region highly sensitive to circulating glucocorticoid levels (Krugers *et al.* 1996; Sapolsky 1996). Similarly, the acute release of stress hormones elicited by very short periods of TSD tends to enhance, not impair synaptic plasticity (De Kloet *et al.* 1999), and is probably unrelated to the loss of plasticity in sleep-deprived cats and the enhancement of plasticity in cats allowed to sleep reported in Frank *et al.* 2001).

Vigilance state specificity

A related issue that complicates the interpretation of some studies occurs when the experimental manipulation alters vigilance states in ways likely to influence both the acquisition of sensory input in wake as well as subsequent processing during REM sleep *and* NREM sleep. For example, REMD increases noradrenergic activity in the central nervous system (CNS); Porrka-Heiskanen *et al.* 1995; Irwin *et al.* 1999) which enhances signal detection in sensory neurons during wake (Smiley 1996; Aston-Jones *et al.* 1999). REMD also profoundly alters NREM sleep architecture (fragmentation, loss of deeper stages of NREM sleep) even in cases when total NREM sleep amounts are preserved (Beersma *et al.* 1990; Brunner *et al.* 1993; Endo *et al.* 1997). Thus, in experimental designs that employ prolonged REMD interspersed with periods of sensory input, the observed behavioral changes may result from numerous factors including REMD, changes in wake neural processing, and disruption of NREM sleep. Determining the cause of developmental effects is also difficult in studies using brainstem lesions. As discussed above, these lesions interrupt ascending pathways that massively innervate subcortical and cortical structures. The impact of these lesions, therefore, is unlikely to be solely restricted to REM sleep.

Theories of sleep function in developing animals

In this section, we analyze more critically the Ontogenetic Hypothesis (Roffwarg *et al.* 1966), and a second view that states that sleep promotes the consolidation of waking experience; a process that begins at certain stages of development, but is retained throughout the lifespan.

The ontogenetic hypothesis

In their classic study of human infants, Roffwarg, Muzio, and Dement proposed that the large amounts of REM sleep in early infancy provide an important source of endogenous neural activity necessary for brain maturation (Roffwarg *et al.* 1966). In the more recent formulations of this hypothesis, it is suggested that REM sleep not only stimulates normal brain development, but also protects the brain from excessive experience-dependent plasticity (Oksenberg *et al.* 1996; Roffwarg and Shaffery 1999). Both functions are believed to be mediated by the PGO waves, or heightened release of acetylcholine during REM sleep (Oksenberg *et al.* 1996; Roffwarg and Shaffery 1999; Shaffery *et al.* 2001).

The Ontogenetic Hypothesis and its variants (Marks *et al.* 1995; Mirmiran and Maas 1999), has intuitive appeal since REM sleep amounts are very high in infants, and decline as the brain matures (Roffwarg *et al.* 1966; Jouvet-Mounier *et al.* 1970). It is supported by several findings that indicate that REMD or REMPD can modify morphological and electrophysiological development of the LGN, and developmentally regulated cortical synaptic plasticity *in situ*. The theory that REM sleep counter-balances or offsets waking experience in early development has less direct support, but is suggested by three find-ings. First, REM sleep PGO waves in adult cats activate all LGN lamina simultaneously, indicating that this activity, in contrast to visual experience, is not eye-specific (Marks *et al.* 1999). Theoretically, such nonspecific activation of neural circuits, if present in developing animals, could offset the more specific, experience-dependent activation of neural circuitry present in wake. Second, in contrast to healthy, adult mammals, latencies to REM sleep in infants are very short, and sleep-onset REM (SOREM) sleeps frequently occur (Jouvet-Mounier *et al.* 1970; McGinty *et al.* 1977). Third, in the study by Frank *et al.* cortical plasticity was negatively correlated with REM sleep amounts in the sleep-ing cats, suggesting that REM sleep may slightly inhibit experience-dependent plasticity (Frank *et al.* 2001). It is therefore possible that the more frequent entries into REM sleep in neonatal animals interfere with the consolidation of experience-dependent changes in neural circuitry.

Despite the appeal of the Ontogenetic Hypothesis, a number of issues remain to be resolved. As discussed above, the interpretation of the experimental support for the Ontogenetic hypothesis is less than straightforward since the effects of stress, and other side effects of the procedures used in REMD and REMPD are not always clear. A second issue is that the neurophysiological phenomena typical of adult REM sleep (e.g. PGO waves) may not occur during early stages of development, when REM sleep might be expected to be most important for brain maturation. For example, REM sleep PGO waves in the kitten are not observed at ages when REM sleep is maximally expressed (Bowe-Anders *et al.* 1974). Nor is it known if other aspects of REM sleep, like heightened cholinergic activity, are present in newborn animals. Given the relatively slow maturation of cholinergic systems (Coyle and Yamamura 1976; Lee *et al.* 1990; Ninomiya *et al.* 2001), and the late appearance of other REM sleep phenomena (Chase 1971), this seems rather unlikely. In fact, the majority of studies suggesting a developmental role for REM sleep have been performed at ages when REM sleep has already declined to near adult levels (Oksenberg *et al.* 1996; Shaffery *et al.* 1998, 1999, 2001; Hogan *et al.* 2001). Thus, while there are data to support predictions of the Ontogenetic Hypothesis, they are limited to a very narrow, developmental period, and their interpretation must await further experiments that more carefully control for indirect effects induced by REMD and REMPD.

Sleep as consolidation

The demonstration that developmental cortical plasticity *in vivo* is enhanced by a period of NREM sleep suggests that NREM sleep may also play an important role in brain development (Frank *et al.* 2001). The enhancement of experience-dependent synaptic plasticity is consistent with findings in adult animals; where NREM sleep has been linked to learning and memory consolidation (Guiditta *et al.* 1995; Gais *et al.* 2000; Stickgold *et al.* 2000), and neuronal processes that may contribute to synaptic remodeling (Wilson and McNaughton 1994; Qin *et al.* 1997; Steriade 1999). A role for NREM sleep in developmental cortical plasticity is further suggested by maturational changes in NREM sleep that coincide with periods of heightened cortical plasticity. In the cat, there is a steep decline in REM sleep and a sharp increase in NREM sleep amounts near the beginning of the critical period for visual development (Jouvet-Mounier *et al.* 1970). In rats, the beginning of the critical period for visual development coincides with the development of NREM sleep homeostasis. Prior to the fourth postnatal week, NREM sleep EEG activity does not intensify following sleep deprivation, indicating that the regulatory relationship between wake and NREM sleep matures in parallel with periods of heightened cortical plasticity (Frank *et al.* 1998). These findings suggest that NREM sleep may consolidate waking experience; a process that begins during critical periods of brain development when the animal is most sensitive to waking experience, but is retained throughout life.

While it appears that one function of NREM sleep may be to consolidate waking experience, it is likely that this sleep stage serves additional functions in the developing brain as well. In altricial species like the rat and cat, the most rapid increase in NREM sleep occurs several weeks before the critical period for visual development (Jouvet-Mounier *et al.* 1970; Frank and Heller 1997). In precocial species like the sheep, NREM sleep amounts are near adult levels *in utero*; a time when exogenous visual experience is minimal (Szeto and Hinman 1985). The full development of visual cortical organization and selectivity also takes place *in utero* in the sheep, and neuronal plasticity is limited in the postnatal period (Clarke *et al.* 1977; Ramachandran *et al.* 1977). Given that the appearance of NREM sleep coincides with periods of explosive neocortical development, and is actively regulated within 24–48 h of its electrographic appearance (Frank *et al.* 1998; Davis *et al.* 1999), it would appear that NREM sleep may have functions in developing animals in addition to its role during critical periods of experience-dependent plasticity.

Summary and concluding remarks

The large amounts of sleep during periods of rapid brain growth and synaptic plasticity suggest a role for sleep in brain development. Experimental support for this view has come primarily from studies in the visual system, where it has been shown that sleep and sleep loss influence developmental events in the LGN and in V1. In particular, REMD and REMPD produce several anatomical and electrophysiological changes in the LGN, and modify cortical plasticity *in situ*. NREM sleep appears to be necessary for the consolidation of visual experience during critical periods of experience-dependent cortical plasticity *in vivo*. These findings indicate that both sleep states may be important for neuronal development, although the contribution of each state is likely to be different.

While the precise role of each sleep state in brain development is still unclear, current findings suggest that the relative amounts of REM sleep and NREM sleep during early life may critically influence brain maturation. REM sleep is maximally expressed at ages when endogenous neuronal activity is critical for the establishment of rudimentary neural circuitry in the visual system. NREM sleep, on the other hand, is present at later stages of development, rapidly matures after eye opening (Gramsbergen 1976; Jouvet-Mounier *et al.* 1970; Frank and Heller 1997) and becomes homeostatically regulated by wake in a manner similar to adult NREM sleep during critical periods of experience-dependent synaptic plasticity (Frank *et al.* 1998). Thus, it seems plausible that while REM sleep helps establish early patterns of neural circuitry, NREM sleep in part consolidates changes in neural circuitry elicited by waking experience.

In conclusion, many phenomena strongly suggest a role for sleep in brain development and plasticity, but we currently know little about the cellular and molecular mechanisms by which sleep exerts its effects. The opportunities afforded by advances in genetic and pharmacological manipulation of specific molecules and signaling pathways, and by chronic recording and manipulation of neural activity, raise the hope that these mechanisms may soon be revealed.

Acknowledgments

This research supported by grants from the US National Institutes of Health.

References

Abraham, I., Harkany, T., Horvath, K. M., Veenema, A. H., Penke, B., Nyakas, C., and Luiten, P. G. M. (2000). Chronic corticosterone administration dose-dependently modulates A(142) and NMDA-induced neurodegeneration in rat magnocellular nucleus basalis. *Journal of Endocrinology*, **12**, 486–494.

Antonini, A. and Stryker, M. P. (1993). Rapid remodeling of axonal arbors in the visual cortex. *Science*, **260**, 1819–1821.

Aston-Jones, G., Rajkowski, J., and Cohen, J. (1999). Role of locus coeruleus in attention and behavioral flexibility. *Biological Psychiatry*, **46**, 1309–1320.

Beersma, D. G. M., Dijk, D. J., Blok, C. G., and Everhardus, I. (1990). REM sleep deprivation during 5 hours leads to an immediate REM sleep rebound and to suppression of non-REM sleep intensity. *Electroencephalography and Clinical Neurophysiology*, **76**, 114–122.

Berardi, N., Pizzorusso, T., and Maffei, L. (2000). Critical periods during sensory development. *Current Opinion in Neurobiology*, **10**, 138–145.

Bowe-Anders, C., Adrien, J., and Roffwarg, H. P. (1974). Ontogenesis of ponto-geniculo-occipital activity in the lateral geniculate nucleus of the kitten. *Experimental Neurology*, **43**, 242–260.

Brunner, D. P., Dijk, D. J., and Borbely, A. A. (1993). Repeated partial sleep deprivation progressively changes EEG during sleep and wakefulness. *Sleep*, **16**, 100–113.

Caillard, O., Moreno, H., Schwaller, B., LLano, I., Celio, M. R., and Marty, A. (2000). Role of the calcium-binding protein parvalbumin in short-term synaptic plasticity. *Proceedings of the National Academy of Science, USA*, **97**, 13372–13377.

Catalano, S. M. and Shatz, C. J. (1998). Activity-dependent cortical target selection by thalamic axons. *Science*, **281**, 559–562.

Cauter, E. V. and Spiegel, K. (1999). Circadian and sleep control of hormonal secretions. In *Regulation of sleep and circadian rhythms*. Vol. 133 (eds P. C. Zee and F. W. Turek), pp. 397–425. Marcel Dekker, Inc., New York.

Chapman, B., Godecke, I., and Bonhoeffer, T. (1999). Development of orientation preference in the mammalian visual cortex. *Journal of Neurobiology*, **41**, 18–24.

Chapman, B. and Stryker, M. P. (1993). Development of orientation selectivity in ferret visual cortex and effects of deprivation. *Journal of Neuroscience*, **13**, 5251–5262.

Chase, M. H. (1971). Brain stem somatic reflex activity in neonatal kittens during sleep and wakefulness. *Physiology and Behavior*, **7**, 165–172.

Chiu, C. and Weliki, M. (2001). Spontaneous activity in developing ferret visual cortex *in vivo*. *Journal of Neuroscience*, **21**, 8906–8914.

Clarke, P. G., Ramachandran, V. S., and Whitteridge, D. (1979). The development of the binocular depth cells in the secondary visual cortex of the lamb. *Proceedings of the Royal Society of London. Series B: Biological Sciences*, **204**, 455–465.

Coyle, J. T. and **Yamamura, H. I.** (1976). Neurochemical aspects of the ontogenesis of cholinergic neurons in the rat brain. *Brain Research*, **118**, 429–440.

Crair, M. C., Gillespie, D. C., and **Stryker, M. P.** (1998). The role of visual experience in the development of columns in cat visual cortex. *Science*, **279**, 566–570.

Crair, M. C., Horton, J. C., Antonini, A., and **Stryker, M. P.** (2001). Emergence of ocular dominance columns in cat visual cortex by 2 weeks of age. *Journal of Comparative Neurology*, **430**, 235–249.

Crowley, J. C. and **Katz, L. C.** (2000). Early development of ocular dominance columns. *Science*, **290**, 1321–1324.

Daniels, J. D., Pettigrew, J. D., and **Norman, J. L.** (1978). Development of single-neuron responses in kitten's lateral geniculate nucleus. *Journal of Neurophysiology*, **41**, 1373–1393.

Davenne, D. and **Adrien, J.** (1984). Suppression of PGO waves in the kitten: anatomical effects on the lateral geniculate nucleus. *Neuroscience Letters*, **45**, 33–38.

Davenne, D., Fregnac, Y., Imbert, M., and **Adrien, J.** (1989). Lesion of the PGO pathways in the kitten. II. Impairment of physiological and morphological maturation of the lateral geniculate nucleus. *Brain Research*, **485**, 267–277.

Davis, F. C., Frank, M. G., and **Heller, H. C.** (1999). Ontogeny of sleep and circadian rhythms. In *Regulation of sleep and circadian rhythms*, Vol. 133 (eds P. C. Zee, and F. W. Turek), pp. 19–80. Marcel Dekker, Inc., New York.

De Kloet, E. R., Oitzl, M. S., and **Joels, M.** (1999). Stress and cognition: are corticosteroids good or bad guys? *Trends in Neuroscience*, **22**, 422–426.

Derrington, A. (2001). The lateral geniculate nucleus. *Current Biology*, **11**, R635–R637.

Endo, T., Schwierin, B., Borbely, A. A., and **Tobler, I.** (1997). Selective and total sleep deprivation: effect on the sleep EEG in the rat. *Psychiatry Research*, **66**, 97–110.

Ferster, D. and **Miller, K. D.** (2000). Neural mechanisms of orientation selectivity in the visual cortex. *Annual Review of Neuroscience*, **23**, 441–471.

Frank, M. G. and **Heller, H. C.** (1997). Development of REM sleep and slow wave sleep in the rat. *American Journal of Physiology*, **272**, R1792–R1799.

Frank, M. G., Issa, N. P., and **Stryker, M. P.** (2001). Sleep enhances plasticity in developing visual cortex. *Neuron*, **30**, 275–287.

Frank, M. G., Morrissette, R., and **Heller, H. C.** (1998). Effects of sleep deprivation in neonatal rats. *American Journal of Physiology*, **275**, R148–R157.

Freeman, R. D. (1979). Effects of brief uniocular "patching" on kitten visual cortex. *Transactions of the Opthalmic Society UK*, **99**, 382–385.

Galli, L. and **Maffei, L.** (1988). Spontaneous impulse activity of rat retinal ganglion cells in prenatal life. *Science*, **242**, 90–91.

Gais, S., Plihal, W., Wagner, U., and **Born, J.** (2000). Early sleep triggers memory for early visual discrimination skills. *Nature Neurosciences*, **3**, 1335–1339.

Gilbert, C. D. and **Wiesel, T. N.** (1983). Clustered intrinsic connections in cat visual cortex. *Journal of Neuroscience*, **3**, 1116–1133.

Gramsbergen, A. (1976). The development of the EEG in the rat. *Developmental Psychobiology*, **9**, 501–515.

Grinvald, A., Lieke, E., Frostig, R. D., Gilbert, C. D., and Wiesel, T. N. (1986). Functional architecture of cortex revealed by optical imaging of intrinsic signals. *Nature*, **324**, 361–364.

Guiditta, A., Amborsini, M. V., Montangnese, P., Mandile, P., Cotugno, M., Zucconi, G. G., and Vescia, S. (1995). The sequential hypothesis of the function of sleep. *Behavioral Brain Research*, **69**, 157–166.

Guillery, R. W. (1972). Binocular competition in the control of geniculate cell growth. The differential effects of unilateral lid closure upon the monocular and binocular segments of the dorsal lateral geniculate nucleus in the cat. *Journal of Comparative Neurology*, **144**, 117–129.

Guillery, R. W. and Stelzner, D. J. (1970). The differential effects of unilateral lid closure upon the monocular and binocular segments of the dorsal lateral geniculate nucleus in the cat. *Journal of Comparative Neurology*, **139**, 413–421.

Hobson, J. A. (1999). Neural control of sleep. In *Regulation of sleep and circadian rhythms*, Vol. 133 (eds F. W. Turek and P. C. Zee), pp. 81–110. Marcel Dekker, Inc., New York.

Hogan, D., Roffwarg, H. P., and Shaffery, J. P. (2001). The effects of 1 week of REM sleep deprivation on parvalbumin and calbindin immunoreactive neurons in central visual pathways of kittens. *Journal of Sleep Research*, **10**, 285–296.

Horton, J. C. and Hocking, D. R. (1996). An adult-like pattern of ocular dominance columns in striate cortex of newborn monkeys prior to visual experience. *Journal of Neuroscience*, **16**, 1791–1807.

Hubel, D. H. and Wiesel, T. N. (1970). The period of susceptibility to the physiological effects of unilateral eye closure in kittens. *Journal of Physiology*, **206**, 419–436.

Hubel, D. H. (1982). Exploration of the primary visual cortex, 1955–78. *Nature*, **299**, 515–524.

Hubel, D. H. (1988). Eye, Brain, and Vision. Scientific American Library. Distributed by W. H. Freeman Co., New York.

Imamura, K. and Kasamatsu, T. (1991). Ocular dominance plasticity restored by NA infusion to aplastic visual cortex of anesthetized and paralyzed kittens. *Experimental Brain Research*, **87**(2), 309–318.

Irwin, M., Thompson, J., Miller, C., Gillin, J. C., and Ziegler, M. (1999). Effects of sleep and sleep deprivation on catecholamine and interleukin-2 levels in humans: clinical implications. *The Journal of Clinical Endocrinology and Metabolism*, **84**, 1979–1985.

Jones, B. (1991). Paradoxical sleep and its chemical/structural substrates in the brain. *Neuroscience*, **40**, 637–656.

Jones, B. E. (1994). Basic mechanisms of sleep-waking states. In *Principles and practice of sleep medicine* (eds M. H. Kryger, T. Roth, and W. C. Dement), pp. 145–162. Saunders, Philadelphia.

Jouvet-Mounier, D., Astic, L., and Lacote, D. (1970). Ontogenesis of the states of sleep in rat, cat and guinea pig during the first postnatal month. *Developmental Psychobiology*, **2**, 216–239.

Kirkwood, A., Lee, H. K., and Bear, M. F. (1995). Co-regulation of long-term potentiation and experience-dependent synaptic plasticity in visual cortex. *Nature*, **375**, 328–331.

Krugers, H. J., Koolhaas, J. M., Medema, R. M., and Korf, J. (1996). Prolonged subordination stress increases Calbindin-D28k immunoreactivity in the rat hippocampal CA1 area. *Brain Research*, **729**, 289–293.

Lauder, J. M. (1983). Hormonal and humoral influence on brain development. *Psychoneuroendocrinology*, **8**, 121–155.

Lauder, J. M. and Schambra, U. B. (1999). Morphogenetic roles of acetylcholine. *Environmental Health Perspective*, **107**, 65–69.

Lee, W., Nicklaus, K. J., Manning, D. R., and Wolfe, B. B. (1990). Ontogeny of cortical muscarinic receptor subtypes and muscarinic receptor-mediated responses in rat. *Journal of Pharmacological Experimental Therapy*, **252**, 284–490.

LeVay, S., Wiesel, T. N., and Hubel, D. H. (1980). The development of ocular dominance columns in normal and visually deprived monkeys. *Journal of Comparative Neurology*, **191**, 1–51.

Maquet, P. (2001). The role of sleep in learning and memory. *Science,* **294**, 1048–1051.

Marks, G. A., Roffwarg, H. P., and Shaffery, J. P. (1999). Neuronal activity in the lateral geniculate nucleus associated with ponto-geniculate-occipital waves lacks lamina specificity. *Brain Research*, **815**, 21–28.

Marks, G. A., Shaffery, J. P., Oksenberg, A., Speciale, S. G., and Roffwarg, H. P. (1995). A functional role for REM sleep in brain maturation. *Behavioral Brain Research*, **69**, 1–11.

McGinty, R. J., Stevenson, M., Hoppenbrouwers, T., Harper, R. M., Sterman, M. B., and Hodgman, J. (1977). Polygraphic studies of kitten development: sleep state patterns. *Developmental Psychobiology*, **10**, 455–469.

Mirmiran, M. and Maas, Y. G. H. (1999). The function of fetal/neonatal REM sleep. In *Rapid eye movement sleep* (eds B. N. Mallick and S. Inoue), pp. 326–335. Narosa Publishing House, New Delhi.

Miller, K. D., Keller J. B., and Stryker, M. P. (1989). Ocular dominance column development: analysis and simulation. *Science*, **245**(4918), 605–615.

Ninomiya, Y., Koyama, Y., and Kayama, Y. (2001). Postnatal development of choline acetyltransferase activity in the rat laterodorsal tegmental nucleus. *Neuroscience Letters*, **308**, 138–140.

Oksenberg, A., Shaffery, J. P., Marks, G. A., Speciale, S. G., Mihailoff, G., and Roffwarg, H. P. (1996). Rapid eye movement sleep deprivation in kittens amplifies LGN cell-size disparity induced by monocular deprivation. *Developmental Brain Research*, **97**, 51–61.

Penn, A. A. and Shatz, C. J. (1999). Brain waves and brain wiring: the role of endogenous and sensory-driven neural activity in development. *Pediatric Research*, **45**, 447–458.

Pompeiano, O., Pompeiano, M., and Corvaja, N. (1995). Effects of sleep deprivation on the postnatal development of visual-deprived cells in the cat's lateral geniculate nucleus. *Archives Italiennes de Biologie*, **134**, 121–140.

Porrka-Heiskanen, T., Smith, S. E., Taira, T., Urban, J. H., Levine, J. E., Turek, F. W., and Stenberg, D. (1995). Noradrenergic activity in rat brain during rapid eye movement sleep deprivation and rebound sleep. *American Journal of Physiology (Regulatory Integrative Comparative Physiology)*, **268**, R1456–R1463.

Qin, Y. L., McNaughton, B. L., Skaggs, W. E., and Barnes, C. A. (1997). Memory reprocessing in corticocortical and hippocampalcortical neuronal ensembles. *Philosophical Transaction of the Royal Society of London Series B: Biological Sciences*, **352**, 1525–1533.

Rakic, P. (1977). Prenatal development of the visual system in rhesus monkey. *Philosophical Transactions of the Royal Society of London Series B: Biological Sciences*, **278**, 245–260.

Ramachandran, V. S., Clarke, P. G., and Whitteridge, D. (1977). Cells selective to binocular disparity in the cortex of newborn lambs. *Nature*, **268**, 333–335.

Ramoa, A. S. and Prusky, G. (1997). Retinal activity regulates developmental switches in functional properties and ifenprodil sensitivity of NMDA receptors in the lateral geniculate nucleus. *Brain Research, Developmental Brain Research*, **18**, 165–175.

Rasmusson, D. D. (2000). The role of acetylcholine in cortical synaptic plasticity. *Behavioral Brain Research*, **115**, 205–218.

Rauschecker, J. P. and Hahn, S. (1987). Ketamine-Xylazine anesthesia blocks consolidation of ocular dominance changes in kitten visual cortex. *Nature*, **326**, 183–185.

Reiter, H. O., Waitzman, D. M., and Stryker, M. P. (1986). Cortical activity blockade prevents ocular dominance plasticity in the kitten visual cortex. *Experimental Brain Research*, **65**, 182–188.

Roffwarg, H. P., Muzio, J. N., and Dement, W. C. (1966). Ontogenetic development of the human sleep-dream cycle. *Science*, 604–619.

Roffwarg, H. P. and Shaffery, J. P. (1999). The ontogenetic hypothesis of REM sleep function: Its history, current status and prospects for confirmation. *Sleep Research Online*, **2**, 714–715.

Ruthazer, E. S. and Stryker, M. P. (1996). The role of activity in the development of long-range horizontal connections in area 17 of the ferret. *Journal of Neuroscience*, **16**, 7253–7263.

Sapolsky, R. M. (1996). Stress, glucocorticoids, and damage to the nervous system: The current state of confusion. *Stress*, **1**, 1–19.

Schmidt, K. E., Galuske, R. A., and Singer, W. (1999). Matching the modules: cortical maps and long-range intrinsic connections in visual cortex during development. *Journal of Neurobiology*, **41**, 10–17.

Sengpiel, F., Godecke, I., Stawinski, P., Hubener, M., Lowel, S., and Bonhoffer, T. (1998). Intrinsic and environmental factors in the development of functional maps in cat visual cortex. *Neuropharmacology*, **37**, 607–621.

Shaffery, J. P., Oksenberg, A., Marks, G. A., Speciale, S. G., Mihailoff, G., and Roffwarg, H. P. (1998). REM sleep deprivation in monocularly occluded kittens reduces the size of cells in LGN monocular segment. *Sleep*, **21**, 837–945.

Shaffery, J. P., Roffwarg, H. P., Speciale, S. G., and Marks, G. A. (1999). Ponto-geniculo-occipital wave suppression amplifies lateral geniculate nucleus cell-size changes in monocularly deprived kittens. *Developmental Brain Research*, **114**, 109–119.

Shaffery, J. P., Sinton, C. M., Bissette, G., Roffwarg, H. P., and Marks. G. A. (2002). Rapid eye movement sleep deprivation modifies expression of long-term potentiation in visual cortex of immature rats. *Neuroscience*, **110**, 431–443.

Shatz, C. J. (1996). Emergence of order in visual system development. *Proceedings of the National Academy of Sciences, USA*, **93**, 602–608.

Shatz, C. J. and **Stryker, M. P.** (1978). Ocular dominance in layer IV of the cat's visual cortex and the effects of monocular deprivation. *Journal of Physiology*, **281**, 267–283.

Shatz, C. J. and **Stryker, M. P.** (1988). Prenatal tetrodotoxin infusion blocks segregation of retinogeniculate afferents. *Science*, **242**, 87–89.

Siegel, J. M. (1994). Brainstem mechanisms generating REM sleep. In *Principles and practice of sleep medicine* (eds M. H. Kryger, T. Roth, and W. C. Dement), pp. 104–138. W. B. Saunders, Philadelphia.

Siegel, J. M. (2001). The REM sleep sleep-memory consolidation hypothesis. *Science*, **294**, 1058–1063.

Singer, W. (1979). Neuronal mechanisms in experience dependent modification of visual cortex function. In *Development and chemical sensitivity of neurons*. Vol. 31 (eds M. Cuenod, G. W. Kreutzberg, and F. E. Bloom), pp. 457–477. Elsevier/North-Holland Biomedical Press, Amsterdam.

Singer, W. (1982). The role of attention in developmental plasticity. *Human Neurobiology*, **1**, 41–43.

Skaggs, W. E. and **McNaughton, B. L.** (1996). Replay of neuronal firing sequences in rat hippocampus during sleep following spatial experience. *Science*, **271**, 1870–1873.

Smiley, J. F. (1996). Monoamines and acetylcholine in primate cerebral cortex: what anatomy tells us about function. *Revisita Brasileira de Biologia*, **56**, 153–164.

Smith, C. (1995). Sleep states and learning: a review of the animal literature. *Behavioral Brain Research*, **69**, 137–145.

Steriade, M. (1996). Arousal: revisiting the reticular activating system. *Science*, **272**, 225–226.

Steriade, M. (1999). Coherent oscillations and short-term plasticity in corticothalamic networks. *Trends in Neuroscience*, **22**, 337–345.

Steriade, M. (2000). Corticothalamic resonance, states of vigilance and mentation. *Neuroscience*, **101**, 243–276.

Steriade, M. and **Amzica, F.** (1998). Coalescence of sleep rhythms and their chronology in corticothalamic networks. *Sleep Research Online*, **1**, 1–10.

Stickgold, R., Hobson, J. A., Fosse, R., and **Fosse, M.** (2001). Sleep, learning and dreams: off-line memory reprocessing. *Science*, **294**, 1052–1057.

Stickgold, R., LaTanya, J., and **Hobson, J. A.** (2000). Visual discrimination learning requires sleep after training. *Nature Neuroscience*, **3**, 1237–1238.

Sretavan, D. W., Shatz, C. J., and **Stryker, M. P.** (1988). Modification of retinal ganglion cell axon morphology by prenatal infusion of tetrodotoxin. *Nature*, **336**, 468–471.

Stryker, M. P. and **Harris, W. A.** (1986). Binocular impulse blockade prevents the formation of ocular dominance columns in cat visual cortex. *Journal of Neuroscience*, **6**, 2117–2133.

Sur, M. and **Leamey, C. A.** (2001). Development and plasticity of cortical areas and networks. *Nature Review Neuroscience*, **2**, 251–262.

Szeto, H. and **Hinman, D. J.** (1985). Prenatal development of sleep–wake patterns in sheep. *Sleep*, **8**, 347–355.

Tieman, S. B. (1985). The anatomy of geniculocortical connections in monocularly deprived cats. *Cellular and Molecular Neurobiology*, **5**, 35–45.

Vertes, R. P. and **Eastman, K. E.** (2000). The case against memory consolidation in REM sleep. *Behavioral and Brain Sciences*, **23**, 867–876.

Wandell, B. A. (1995). *Foundations of vision.* Sinauer Associates, Inc., Sunderland.

Weliky, M. and **Katz, L. C.** (1999). Correlational structure of spontaneous neuronal activity in the developing lateral geniculate nucleus *in vivo. Science*, **285**, 599–604.

White, L. E., Coppola, D. M., and **Fitzpatrick, D.** (2001). The contribution of sensory experience to the maturation of orientation selectivity in ferret visual cortex. *Nature*, **411**, 1049–1052.

Wiesel, T. N. and **Hubel, D. H.** (1965). Comparison of the effects of unilateral and bilateral eye closure on cortical unit responses in kittens. *Journal of Neuophysiology*, **28**, 1029–1040.

Wiesel, T. N. (1982). Postnatal development of the visual cortex and the influence of environment. *Nature*, **299**, 583–591.

Williams, A. L. and **Jeffery, G.** (2001). Growth dynamics of the developing lateral geniculate nucleus. *Journal of Comparative Neurology*, **430**, 332–342.

Wilson, M. A. and **McNaughton, B. L.** (1994). Reactivation of hippocampal ensemble memories during sleep. *Science*, **265**, 676–682.

Wong, R. O. L. (1999). Retinal waves and visual system development. *Annual Review of Neuroscience*, **22**, 29–47.

Yusim, A., Ajilore, O., Bliss, T., and **Sapolsky, R.** (2000). Glucocorticoids exacerbate insult-induced declines in metabolism in selectively vulnerable hippocampal cell fields. *Brain Research*, **870**, 109–117.

SYSTEMS LEVEL

This section reviews data obtained at the systems level. Macroscopic systems correspond to networks of brain areas. Their activity can be estimated in humans as in animals by functional neuroimaging techniques. At the microscopic systems level, multiunit recordings allow the description of neural firing patterns and interneuronal interactions.

One important theme of this section is to provide evidence that the neuronal firing patterns during sleep promote changes in neural responsiveness. In Chapter 14, Steriade and Timofeev (University Laval, Montréal) provide evidence that brain rhythms during SWS can produce plastic changes in thalamic and neocortical networks. Using an experimental model of spindles in thalamo-cortical circuits, they show that by eliciting augmenting responses, oscillations during SWS modify the neuronal responsiveness for up to 15 min. These changes might lead to consolidation of memory traces.

A second theme in this section pertains to the experience-dependent neuronal activities during sleep. Understanding these processes in terms of cellular firing patterns is essential to the comprehension of sleep and its putative involvement in memory processing. If memory traces are processed during sleep, there should be some changes in neural activity that modify local synaptic functions, or the intrinsic properties or the structure of the neurones.

It appears that reactivation of neuronal populations during post-exposure sleep have been reported in at least two different systems: in the rat hippocampus (see Chapters 12 and 13) and in the song areas of young zebra finches (Dave and Margoliash 2000). At the macroscopic systems level, experience-dependent reactivation has also been reported in human cortex (see Chapter 11).

The data presented in this section suggest that these reactivations correspond to the off-line replay of the information previously acquired during active wakefulness and might play an important role in the processing of memory traces. McNaughton *et al.* (University of Arizona, Tucson) review the computational necessity of this off-line reprocessing of memory traces in a sparsley connected modular brain. They would allow the progressive formation of direct associative connections between lower-level modules and decrease the demand on the indexing system.

In the rat hippocampus, as reviewed in Chapters 12 and 13, neuronal firing is shaped by two separate activities: sharp waves (SPW) and ripples occurring in a state of large irregular activity (LIA) on the one hand, and theta and gamma oscillations on the other hand. The former activities are recorded in restful waking, consummatory behaviors and slow wave sleep. The latter are observed during active wakefulness and REM sleep.

McNaughton and Buzsáki emphasize the role of the LIA state in processing of memory traces.

The off-line processing of memory traces has first been suggested by the similarity in the correlation matrix structure of hippocampal firing patterns between the exposure to a familiar environment and the post-exposure sleep. The replay of temporal sequences of discharges is an even more convincing marker of this off-line processing of memory traces. First, an asymmetry of cross correlograms was shown to be similar in post-exposure sleep to that observed during the preceding task phase. Likewise the replay of sequences involving more than 2 neurons were demonstrated.

Buzsáki *et al.* (Rutgers, The State University of New Jersey) insist on the importance of studying the effect of a *novel* environment on the firing pattern during subsequent sleep. This experimental situation is directly related to learning and memory. They show that, as with familiar environment, the correlation structure observed during the novel task is preserved during post-exposure sleep.

As mentioned in the introduction, further research is needed to confirm the hypothesis that the off-line processing of memory traces is related to their consolidation. Especially, it would be important to relate these reactivations to a change in subsequent behavior.

Reference

Dave, A. S. and **Margoliash, D.** (2000). Song replay during sleep and computational rules for sensorimotor vocal learning. *Science*, **290**, 812–816.

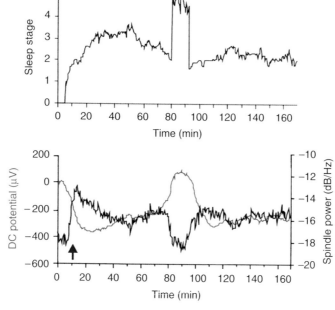

Plate 1 Sleep stages and related changes in DC potentials and spindle power.

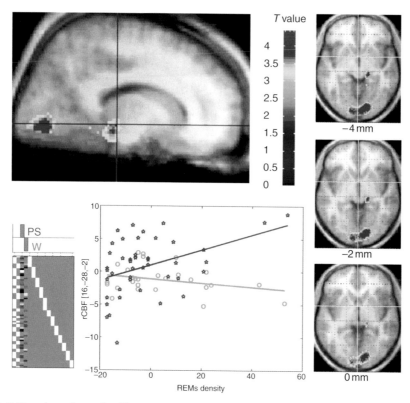

Plate 2 Neural correlates of rapid eye movements during human REM sleep.

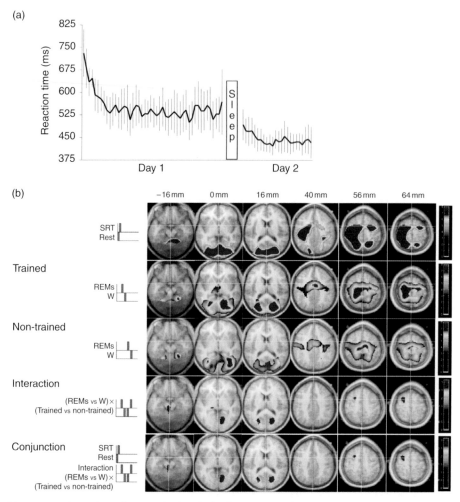

Plate 3 Experience-dependent reactivation during human REM sleep.

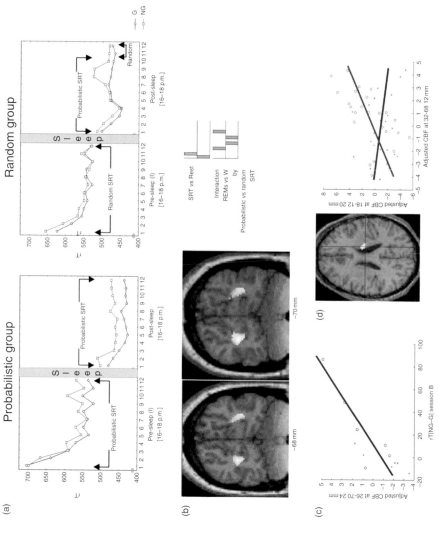

Plate 4 Experience-dependent reactivation during human REM sleep.

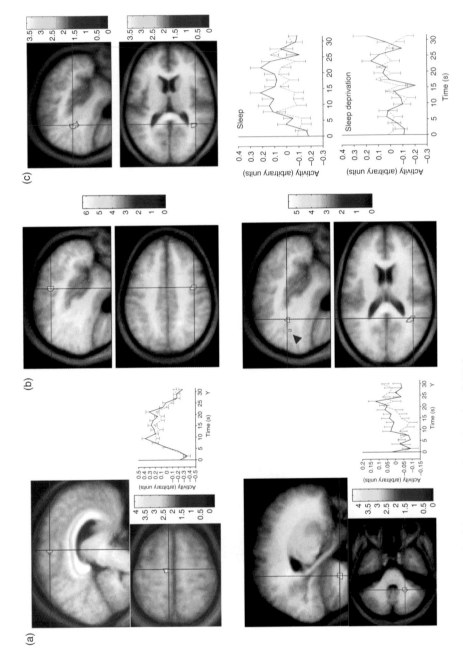

Plate 5 Effects of sleep and lack of sleep on pursuit task learning. fMRI data.

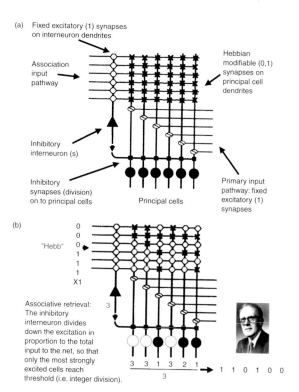

(a) Fixed excitatory (1) synapses on interneuron dendrites

Association input pathway

Hebbian modifiable (0,1) synapses on principal cell dendrites

Inhibitory interneuron (s)

Inhibitory synapses (division) on to principal cells

Principal cells

Primary input pathway: fixed excitatory (1) synapses

(b)

0
0
0
1
1
1
X1

"Hebb"

Associative retrieval: The inhibitory interneuron divides down the excitation in proportion to the total input to the net, so that only the most strongly excited cells reach threshold (i.e. integer division).

3

3 3 1 3 2 1
3

1 1 0 1 0 0

Plate 6 Principles of associative memory.

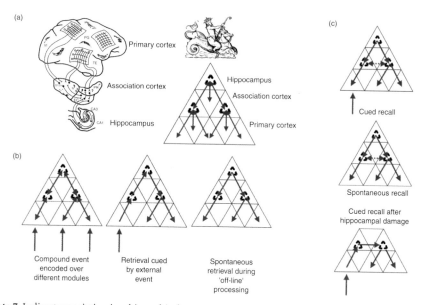

(a)

Primary cortex

Association cortex

Hippocampus

Hippocampus
Association cortex
Primary cortex

(b)

Compound event encoded over different modules

Retrieval cued by external event

Spontaneous retrieval during 'off-line' processing

(c)

Cued recall

Spontaneous recall

Cued recall after hippocampal damage

Plate 7 Indirect association in a hierarchical system.

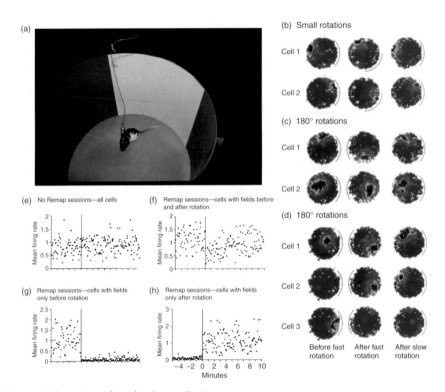

Plate 8 An illustration of rapid orthogonalization.

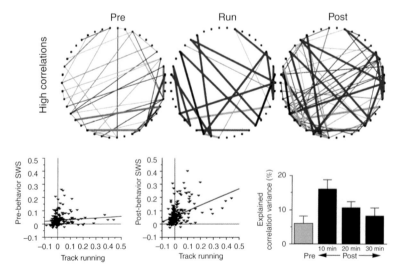

Plate 9 Neurophysiological evidence of memory reactivation.

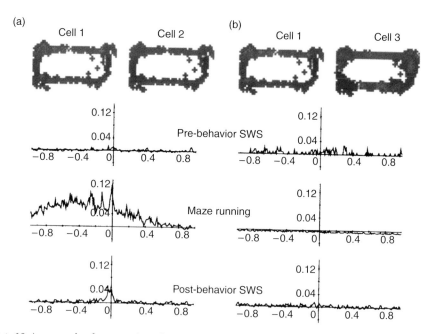

Plate 10 An example of preservation of temporal order of firing during SWS related reactivation of hippocampal activation patterns.

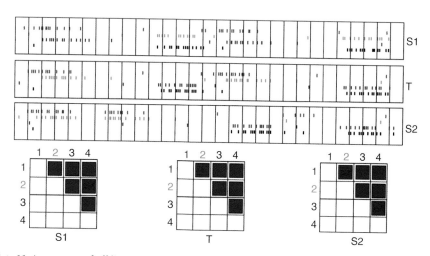

Plate 11 Assessment of off-line memory retrieval in neuronal ensemble recording.

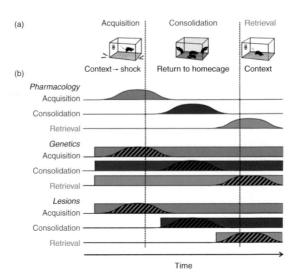

Plate 12 Three stages of memory.

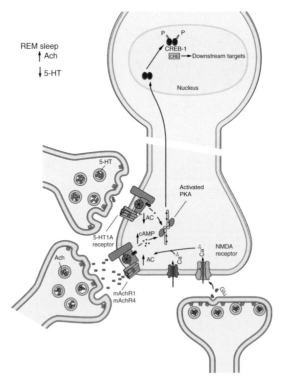

Plate 13 Molecular mechanisms by which REM sleep might mediate memory consolation within the hippocampus.

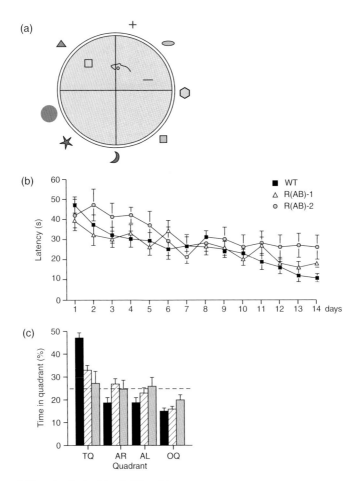

Plate 14 Spatial learning in the Morris Water Maze.

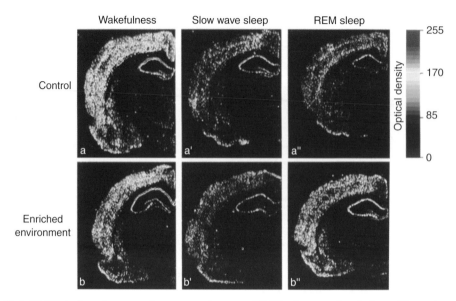

Plate 15 Effect of previous sensorimotor experience on *zif-268* brain expression during waking and sleep states.

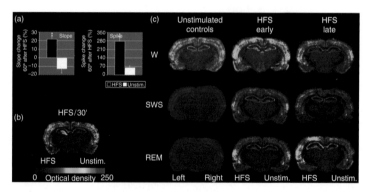

Plate 16 (a) HFS produced significant LTP that was long-lasting and unilateral to the stimulated (ipsilateral) hemisphere. (b) Phosphorimager autoradiogram of a representative *zif-268*-hybridized section. (c) *Zif-268* brain expression levels during early and late WK, SW, and REM sleep depend on prior waking stimulation.

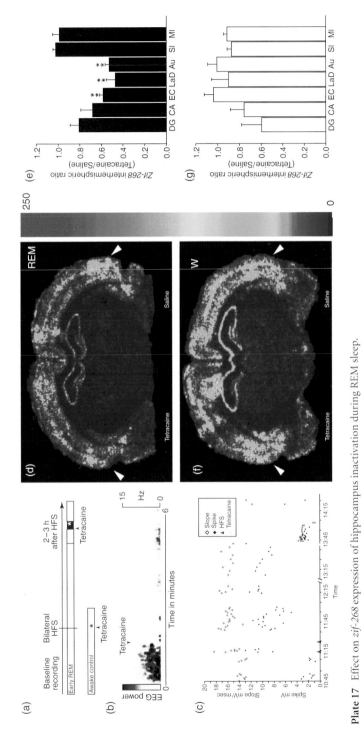

Plate 17 Effect on *zif-268* expression of hippocampus inactivation during REM sleep.

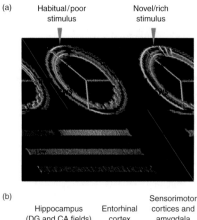

(a)

Habitual/poor
stimulus

Novel/rich
stimulus

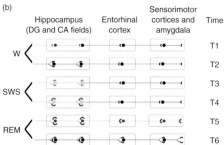

Plate 18 A model of memory consolidation across the wake–sleep cycle.

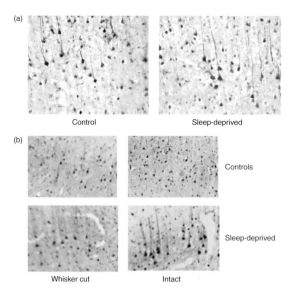

Plate 19 NGF immunoreactivity increases in layer V of the somatosensory cortex after 6 h of sleep deprivation of rats with no whisker cut.

CHAPTER 11

CEREBRAL CORRELATES OF MEMORY CONSOLIDATION DURING HUMAN SLEEP: CONTRIBUTION OF FUNCTIONAL NEUROIMAGING

PHILIPPE PEIGNEUX, STEVAN LAUREYS, AXEL CLEEREMANS, AND PIERRE MAQUET

Introduction

At the level of macroscopic cerebral systems, it is now possible to explore the brain dynamics in humans with a wide variety of non-invasive neuroimaging techniques: electroencephalography (EEG), magnetoencephalography (MEG), near infrared spectroscopy (NIRS), single photon emission tomography (SPECT), positron emission tomography (PET), and functional magnetic resonance imaging (fMRI). Each technique is based on a particular signal and has its own characteristics in terms of temporal and spatial resolution, safety and cost (Toga and Mazziotta 1996). Although most of them have been successfully applied to sleep studies, this chapter will concentrate on the contributions of PET and fMRI. Many aspects of human sleep have been recently reported, but we will focus on two main topics. First, the pattern of regional brain activity during sleep is consistent with the mechanisms described in animals at the microscopic systems level for the generation and maintenance of sleep states. A comprehensive overview of these results can be found in Maquet (2000). This aspect is important because if sleep processes are similar in humans and in animals, the links between sleep and memory processes described in the latter are potentially valid in the former. Second, far from being fixed and stereotyped, regional brain function during sleep is modulated by the individual experience acquired during the previous waking period. We present evidence that these experience-dependent changes in regional brain activity are related to the amount of learning achieved by the subjects prior to sleep and also depend on the material to which the subjects have been exposed. These experiments provide the first experimental evidence in humans for a link between learning, as measured by behavioral methods, and the activity of neuronal populations during sleep.

Functional neuroanatomy of human "canonical" sleep

Here, we use the term canonical to describe all the features of regional brain activity which characterize the typical sleep of normal young humans, irrespective of any circumstantial modulatory factor (previous sleep deprivation, previous waking experience, external stimuli, pharmacological agents . . .).

NREM sleep

For our present purposes, three main points should be emphasized. First, in mammals, the decreased firing in the activating structures of the brainstem tegmentum plays a permissive role in the generation of non-rapid eye movement (NREM) sleep. It is the first move which allows a cascade of events to take place in the thalamo-neocortical networks, eventually leading to the generation of NREM sleep oscillations. Second, the thalamus plays a central and executive role in the generation of NREM sleep rhythms, due to the intrinsic properties of its neurones and to the intrathalamic and thalamo-cortico-thalamic connectivity. The role of the cortex is equally important and begins to be better understood. However, the respective contribution of the different parts of the neocortex in NREM sleep rhythms generation is still unknown at the microscopic level. Third, NREM sleep oscillations (spindles, theta, slow rhythms) are characterized by bursting patterns which alternate short bursts of firing with long periods of hyperpolarization. The latter have a major impact on the regional blood flow, which on the average decreases in the areas where these oscillations are expressed. These points easily explain the basic features of NREM sleep functional neuroanatomy.

As compared to wakefulness, the average cerebral metabolism and blood flow begin to decrease in light (stage 2) sleep (Maquet *et al.* 1992), and their nadir is observed in deep (stages 3 and 4) NREM sleep or slow wave sleep (SWS) (Maquet *et al.* 1990). Regionally, the brainstem blood flow is decreased in light NREM sleep as in SWS (Madsen *et al.* 1991*a,b*; Braun *et al.* 1997; Kajimura *et al.* 1999). In light NREM sleep, the pontine tegmentum is specifically deactivated whereas the mesencephalon retains an activity which is not significantly different from wakefulness (Kajimura *et al.* 1999). In SWS, both pontine and mesencephalic tegmenta are deactivated (Braun *et al.* 1997; Maquet *et al.* 1997; Kajimura *et al.* 1999). The thalamus is deactivated in both light and deep NREM sleep (Braun *et al.* 1997; Maquet *et al.* 1997; Kajimura *et al.* 1999), in proportion respectively to the power density in the spindle and delta frequency range (Hofle *et al.* 1997). The deactivation of the cortex is not homogeneous. The most deactivated areas are located in associative cortices of the frontal, parietal—and to a lesser extent temporal and insular—lobes (Braun *et al.* 1997; Maquet *et al.* 1997; Andersson *et al.* 1998; Kajimura *et al.* 1999). The explanation of this cortical activity pattern is still unclear at the microscopic level (for further discussion, as well as details concerning other structures like the cerebellum, the basal ganglia or the basal forebrain, see Maquet 2000).

It is important to point out here that one of the most deactivated areas is the hippocampal formation and neighboring parahippocampal gyrus (Maquet *et al.* 1997;

Andersson *et al.* 1998). This may be of interest, given the role suspected to be played by these structures in the processing of recent memories during sleep in rodents (see Chapters 12, 13, and 16). However, discrepant results were recently published with glucose metabolism (Nofzinger *et al.* 2002) and further research is needed to specify the metabolic pattern of mesio-temporal areas during NREM sleep in humans.

REM sleep

Details about the generation of REM sleep can be found in Box 7.1 in Chapter 7. A key role is played by neuronal populations of the mesopontine tegmentum. These structures activate the thalamic nuclei which in turn forward this activation to the cortex. The activation of mesopontine tegmentum and thalamic nuclei has been systematically reported in PET studies of human REM sleep (Maquet *et al.* 1996; Braun *et al.* 1997; Nofzinger *et al.* 1997).

In the forebrain, early studies suggested that limbic areas were particularly active during REM sleep. The PET studies definitively confirmed that limbic and paralimbic areas (amygdala, hippocampal formation, anterior cingulate, orbito-frontal, insular cortices) were among the most active areas in REM sleep. Temporal and occipital cortices were also shown to be very active, although this result is less reproducible. The functional interaction between the amygdala and these posterior cortices were also shown to be different in REM sleep than during wakefulness or SWS. These results are in keeping with an interaction between limbic and neocortical areas during REM sleep (see Chapters 12, 13, and 16).

As discussed in Chapter 7, a distinguishing feature of REM sleep in animals is the recording of pontine or ponto-geniculo-occipital (PGO) waves, that is, prominent phasic bioelectrical potentials that occur in isolation or in bursts just before and during REM sleep (Mouret *et al.* 1963). In several mammal species, including nonhuman primates, PGO waves seem to represent a fundamental process of REM sleep, at least to its phasic aspects (Callaway *et al.* 1987), and PGO waves have been implicated, along with various nonexclusive processes, in the facilitation of brain plasticity (Datta 1999).

Animal studies have shown (Datta 1999) that PGO waves are closely related to the generation of rapid eye movements (REMs). Therefore, a plausible hypothesis would be that REMs are generated in humans by mechanisms similar to PGO waves in animals during REM sleep (Salzarulo *et al.* 1975; McCarley *et al.* 1983; Inoué *et al.* 1999). In neuroanatomical terms, this implies that the neural activity of the brain regions from which PGO are the most easily recorded in cats, that is, the mesopontine tegmentum (Jouvet and Michel 1959), the lateral geniculate bodies (Mikiten *et al.* 1961) and the occipital cortex (Mouret *et al.* 1963), should be more closely related to spontaneous ocular movements during REM sleep than during wakefulness. According to this prediction, regional blood flow changes in the lateral geniculate bodies and in the striate cortex are significantly more correlated to ocular movement density during REM sleep than during wakefulness (Peigneux *et al.* 2001*b*, Fig. 11.1). Hence, mechanisms for spontaneous ocular movement generation differ during REM sleep and during wakefulness, and brain

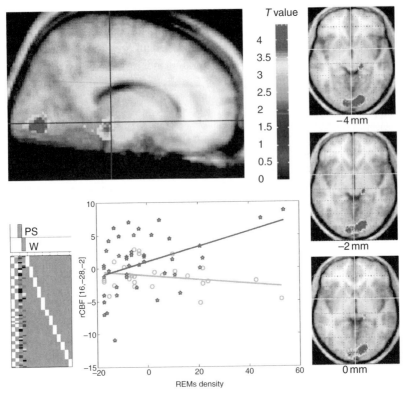

Figure 11.1 Neural correlates of rapid eye movements during human REM sleep. Right geniculate body and striate cortex are more active in relation to REMs during PS than during wakefulness. The significant results are overlaid on a standard MRI scan coregistered to the same sterotaxic space. Upper left panel: sagittal section 16 mm to the right of the midline. Right panel: transverse sections from −4 to 0 mm from the bi-commissural plane. Left bottom panel: statistical design matrix. Middle bottom panel: plot of the regional adjusted cerebral blood flow (CBF) in the right geniculate body in relation to the REM counts. The geniculate CBF is correlated to the REM counts more during PS (in red) than during wakefulness (in green). (Data from Peigneux *et al.* 2001. Reproduced with permission from NeuroImage.) (See Plate 2.)

regions known to be involved in the generation of PGO waves in animals are involved in this phenomenon.

Experience-dependent cerebral reactivations during human REM sleep

If sleep plays a role in memory trace processing, changes in activity should be observed during post-training sleep in the neuronal populations involved in the learning of a particular task. At the time this experiment was designed, animal studies already suggested the replay of waking activity during subsequent sleep in rodent hippocampus.

Based on literature available at that time, we chose an implicit learning task, the probabilistic serial reaction time task (SRT), which allowed both a quantitative measure of implicit learning and massive training of the participants without any ceiling effect (Cleeremans and McClelland 1991). In this task, participants face a computer screen where 6 permanent position markers are displayed above 6 spatially compatible response keys. On each trial, a black circle appears below one of the position markers, and the task consists of pressing as fast and as accurately as possible on the corresponding key. The next stimulus is displayed at another location after a 200-ms response–stimulus interval. Unknown to participants, the sequential structure of the material is manipulated by generating series of stimuli based on a probabilistic finite-state grammar that defines legal transitions between successive trials. To assess learning of the probabilistic rules of the grammar, there is a 15 percent chance, on each trial, that the stimulus generated based on the grammar (grammatical stimuli, G) is replaced by a nongrammatical (NG), random stimulus. Assuming that response preparation is facilitated by high predictability, predictable G stimuli should thus elicit faster responses than NG stimuli, but only if the context in which stimuli may occur has been encoded by participants. In this task, contextual sensitivity emerges through practice as a gradually increasing difference between the reaction times (RTs) elicited by G and NG stimuli occurring in specific contexts set by two to three previous trials at most (Cleeremans and McClelland 1991).

In order to observe the reactivation of brain areas during post-training sleep, we designed a multigroup experiment (Maquet *et al.* 2000). A first group of 7 subjects (group 1) were scanned during wakefulness both while they were performing the SRT task and at rest. The comparison provided a list of the brain areas that are activated during the execution of the SRT task. A second group of 6 subjects (group 2) were trained on the task in the afternoon, then scanned during the post-training night, both during waking and in various sleep stages (i.e. SWS, stage 2 and REM sleep). A post-sleep training session verified that learning had occurred overnight (Fig. 11.2). Here, the analysis of PET data identified the brain areas more active in REM sleep than during resting wakefulness. To ensure that the post-training REM sleep regional cerebral blood flow (rCBF) distribution differed from the pattern of "typical" REM sleep, a third group of 5 subjects (group 3), not trained to the task, were similarly scanned at night, both awake and during sleep. The analysis was aimed at detecting the brain areas that would be more active in trained versus non trained subjects, and in REM sleep as compared to resting wakefulness. Finally, to formally test that these brain regions, possibly reactivated during REM sleep, would be among the structures that had been engaged by executing and learning the task, a conjunction analysis was performed. This analysis identified those regions that would be *both* more active during REM sleep in the trained subjects (group 2) compared to the non-trained subjects (group 3) *and* activated during the execution of the task during waking (group 1). Our results showed (Fig. 11.2) that the bilateral cuneus and adjacent striate cortex, mesencephalon and left premotor cortex were both activated during the practice of the SRT task and during post-training REM sleep in subjects previously trained on the task, significantly more than in control subjects

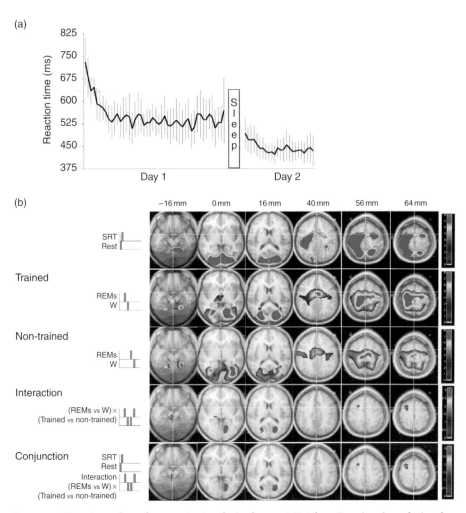

Figure 11.2 Experience-dependent reactivation during human REM sleep. Reaction times during the training and retest session (mean and SEM). Statistical parametric map (SPM) of different contrasts, displayed on transverse planes at 6 different brain levels (from 16 mm below to 64 mm above the bicommissural plane) and superimposed on the average MRI image of the sleeping subjects. First row: SPMs of the brain regions activated during practice of the SRT task during wakefulness, as compared to rest. Second row: Brain regions activated during REM sleep after SRT task practice (trained group), as compared to wakefulness. Third row: Brain regions activated during REM sleep in subjects without prior experience (non-trained group). Fourth row: Brain regions that activated more during REM sleep in subjects trained (b) than non-trained (c) to the task. Fifth row: Brain regions that showed a common activation in subjects scanned while performing the task during wakefulness (a) and that activated more in trained (b) than in non-trained (c) subjects scanned during REM sleep. (Data from Maquet *et al.* 2000. Reproduced with permission from Nature Neuroscience.) (See Plate 3.)

without prior training, suggesting a reactivation process which may have contributed to overnight performance improvement in the SRT task.

Moreover, we further reasoned that, if the reactivated regions participate in the processing of memory traces during REM sleep, they should establish or reinforce functional connections between parts of the network activated during the task. Consequently, such connections should be stronger, and the synaptic trafficking between network components more intense during post-training REM sleep than during the "typical" REM sleep of non-trained subjects. Accordingly, we found that among the reactivated regions, the rCBF in the left premotor cortex was significantly more correlated with the activity of the pre-supplementary motor area (SMA) and posterior parietal cortex during post-training REM sleep than during REM sleep in subjects without any prior experience with the task (Laureys *et al.* 2001). Hence, the demonstration of a differential functional connectivity during REM sleep between remote brain areas engaged in the practice of a previously experienced visuo-motor task gave further support to the hypothesis that memory traces are replayed in the cortical network and contribute to the optimization of the performance.

However, in this first experiment, our conclusions were limited by the fact that we could not specify whether this experience-dependent reactivation during REM sleep was related to the simple optimization of a visuo-motor skill or to the high-order acquisition of the probabilistic structure of the learned material, or both. To test the hypothesis that cerebral reactivation during post-training REM sleep reflects the reprocessing of high-order information about the sequential structure of the material to be learned, a new group of subjects (group 4) was scanned during sleep after practice on the same SRT task, but using a completely random sequence (Peigneux *et al.* submitted). The experimental protocol was identical in all respects to the trained group in our original study (Maquet *et al.* 2000), except for the absence of sequential rules. Therefore, post-training regional cerebral blood flow differences during REM sleep between the subjects trained respectively to probabilistic SRT or to its random version, should be related specifically to the reprocessing of the high-order sequential information. Moreover, during REM sleep, functional connections should be reinforced between the reactivated areas and cerebral structures specifically involved in sequence learning only after the practice of the probabilistic version of the task.

We found a gradual implicit learning of the temporal context set by the prior stimulus through practice in the group trained on the probabilistic sequence (Fig. 11.3). In the group trained to the random sequence, grammaticality effects were not significant during the training session, as expected given the absence of temporal context. During the post-sleep session, in which all subjects were exposed to the probabilistic sequence, grammaticality effect was significant in both groups. Demonstration of increasing sensitivity to sequential regularities during the post-sleep session in the group submitted to the random sequence rules out the possibility that differences between groups in post-training cerebral reactivation during REM sleep could be due to unequal high-order learning abilities.

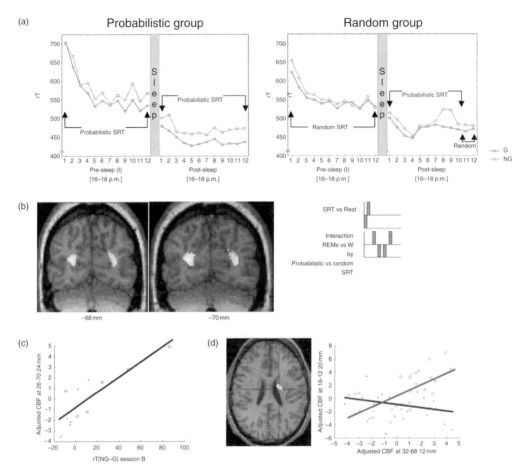

Figure 11.3 Sequence-dependent reactivations during human REM sleep. (a) Average reaction times (and standard errors) per block for grammatical (G; red lines) and non-grammatical (NG; blue lines) stimuli during pre- and post-sleep sessions in Probabilistic (left panel) and Random (right panel) groups. Subjects in the random group were exposed to the random sequence in pre-sleep sessions and to the probabilistic sequence in blocks 1–20 of post-sleep session. (b) Statistical parametric maps of the brain regions that both activated during SRT practice (vs rest) and activated more during REM sleep (vs wakefulness; W) in Probabilistic rather than Random group, superimposed on the coronal section of a subject's normalized MRI at 68 and 70 mm behind the anterior commissure. Activations are displayed at $p < 0.001$, uncorrected. (c) Regression of pre-sleep high-order performance on post-training REM sleep CBF (centered) in the right parieto–occipital fissure (coordinates 26, −70, 24 mm in standard anatomical space), in probabilistic SRT (circles) and random SRT (stars) subjects. (d) Plot of the regression of centered CBF in the right cuneus (32, −68, 12 mm) and right caudate nucleus (18 −12, 20 mm) during post-training REM sleep in subjects trained to the probabilistic SRT task (red circles) and subjects trained to the random SRT task (blue stars). A similar regression is observed between cuneus and caudate nucleus in the left hemisphere. The left panel shows the location of the peak voxel superimposed on a subject's normalized MRI transverse section (displayed at $p < 0.001$, uncorrected. (Data from Peigneux et al. submitted.) (See Plate 4.)

During post-training REM sleep, blood flow in left and right cuneus increased more in subjects previously trained to a probabilistic sequence of stimuli than to a random one (Fig. 11.3). Both groups were exposed prior to sleep to identical SRT tasks that differed only in the sequential structure of the stimuli. In consequence, our results suggest that reactivation of neural activity in the cuneus during post-training REM sleep is not merely due to the acquisition of basic visuo-motor skills. Rather, it corresponds to the reprocessing of elaborated information about the sequential contingencies contained in the learned material.

The processing of recent memories during post-training sleep does not seem to be initiated unless the material to be learned is structured. If the material does not contain any structure, as it is the case in the random SRT task, post-training REM sleep reactivation does not occur, or at least to a significantly lesser extent. These results are in keeping with previous experiments. At the behavioral level, increase in REM sleep duration is observed in rats following aversive conditioning in which a tone is paired with a footshock, but not after pseudo-conditioning in which the tone and the footshock are not paired (Bramham *et al.* 1994). Using a similar procedure at the systems level, tone-evoked responses are obtained in the medial geniculate nucleus (Hennevin *et al.* 1993) and in the hippocampus (Maho *et al.* 1991) during REM sleep after a conditioning procedure initiated at wake, but not after pseudo-conditioning. Likewise in humans, REM sleep percentage increases after learning textbook passages, but only when they are meaningful (Verschoor and Holdstock 1984). A similar situation occurs when the material to learn is so complex that its underlying structure cannot be extracted through practice. For instance, post-training modifications of the sleep architecture (in this case, increases of stage 2 sleep duration) have been reported in humans after virtual maze exploration only when the complexity of the maze allowed subjects to learn their way and form a cognitive map (Meier-Koll *et al.* 1999).

Furthermore, we observed that as compared to the practice of the random sequence, the cuneus establishes or reinforces functional connections with the caudate nucleus during REM sleep following probabilistic SRT practice (Fig. 11.3). The cuneus, which participates in the processing of the probabilistic sequence both during SRT practice and post-training REM sleep, has been previously shown to be activated during sequential information processing in the waking state (Schubotz and von Cramon 2001). However, it is not commonly seen as a critical component of sequence learning. In contrast, the striatum is known to participate in implicit sequence learning (Grafton *et al.* 1995; Rauch *et al.* 1995, 1997) and specifically in the encoding of the temporal context set by the previous stimulus in the probabilistic SRT task (Peigneux *et al.* 2000). The finding that the strength of the functional connections between cuneus and striatum is increased during post-training REM sleep suggests the involvement of the basal ganglia in the off-line reprocessing of implicitly acquired high-order sequential information (Fig. 11.3).

All these results are only indirectly related to learning. We infer that the reactivated areas process the high level material recently encoded because the experimental design contrasted subjects trained to the probabilistic SRT to subjects trained to the random version of the task. We looked for a more direct relationship between learning performance and regional blood flow. We found that in the cuneus, regional blood flow during post-training REM sleep is modulated by the level of high-order, but not low-order, learning attained prior to sleep (Fig. 11.3). In other words, the neural activity during REM sleep in brain areas already engaged in the learning process during wakefulness is related to the *amount of high-order learning* achieved prior to sleep. This result strongly supports the hypothesis that sleep is actively involved in the processing of recent memory traces.

Influence of sleep versus sleep deprivation on recent memory traces

If sleep processes favor plastic brain changes and consolidate memory (Peigneux *et al.* 2001*a*), sleep deprivation should hamper the off-line processing of recent memory traces. We ran a fMRI study where we compared learning-dependent changes in regional brain activity after sleep or sleep deprivation using a pursuit task (PT; Maquet *et al.* in press). We trained the participants on a particular version of the PT (Frith 1973) in which the target trajectory was predictable on the horizontal but not on the vertical axis. Half of the subjects were totally sleep-deprived during the first post-training night (Fig. 11.4). Three days later, during a fMRI scanning session, they were exposed to the previously learned trajectory and also to a new one in which the predictable axis was vertical. This experimental design allowed for the assessment of the effects of learning on brain activity, using within-subject comparisons between learned and new conditions.

Our objective was to provide evidence that sleep deprivation disrupts the slow processes that lead to memory consolidation. In contrast to others (e.g. Drummond *et al.* 2000), we were not aiming to characterize the immediate effect of sleep-deprivation on human performance or cognition. This is the reason why we adopted an experimental protocol where both sleeping and sleep-deprived subjects were retested after at least two complete nights of sleep, that is, in a state of arousal that was similar across the two groups, and between the training and retest sessions (Stickgold *et al.* 2000).

Behaviourally, the time on target was used as the metric of subjects' performance. The time on target was comparable for the two groups during the scanning session, irrespective of the trajectory. The time on target was larger for the learned trajectory than for the new one in both groups. However, the difference in time on target was significantly larger in the group of subjects who slept than in the subjects who were sleep-deprived on the first post-training night (Fig. 11.4). These results suggest that performance gain is maximal only in subjects allowed to sleep on the first post-training night.

The analysis of fMRI data showed a significant effect of learning (irrespective of the group) in the left supplementary eye field and in the right dentate nucleus. The group by trajectory interaction was significant in the right superior temporal sulcus (STS). This suggests that STS is more active for the learned than the new trajectory, and more so in subjects allowed to sleep on the first post-training night than in subjects deprived of sleep during this night (Fig. 11.5). Interestingly, the functional connectivity of the dentate nucleus and the supplementary eye field was different in the two groups of

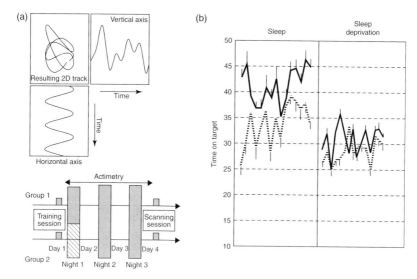

Figure 11.4 Pursuit task: experimental design and behavioral results. (a) Experimental design. Upper panel: The bidimensional trajectory followed by the target during the training session combined a regular movement on the horizontal axis and an irregular movement on the vertical axis. Lower panel: Two experimental groups were compared: half of the subjects were totally sleep deprived during the first night after training on the PT and half were allowed to sleep normally. All subjects continuously wore an actimeter and were scanned while doing the PT on the third day post-training. (b) Behavioral data. Time on target (arbitrary units) during the scanning sessions, in the sleeping and sleep-deprived group, for the learned (continuous line) and new (dotted line) trajectories. Mean time on targets are shown for successive 15-s blocks; error bars are standard error of the mean. Units are the number of 40 ms intervals spent on the target.

subjects (Fig. 11.5). The dentate nucleus was more tightly linked to the STS, and the supplementary eye field to the frontal eye field for the learned than for the new trajectory, and more so in subjects who slept during the first post-training night.

Taken together, these data suggest that the performance on the PT heavily relies on the subject's capacity to learn the motion patterns of the trajectory in order to program the optimal pursuit eye movements. Indeed, interactions between temporal cortex and the cerebellum as well as between the frontal eye field and the supplementary eye field are both implicated in conventional pursuit eye movement pathways (Krauzlis and Stone 1999). More importantly, our data suggest that sleep deprivation during the first post-training night disturbs the slow processes that lead to the acquisition of this procedural skill and hampers the related changes in connectivity that are usually reinforced in subjects allowed to sleep on the first post-training night.

Conclusions

Functional neuroimaging during post-training sleep provides direct evidence for experience-dependent changes in regional brain activity. These changes are likely to be task-dependent. They were shown to be related to the processing of high-level

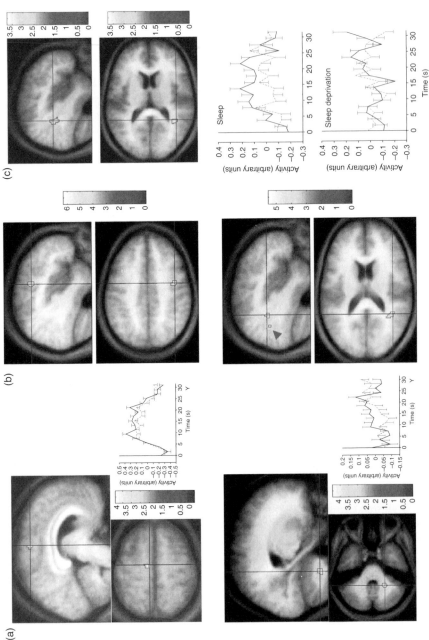

Figure 11.5 Effects of sleep and lack of sleep on pursuit task learning. fMRI data. (a) Main effect of learning. Activation foci (supplementary eye field on the upper panel, dentate nucleus on the lower panel), superimposed on the average normalized structural MR image of the group. Insets show the peri-stimulus time course of the response in the corresponding area (continuous line, responses to the learned trajectory; dotted line, for the new trajectory). Error bars represent standard error of the mean across subjects. (b) Results of the second level analysis based on psychophysiological interactions. On the upper and lower panels, brain areas that are connected respectively with the supplementary eye field and dentate nucleus more tightly for learned than new trajectories, and more so in sleeping subjects than in the sleep deprived group. The red arrowhead shows a second area detected in the STS. Displays are thresholded at $p < 0.001$. (c) Trajectory by group interaction. Upper panel. The superior temporal sulcus is significantly more active in the learned condition in sleeping subjects. The statistical results, displayed at $p < 0.001$ are superimposed on the average normalized structural MR image of the group. Lower panel. Peri-stimulus time courses of STS response (continuous line, responses to the learned trajectory; dotted line, for the new trajectory; top row: sleep group; bottom row: sleep-deprivation group). Error bars represent standard error of the mean across subjects. (See Plate 5.)

material and to be modulated by the amount of learning achieved during the training session. These changes do not involve isolated brain areas but entire macroscopic cortico-subcortical networks. In contrast, sleep deprivation disrupts the processing of recent memory traces and hampers the changes in functional connectivity which underpin the gain in performance usually observed in subjects allowed to sleep on the first post-training night.

References

Andersson, J. L. R., Onoe, H., Hetta, J., Lidstrom, K., Valind, S., Lilja, A., Sundin, A., Fasth, K. J., Westerberg, G., Broman, J. E., Watanabe, Y., and **Langstrom, B.** (1998). Brain networks affected by synchronized sleep visualized by positron emission tomography. *Journal of Cerebral Blood Flow and Metabolism*, **18**, 701–715.

Bramham, C. R., Maho, C., and **Laroche, S.** (1994). Suppression of long-term potentiation induction during alert wakefulness but not during "enhanced" REM sleep after avoidance learning. *Neuroscience*, **59**, 501–509.

Braun, A. R., Balkin, T. J., Wesensten, N. J., Carson, R. E., Varga, M., Baldwin, P., Selbie, S., Belenky, G., and **Herscovitch, P.** (1997). Regional cerebral blood flow throughout the sleep-wake cycle—an (H2O)-O-15 PET study. *Brain*, **120**, 1173–1197.

Callaway, C. W., Lydic, R., Baghdoyan, H. A., and **Hobson, J. A.** (1987). Pontogeniculooccipital waves: spontaneous visual system activity during rapid eye movement sleep. *Cellular and Molecular Neurobiology*, **7**, 105–149.

Cleeremans, A. and **McClelland, J. L.** (1991). Learning the structure of event sequences. *Journal of Experimental Psychology General*, **120**, 235–253.

Datta, S. (1999). PGO wave generation: mechanism and functional significance. In *Rapid eye movement sleep* (eds B. N. Mallick and S. Inoue), pp 91–106. Narosa Publishing House, New Delhi.

Drummond, S. P., Brown, G. G., Gillin, J. C., Stricker, J. L., Wong, E. C., and **Buxton, R. B.** (2000). Altered brain response to verbal learning following sleep deprivation. *Nature*, **403**, 655–657.

Frith, C. (1973). Learning rhythmic hand movements. *Quarterly Journal of Experimental Psychology*, **25**, 253–259.

Grafton, S. T., Hazeltine, E., and **Ivry, R.** (1995). Functional mapping of sequence learning in normal humans. *Journal of Cognitive Neuroscience*, **7**, 497–510.

Hennevin, E., Maho, C., Hars, B., and **Dutrieux, G.** (1993). Learning-induced plasticity in the medial geniculate nucleus is expressed during paradoxical sleep. *Behavioral Neuroscience*, **107**, 1018–1030.

Hofle, N., Paus, T., Reutens, D., Fiset, P., Gotman, J., Evans, A. C., and **Jones, B. E.** (1997). Regional cerebral blood flow changes as a function of delta and spindle activity during slow wave sleep in humans. *Journal of Neuroscience*, **17**, 4800–4808.

Inoué, S., Saha, U. K., and **Musha, T.** (1999). Spatio-temporal distribution of neuronal activities and REM sleep. In *Rapid eye movement sleep* (eds B. N. Mallick and S. Inoue), pp. 214–220. Narosa Publishing, New Delhi.

Jouvet, M. and Michel, F. (1959). Corrélations électromyographiques du sommeil chez le Chat décortiqué et mésencéphalique chronique. *Comptes Rendus de la Société de Biologie Paris*, **153**, 422–425.

Kajimura, N., Uchiyama, M., Takayama, Y., Uchida, S., Uema, T., Kato, M., Sekimoto, M., Watanabe, T., Nakajima, T., Horikoshi, S., Ogawa, K., Nishikawa, M., Hiroki, M., Kudo, Y., Matsuda, H., Okawa, M., and Takahashi, K. (1999). Activity of midbrain reticular formation and neocortex during the progression of human non-rapid eye movement sleep. *Journal of Neuroscience*, **19**, 10065–10073.

Krauzlis, R. J. and Stone, L. S. (1999). Tracking with the mind's eye. *Trends in Neuroscience*, **22**, 544–550.

Laureys, S., Peigneux, P., Phillips, C., Fuchs, S., Degueldre, C., Aerts, J., Del Fiore, G., Petiau, C., Luxen, A., van der Linden, M., Cleeremans, A., Smith, C., and Maquet, P. (2001). Experience-dependent changes in cerebral functional connectivity during human rapid eye movement sleep. *Neuroscience*, **105**, 521–525.

Madsen, P. L., Schmidt, J. F., Holm, S., Vorstrup, S., Lassen, N. A., and Wildschiodtz, G. (1991*a*). Cerebral oxygen metabolism and cerebral blood flow in man during light sleep (stage 2). *Brain Research*, **557**, 217–220.

Madsen, P. L., Schmidt, J. F., Wildschiodtz, G., Friberg, L., Holm, S., Vorstrup, S., and Lassen, N. L. (1991*b*). Cerebral O_2 metabolism and cerebral blood flow in humans during deep sleep and rapid-eye-movement sleep. *Journal of Applied Physiology*, **70**, 2597–2601.

Maho, C., Hennevin, E., Hars, B., and Poincheval, S. (1991). Evocation in paradoxical sleep of a hippocampal conditioned cellular response acquired during waking. *Psychobiology*, **19**, 193–205.

Maquet, P. (2000). Functional neuroimaging of normal human sleep by positron emission tomography. *Journal of Sleep Research*, **9**, 207–231.

Maquet, P., Schwartz, S., Passingham, R., and Frith, C. D. (in press) Sleep-related consolidation of a visuo-motor skill: brain mechanisms as assessed by fMRI. *The Journal of Neuroscience*.

Maquet, P., Dive, D., Salmon, E., Sadzot, B., Franco, G., Poirrier, R., and Franck, G. (1992). Cerebral glucose utilization during stage 2 sleep in man. *Brain Research*, **571**, 149–153.

Maquet, P., Degueldre, C., Delfiore, G., Aerts, J., Péters, J. M., Luxen, A., and Franck, G. (1997). Functional neuroanatomy of human slow wave sleep. *Journal of Neuroscience*, **17**, 2807–2812.

Maquet, P., Péters, J. M., Aerts, J., Delfiore, G., Degueldre, C., Luxen, A., and Franck, G. (1996). Functional neuroanatomy of human rapid eye movement sleep and dreaming. *Nature*, **383**, 163–166.

Maquet, P., Dive, D., Salmon, E., Sadzot, B., Franco, G., Poirrier, R., von Frenckell, R., and Franck, G. (1990). Cerebral glucose utilization during sleep–wake cycle in man determined by positron emission tomography and [18F]2-fluoro-2-deoxy-D-glucose method. *Brain Research*, **513**, 136–143.

Maquet, P., Laureys, S., Peigneux, P., Fuchs, S., Petiau, C., Phillips, C., Aerts, J., Del Fiore, G., Degueldre, C., Meulemans, T., Luxen, A., Franck, G., van der Linden, M., Smith, C., and

Cleeremans, A. (2000). Experience-dependent changes in cerebral activation during human REM sleep. *Nature Neuroscience,* **3**, 831–836.

McCarley, R. W., Winkelman, J. W., and **Duffy, F. H.** (1983). Human cerebral potentials associated with REM sleep rapid eye movements: links to PGO waves and waking potentials. *Brain Research,* **274**, 359–364.

Meier-Koll, A., Bussman, B., Schmidt, C., and **Neuschwander, D.** (1999). Walking through a maze alters the architecture of sleep. *Perceptual and Motor Skills,* **88**, 1141–1159.

Mikiten, T. H., Niebyl, P. H., and **Hendley, C. D.** (1961). EEG desynchronization during behavioral sleep associated with spike discharges from the thalamus of the cat. *Federation Proceedings,* **20**, 327.

Mouret, J., Jeannerod, M., and **Jouvet, M.** (1963). L'activité électrique du système visuel au cours de la phase paradoxale du sommeil chez le chat. *Journal of Physiology (Paris),* **55**, 305–306.

Nofzinger, E. A., Buysse, D. J., Miewald, J. M., Meltzer, C. C., Price, J. C., Sembrat, R. C., Ombao, H., Reynolds, C. F., Monk, T. H., Hall, M., Kupfer, D. J., and **Moore, R. Y.** (2002). Human regional cerebral glucose metabolism during non-rapid eye movement sleep in relation to waking. *Brain,* **125**, 1105–1115.

Nofzinger, E. A., Mintun, M. A., Wiseman, M., Kupfer, D. J., and **Moore, R. Y.** (1997). Forebrain activation in REM sleep: an FDG PET study. *Brain Research,* **770**, 192–201.

Peigneux, P., Maquet, P., Meulemans, T., Destrebecqz, A., Laureys, S., Degueldre, C., Delfiore, G., Luxen, A., Franck, G., van der Linden, M., and **Cleeremans, A.** (2000). Striatum forever despite sequence learning variability: a random effect analysis of PET data. *Human Brain Mapping,* **10**, 179–194.

Peigneux, P., Laureys, S., Fuchs, S., Collette, F., Delbeuck, X., Phillips, C., Aerts, J., Del Fiore, G., Degueldre, C., Luxen, A., Cleeremans, A., and **Maquet, P.** (submitted). Learned material content and acquisition level modulate cerebral reactivations during post-training REM sleep.

Peigneux, P., Laureys, S., Delbeuck, X., and **Maquet, P.** (2001*a*). Sleeping brain, learning brain. The role of sleep for memory systems. *Neuroreport,* **12**, A111–124.

Peigneux, P., Laureys, S., Fuchs, S., Delbeuck, X., Degueldre, C., Aerts, J., Delfiore, G., Luxen, A., and **Maquet, P.** (2001*b*). Generation of rapid eye movements during paradoxical sleep in humans. *Neuroimage,* **14**, 701–708.

Rauch, S. L., Savage, C. R., Brown, H. D., Curran T., Alpert, N. M., Kendrick, A., Fischman, A. J., and **Kosslyn, S. M.** (1995). A PET investigation of implicit and explicit sequence learning. *Human Brain Mapping,* **3**, 271–286.

Rauch, S. L., Savage, C. R., Alpert, N. M., Dougherty, D., Kendrick, A., Curran, T., Brown, H. D., Manzo, P., Fischman, A. J., and **Jenike, M. A.** (1997). Probing striatal function in obsessive compulsive disorder using PET and a sequence learning task. *The Journal of Neuropsychiatry and Clinical Neurosciences,* **9**, 568–573.

Salzarulo, P., Lairy, G. C., Bancaud, J., and **Munari, C.** (1975). Direct depth recording of the striate cortex during REM sleep in man: are there PGO potentials? *Electroencephalography and Clinical Neurophysiology,* **38**, 199–202.

Schubotz, R. I. and von Cramon, D. Y. (2001). Interval and ordinal properties of sequences are associated with distinct premotor areas. *Cereberal Cortex*, **11**, 210–222.

Stickgold, R., James, L., and Hobson, J. A. (2000). Visual discrimination learning requires sleep after training. *Nature Neuroscience*, **3**, 1237–1238.

Toga, A. W. and Mazziotta, J. C. (1996). *Brain mapping. The methods*. Academic Press, San Diego.

Verschoor, G. J. and Holdstock, T. L. (1984). REM bursts and REM sleep following visual and auditory learning. *South African Journal of Psychology*, **14**, 69–74.

CHAPTER 12

OFF-LINE REPROCESSING OF RECENT MEMORY AND ITS ROLE IN MEMORY CONSOLIDATION: A PROGRESS REPORT

B. L. MCNAUGHTON, C. A. BARNES, F. P. BATTAGLIA,

M. R. BOWER, S. L. COWEN, A. D. EKSTROM,

J. L. GERRARD, K. L. HOFFMAN, F. P. HOUSTON,

Y. KARTEN, P. LIPA, C. M. A. PENNARTZ, AND

G. R. SUTHERLAND

It was pointed out in #4.3.3 that when afferent synapses to codon cells are modifiable, only that information for which new evidence functions are required should be allowed to reach these cells. In #4.3.5, it was shown that information from which a new classificatory unit is to be formed will often come from a simple associative store (au add: the hippocampus), not directly from the environment. In #5.1.1 it was argued that the most natural way of selecting the location of a new classificatory unit was to allow one to form wherever enough of the relevant fibers converge. This requires that potential codon cells over the whole cerebral cortex should simultaneously allow their afferent synapses to become modifiable. Hence, at such times, ordinary sensory information must be rigorously excluded. The only time when this exclusion condition is satisfied is during certain phases of sleep.

David Marr (1970), *A Theory for Cerebral Neocortex.*

Introduction

The idea that the brain makes use of "off-line" periods such as sleep to "sort-out" and consolidate memories has a long history, probably as long as humans have wondered about the meaning of their dreams. Computationally principled suggestions for why such post-experience reprocessing should be necessary, however, have a much more modern history (Marr 1970, 1971; Ackley *et al.* 1985), and were at least partly inspired by the phenomenon of temporally limited retrograde amnesia, the so-called Ribot gradient, following damage to the hippocampus and surrounding cortex. In this chapter, we review briefly the theoretical considerations for why the brain might require an active reprocessing of memories during periods when it is relatively "disconnected" from external input, and summarize our perspective on the current understanding of the phenomenon based on neurophysiological investigations in animals.

Cortical hierarchies, indirect association, and the need for off-line reprocessing

The fundamental necessity for off-line reprocessing derives from the most basic model for associative memory: a network of neurons containing a primary (e.g. sensory) input that determines the output pattern, and an association input pathway that is exhaustively (i.e. all-to-all) connected via Hebbian synapses (Fig. 12.1(a)). In the simplest scheme, the modifiable synapses have binary weights that are initially 0 and convert permanently to 1 following Hebb's principle of association. Input vectors (also binary) are of a fixed length, and retrieval of the paired-associate of a given pattern (or pattern fragment) on the association input is accomplished by summing the net synaptic current to each cell and dividing by the number of active axons. The latter operation, which ensures that only those output neurons fire which contain a maximum proportion of already potentiated synapses in the current input pattern, was proposed by Marr to be accomplished by inhibitory interneurons (Fig. 12.1(b)). The physiological and anatomical properties of at least one class of gamma-amino-butyric-acidergic (GABAergic) interneurons are surprisingly consistent with this hypothesis (McNaughton and Nadel 1990). Similar fundamental principles apply to the recurrent version of the "Hebb–Marr" (McNaughton and Morris 1987) net, which can implement the more general case, known as "autoassociation," as well as a simple form of sequence encoding.

The three primary factors that determine the storage capacity (in terms of number of patterns) of such networks are well understood (Marr 1971; Gibson and Robinson 1992; Treves and Rolls 1992): connectivity density, coding sparsity, and "orthogonality". It is the first of these constraints that provides a basis for understanding both the hierarchical organization of cortical association areas and the fundamental necessity for a memory consolidation phase involving off-line reprocessing. In fact, the average connectivity within the neocortex is vanishingly small and thus could not possibly support the encoding of arbitrary associations according to the Hebb–Marr scheme (O'Kane and Treves 1992). In humans, the cortical mantle contains on the order of 10^{10} neurons, but the typical cortical principal neuron receives only about 10^4 connections. Thus, the connection probability on average is only about *one in a million*. To a first approximation, the average connectivity density is closer to zero than to one.

The solution to the problem is to create a modular, hierarchical cortex, in which connectivity is locally dense but the intermodular connectivity is even more sparse. Modularity, in this case, is a relative concept and may pertain to the separation of sensory modalities, the separation of within-modality "feature" maps and even possibly local columnar distinctions. In general, according to this scheme (Fig. 12.2), the individual modules are each capable of storing arbitrary associations within the domain of the inputs they receive; however this makes it even more difficult to support intermodular

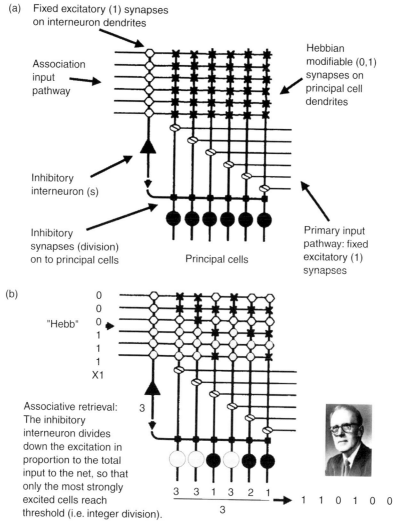

(a) Fixed excitatory (1) synapses on interneuron dendrites

Association input pathway

Hebbian modifiable (0,1) synapses on principal cell dendrites

Inhibitory interneuron (s)

Inhibitory synapses (division) on to principal cells

Principal cells

Primary input pathway: fixed excitatory (1) synapses

(b)

0
0
"Hebb" 0
1
1
1
X1

Associative retrieval: The inhibitory interneuron divides down the excitation in proportion to the total input to the net, so that only the most strongly excited cells reach threshold (i.e. integer division).

3

$\dfrac{3\quad 3\quad 1\quad 3\quad 2\quad 1}{3}$ → 1 1 0 1 0 0

Figure 12.1 Principles of associative memory. (a) The basic network architecture (upper figure) consists of a set of principal neurons that receive a set of primary inputs that impose the output patterns, and a set of binary Hebb-modifiable synapses from an association input. (b) In addition, inhibitory interneurons receive non-modifiable connections from the association input and supply a signal to the principal neurons that is proportional to how many, but not which, association inputs are active. This signal acts as a division (consistent with GABA-mediated shunting inhibition). Associative retrieval in a network in which several associations have been superimposed is illustrated in the lower part of the figure. A stored pattern is presented on the association pathway, but the primary input is omitted. Each principal neuron receives excitatory currents proportional to the sum of the products of the input activity and its synaptic weights. These currents are divided by the inhibitory conductance, and if the result is one or greater, the neuron fires. Provided not too many associations have been stored, only those neurons fire which were part of the original output pattern, because only these have potentiated synapses at all of their active inputs. This scheme depends strongly on the existence of a high connectivity between the association inputs and the principal cells. (See Plate 6.)

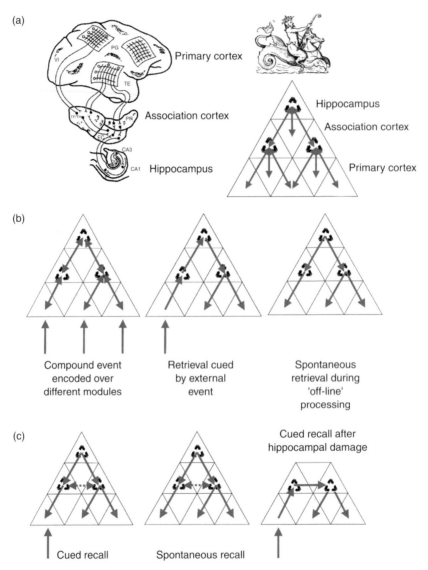

Figure 12.2 Indirect association in a hierarchical system. There are vastly too few neocortical connections to support arbitrary associations in a single layered network. (a) The solution that has evolved is apparently to link lower-level modules, which may have locally dense connectivity, using modifiable bidirectional connections with common higher-level modules. (b) This organization permits both cued and spontaneous pattern completion in lower-level modules. (c) Repeated reactivation of a stored event presumably allows specific horizontal connections to develop in lower modules that ultimately may support the association directly, even after damage to the higher modules. Drawing at upper left from Squire and Zola-Morgan 1991, with permission. (See Plate 7.)

associations. It is possible that the cortex evolved its hierarchical organization to over-come the problem of intermodular associations. If, as appears to be the case, lower level modules are reciprocally connected via Hebbian synapses with one or more higher level modules, then a given pair of patterns encoded in two separate low-level modules would generate a unique pattern in the next higher module. The higher-level pattern would be both stored associatively at that level and fed back to the lower levels via modifiable synapses. The top-down pattern thus would add an extra dimension to the lower level which would serve to "index" (Squire *et al.* 1984; Teyler and Discenna 1986; Treves and Rolls 1991) the corresponding low-level event. Activation of a subevent in one of the lower-level modules would result in associative retrieval of the index pattern, which would then enable associative retrieval of the complementary subevents in the other low-level modules. This *indirect association* thus could enable pattern completion within the set of low-level modules which themselves are far too sparsely connected to accomplish such completion directly.

The principle of indirect association might well suffice, except that it places high demands on the capacity of the indexing system. It would be more efficient to generate the specific intermodular connections that are necessary to support the associations that have already been stored via the indexing system and thus free-up indexing capacity for new memories. This is, presumably, the primary purpose of off-line memory reprocessing. Repeated, spontaneous, retrieval of the index codes would provide the opportunity for growth and selection of the specific intermodular connections necessary to sustain the corresponding association, without the necessity of exhaustive intermodular con-nectivity. In addition, as pointed out by Marr (1971) and others (Alvarez and Squire 1994; McClelland *et al.* 1995), such a gradual selection of connections would also enable the neocortex to develop a more economical, and generalized internal representation of the raw sensory inputs, using some form of gradient descent optimization of the synaptic weights. Such an optimization requires a period of repeated, interleaved activ-ation of the set of memories to be stored, in order to extract and exploit its global correlation structure. As pointed out by McClelland *et al.* (1995), whenever an external event occurs repeatedly, there is no necessity of using the indirect association scheme (e.g. Corkin 2002); however, most experiences occur rarely or only once (Marr 1971), and in these cases, spontaneous retrieval of index codes in the higher modules could guide the gradual development of the requisite horizontal connections among the lower modules. Once these connections are established, the top-down connections are redund-ant and the memory may become resistant to their loss (Fig. 12.2(c)). This explains the Ribot gradient phenomenon.

What do hippocampal neural ensembles "encode": evidence for the index theory

What characteristics should an indexing code exhibit? In many respects, the optimal strategy for an indexing system would be to allocate an arbitrary, random pattern to each event. This "orthogonalization" (Marr 1969) would optimize the indexing capacity and minimize the interference between similar experiences whose identity needs to be kept separate; however, an indexing system has two incompatible requirements: it must be noise tolerant and capable of pattern completion from an appropriate subevent, yet it must also create nonoverlapping patterns for similar events. Neurophysiological studies of hippocampal neurons suggest that this system satisfies these conflicting constraints.

Since the discovery of hippocampal "place cells" (O'Keefe and Dostrovsky 1971) and the subsequent development of the theory that the hippocampus embodies the neural substrate of a cognitive map (O'Keefe and Nadel 1978), there has been much debate as to which of these two theories (index vs place) best accounts for the observed dynamics of hippocampal neuronal populations. The two theories, however, are by no means mutually exclusive. An index code can be viewed as the neural correlate of what psychologists would refer to as a contextual tag (e.g. Gabriel *et al.* 1980), and spatial location constitutes nature's most pervasive context (Nadel *et al.* 1985). A spatial coordinate, represented as an ensemble activity pattern (Wilson and McNaughton 1993) would make an ideal index code, except in those relatively rare cases that important distinctions must be made among events that occur at the same location. There is now abundant evidence that in such cases, the hippocampus is able to generate distinct, sometimes completely uncorrelated "maps" for the same space. It can thus provide unambiguous indices for the separate events (Bostock *et al.* 1991; Markus *et al.* 1995; Sharp *et al.* 1995; Knierim *et al.* 1998). An illustration of this phenomenon is presented in Fig. 12.3. This "index orthogonalization" process is poorly understood at present. In some cases, a change in a single variable, such as the reorientation of the internal directional system, can cause complete "remapping" in the absence of any persistent change in sensory inputs or behavior, whereas in other cases, such as extinguishing the lights, there may be no change whatsoever (Quirk *et al.* 1990; Hoffman *et al.* 1998). This effect represents one of the most important areas of further study. Nevertheless, its existence leads to the inescapable conclusion that hippocampal neurons cannot be said to "represent" anything at all in the traditional sense that we understand the term. Unlike lower cortical areas, there appears, in general, to be no possibility of a priori decoding of hippocampal activity in an unknown context on the basis of observations in previous different contexts. The "meaning" of a hippocampal activity pattern can only be retrieved from the activity that it induces in lower cortical modules, which store the actual data, and are at least in principle, decodable. These are the characteristics predicted by the index theory as outlined in the preceding sections.

Quantification of memory trace reactivation

The first neurophysiological evidence for spontaneous memory trace reactivation in sleep *per se* came from Pavlides and Winson's (1989) study in rats. If a rat was confined to a restricted region of space for 10 min or so, in an alert behavioral state (i.e. probably exhibiting theta in its hippocampal EEG), then "place" cells that were

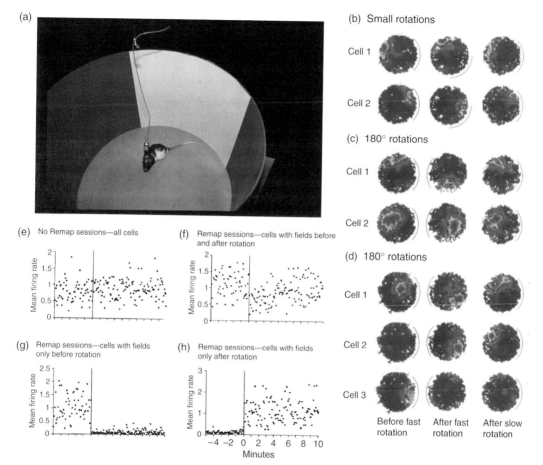

Figure 12.3 An illustration of rapid orthogonalization (Knierim *et al.* 1998). (a) Rats foraged for food in a cylindrical environment (Muller *et al.* 1987) with a single polarizing cue card. The whole cylinder was mounted on a turntable, that could be rotated either rapidly (i.e. above vestibular threshold) or slowly (below vestibular threshold) while the rat was in the environment. During fast rotations, the animal thus experienced a dissociation between vestibular and visual motion cues. Fast rotations were followed (after several minutes) by slow rotations back to the original orientation, to control for possible external influences. (b) After small fast rotations, place fields of simultaneously recorded hippocampal CA1 pyramidal cells always remained aligned with the visual cues in the cylinder. (c) and (d) After fast rotations of 180°, place fields either remained aligned with the visual cues as a group (c) or there was a "remapping" of the cylinder such that the ensemble pattern after the rotation was completely uncorrelated with the pattern before the rotation. Some cells that had place fields originally exhibited different fields; other cells that had been silent originally developed a field; some cells that had place fields originally became silent. These changes persisted after the slow rotations back to the original orientation, demonstrating that they were not due to external cues. Nor was there any change in the animals' behavior. The only altered variable was a change in the relationship between the internal directional sense represented by the directional tuning of head-direction cells, relative to the cue card. The altered hippocampal activity map appeared essentially instantaneously as shown in (f)–(h), in which the average firing rates of the groups of cells that exhibited a change (f), a loss (g), or the appearance (h) of a place field are shown relative to the time of the fast rotation (vertical line). Mean firing rates during sessions in which the place fields reoriented with the cylinder did not change (e). This sudden and complete alteration of the hippocampal code after changing a single internal variable illustrates the fact that the hippocampal activity pattern cannot be thought of as "representing," in the usual sense of the term, anything. Its meaning can only be understood in terms of the corresponding collective activity patterns in the lower modules. (See Plate 8.)

robustly active in this region were selectively more active during subsequent SWS and REM sleep. The observation that the same set of neurons is selectively more active during a sleep session, however, is necessary but not sufficient grounds for concluding that there is coherent reactivation. This would require the demonstration that the same overall pattern of correlations among the discharges within the set of neurons is present during sleep as during behavior. The latter would be the statistical signature of accurate reactivation of the preceding sets of states in the same proportions as occurred during the encoding phase (McNaughton 1998; Kudrimoti *et al.* 1999). The next evidence for reactivation of memory in sleep came from the demonstration by Wilson and McNaughton (1994) that neurons which had strong correlations during the encoding phase (T), by virtue of their spatio-temporal overlap while the rat performed a simple task, were significantly more correlated during subsequent sleep (S2) than the bulk of the other pairwise comparisons, and also more correlated than they had been in the control sleep period (S1). A more complete method for quantifying this phenomenon is the so-called "explained variance" method (EV) developed by Kudrimoti *et al.* (1999), which makes use of the entire correlation matrix (Box 12.1) of the recorded ensemble to provide a quantitative measure of reactivation on a 0–1 scale (Fig. 12.5). If a partial regression is performed, controlling for the S1 distribution of correlations, then the measure reflects how much more similar the T and S2 distributions are, and hence how much T has contributed to shaping the subsequent state-space occupancy distribution of the ensemble. Because this measure ranges from zero to one, its expected value in the null case is nonzero and hence a suitable control measure is required: two candidates are the square of the simple correlation coefficient between S1 and T, and the "reverse explained variance," which exchanges the positions of S1 and S2 in the partial regression. These two measures mean slightly different things, but should both tend to zero if the S1 and T state distributions are completely nonoverlapping.

As discussed elsewhere (McNaughton 1998), an alternative measure would use the similarity of the distributions of the actual state-vectors. Neither measure in its simple form takes into account the sequential order of the states (at whatever bin size they are defined), a fact which enables comparison of the extent of reactivation in different dynamic states of the global network (as discussed below). In addition, with the limited numbers of neurons that can currently be recorded from simultaneously, neither method can discriminate between the case of a memory retrieved frequently but noisily during the reactivation period, and a memory that is retrieved rarely but accurately. The state-vector approach could, in principle, make such a distinction. In any distributed representation, in which neurons each participate in many events, the distinction between related states increases in proportion to the number of recorded neurons. The apparent distance between a given pair of arbitrary memories (pattern-vectors in neuronal state space) increases with the number of recorded neurons, whereas the intrinsic noise of the patterns due to random fluctuations in neuronal dynamics, may remain relatively constant.

Box 12.1 The "Explained Variance" method

The "explained variance" method for assessment of off-line memory retrieval in neuronal ensemble recording can be easily understood by considering the spike trains of simultaneously recorded neurons during three epochs: control sleep (S1), a period during which the animal performs a behavioral task (T), and a subsequent period of sleep (S2) (Fig. 12.4). The firing rates from each neuron during each time bin are determined and then the rate correlations among all pairs of neurons are computed for each epoch. For N neurons, there are are $N(N-1)/2$ unique pairs (i.e. one diagonal of the correlation matrix for the firing rates of the N cells). In the present example, there are four neurons and hence 6 pairs. Notice that exactly which pairs of neurons tend to fire together is dissimilar for S1 and T, but similar for T and S2. Therefore, knowing the distribution of correlations for S1 predicts little about the distribution for T; however, knowing the distribution for T predicts well the distribution for S2. Therefore, the variance among the correlations during S2 is partially "explained" (in the statistical sense) by the pattern in T. By using standard partial regression methods, any similarity that may have existed between S1 and T can be factored out. What remains is a measure of how much memory for the instantaneously occurring spike patterns expressed during the Tepoch is replayed during S2. In the extreme case, if S1 and T are completely independent, and T and S2 are identical, then memory retrieval is perfect. A subtle difficulty occurs when retrieval is less than perfect (as is always the case). An explained variance measure less than one, say 0.5, can arise because the network spends all of S2 retrieving T with 50 percent error, or because it spends only half of the time retrieving T perfectly, and the other half of the time retrieving some completely unrelated set of events, or something in between these extremes. Resolving this ambiguity is a thorny statistical problem. Notice also that the temporal order of the time bins used to compute the spike rates does not enter into the equation for correlation. Thus, the explained variance in the sense defined here does not contain information about the effectiveness of retrieval of sequences in their correct order.

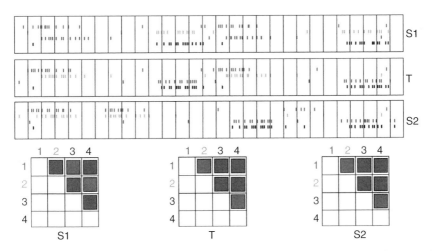

Figure 12.4 Assessment of off-line memory retrieval in neuronal ensemble recording. Spike trains of simultaneously recorded neurons during three epochs: control sleep (S1), a period during which the animal performs a behavioral task (T), and a subsequent period of sleep (S2). (See Plate 11.)

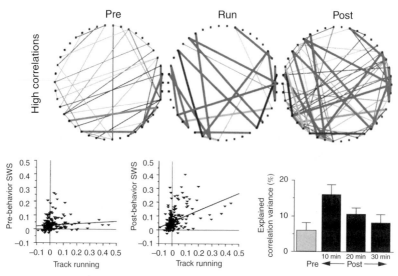

Figure 12.5 Neurophysiological evidence of memory reactivation. The typical protocol for assessing the spontaneous reactivation of recent neural ensemble activity patterns involves an initial period of rest or sleep, a period of behavioral activity, and a subsequent rest or sleep phase (upper row). In the initial studies of Wilson and McNaughton (1994) cells with place fields during the behavior period (Run) were represented as nodes around a circle. The thick lines connecting the nodes represent cells whose activity was highly correlated during Run (due to overlap of their place fields). It is clear that many of these strong correlations were preserved in the activity recorded in subsequent SWS (Post), whereas the correlation pattern during the control SWS period (Pre) were very different. Kudrimoti *et al.* (1999) devised a method of quantifying this effect that takes into account the entire distribution of cell-pair correlations (lower row). In this analysis, all pairwise correlation values are entered into a partial regression analysis that computes how much of the variance of the distribution of correlations in the second sleep episode is accounted for by the distribution observed during behavior, after taking into account the pattern that existed prior to the experience. The simple regression diagrams are illustrated in the first two panels, and the quantitative values of the explained variance are shown in the third panel as a function of time after the end of the behavior session. The first histogram in this panel (gray) represents the square of the simple regression coefficient of sleep 1 correlations vs behavior correlations, whereas the black bars represent the residual explained variance, which is initially high, but declines over 20–30 min. (See Plate 9.)

The LIA state and the role of hippocampal sharp-waves

To a first approximation, the rodent hippocampus exhibits two dynamically different states that are readily observable in their electroencephalogram (EEG) correlates: the theta state occurs during organized, externally-directed behavior and during REM sleep, whereas the LIA state (for large irregular activity; Vanderwolf *et al.* 1975) occurs during restful waking, consummatory behaviors, and SWS. There are identifiable intermediate sleep states (e.g. Skaggs 1995) in which theta is absent, but the neuronal ensemble activity dynamics more closely resemble the theta state, but these occupy a relatively small proportion of the total sleep time. The bulk of the sleep period is taken up by SWS, and 10–20 min of slow wave sleep (SWS) typically precedes rapid eye movement (REM) sleep. Because there is more SWS, and because a recent memory may be to some extent "fresher" during the initial transition from waking to sleep, this would appear to be a useful time for memory processing. Moreover, the presence of sleep *per se*, as defined by other indices such as the initiation by a bout of neocortical spindling and/or a protracted period of resting posture with closed eyes, is not the necessary determinant of reactivation. It appears that the LIA state is sufficient. In contrast, there is no evidence for reactivation during the theta state in waking animals, and, on average, we have obtained very little evidence of reactivation during REM sleep using the explained variance method on rat hippocampal ensembles, following repetitive spatial behavior. Whether the latter failure reflects the ongoing decay of the heightened reactivation, a statistical detection problem, or an intrinsic state effect remains to be determined. Pavlides and Winson (1989) did observe a selective increase in burst discharge in both SWS and REM sleep, in their animals with restricted spatial experience. As discussed presently, this may reflect an overall stronger reactivation measure when the complexity of the state space occupancy distribution is minimized during the T phase. More recently Louie and Wilson (2001), using a vector sequence template matching algorithm have obtained evidence for sequence reactivation or "anticipation" during REM sleep before or after a highly familiar behavioral task.

What dynamics govern hippocampal memory reactivation during LIA? The LIA state is characterized by large fluctuations in total ensemble activity that occur during a recognizable event characterized as a "ripple oscillation" for stratum pyramidale recordings (O'Keefe and Nadel 1978) and a sharp-wave (SPW) for stratum lacunosum recordings (Buzsáki 1986). These signals correspond to the same global event, a large synaptically induced depolarization of the dendrites and a high frequency, but not necessarily synchronous burst discharge of many pyramidal neurons (Buzsáki 1986). The two terms are often used interchangeably. Ripples are somewhat coherent over the hippocampus, have a mean duration of about 50–100 ms, but are locally quite variable in amplitude and duration (Fig. 12.6).

If the ensemble record is parsed into SPW and inter-SPW epochs, the EV measure is observed to be substantially greater during SPWs and may fail to reach significance in the intervening segments (Kudrimoti *et al.* 1999). Thus, reactivation is predominantly a correlate of the SPW event. This is consistent with the behavior of a simulated autoassociative network with stored attractors. Assuming a mechanism for terminating high activity states, such networks, when presented random weak inputs, may exhibit fluctuations between a low-activity "ground" state and a high-activity "memory" state (Shen and McNaughton 1996). Recent *in vitro* neurophysiological and simulation studies (Staley *et al.* 1998) suggest that the high-activity state of the ripple is terminated by the accumulation of presynaptic depression which occurs in most hippocampal excitatory synapses (McNaughton 1982). Although it appears that the ripple is initiated in the CA3 field (Chrobak and Buzsáki 1994) as would be expected if CA3 were the primary

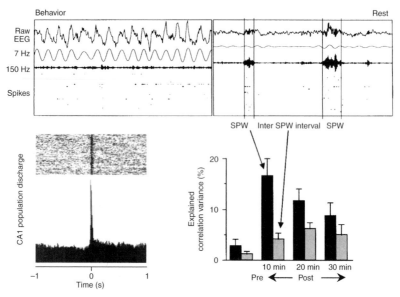

Figure 12.6 Reactivation is strongly focused to the sharp-wave/ripple complex. The upper row illustrates hippocampal EEG (raw and filtered around 7 or 150 Hz) and corresponding ensemble spike rasters during active behavior (left) and during rest (right). The vertical lines designate the SPW/ripple complexes. At the lower left, the sum of the ensemble activity for a period of one second around each sharp wave is shown in raster and histogram form. This illustrates the sharp increase in population discharge during the SPW/ripple events. Because the zero-lag correlations do not involve temporal order, it is possible to parse a data record into SPW and inter-SPW epochs and compute the explained variance due to the behavior patterns separately for the two classes of EEG states. This analysis shows that most if not all of the reactivation occurs during the SPW events themselves (lower right adapted from Kudrimoti *et al.* 1999).

autoassociator of the hippocampus (Marr 1971; McNaughton and Morris 1987; Treves and Rolls 1992), it cannot be ruled out that the recall event is triggered by spontaneous reactivation of a partial event in lower cortical structures, many of which almost certainly express attractor dynamics. Reactivation can be observed for example in the dentate gyrus (Shen *et al.* 1998), and in the rat posterior parietal neocortex (Qin *et al.* 1997). Although the exact temporal relationships of reactivation in these areas to CA3 ripples has not been studied, recent experiments using large scale ensemble recordings in the rat neocortex have revealed widespread modulation of excitability correlated with the peak of hippocampal sharp wave events (Battaglia *et al.* 2001).

Aging, NMDA receptor blockade, and the possible mechanism of reactivation

According to the Hebbian scheme outlined above, a likely basis for the reactivation phenomenon is the associative modification of the synapses involved in encoding the stored state, possibly via LTP, which exhibits the requisite associative properties (McNaughton *et al.* 1978). Two observations suggest that, at least within the hippocampus, this is either not the case or at least not the whole story. Aged, spatial memory-impaired rats exhibit some deficits in LTP induction and maintenance but exhibit no difference from young animals in EV defined reactivation following spatial foraging tasks in familiar environments (Gerrard *et al.* 2001*b*). Likewise, a dose of the systemically administered *N*-methyl-*D*-aspartate (NMDA) receptor antagonist 3-C2-carboxy piperazin-4-yl-propyl-1-phosphoric acid (CPP), sufficient to impair both artificially-induced LTP and experience-dependent place field plasticity *in vivo* (Mehta *et al.* 1997), does not result in a detectable impairment of the EV expression (Ekstrom *et al.* 2000). This may implicate some other associative mechanism underlying the induction of reactivation, that is not NMDA receptor dependent (e.g. Cavus and Teyler 1996).

The experiments to date, however, have been carried out only in highly familiar places and behavioral contexts, and hence it must be assumed that associative synaptic modifications among the relevant neurons had already taken place. This leads to two other alternative explanations for reactivation under these conditions. First, spontaneous reactivation of recently active patterns is possible through nonassociative plasticity mechanisms, if the attractor already exists in the synaptic matrix (Shen and McNaughton 1996). This mechanism involves a nonassociative enhancement of the excitability of this set of neurons, and works only when a relatively small fraction of the neurons was activated in the task phase. Such a selective excitability change biases the retrieval events to those involving the overall ensemble of active neurons (i.e. those which recently expressed a place field) and can produce results that are indistinguishable from a synaptic weight bias. There is at least one candidate mechanisms for such a bias, the persistent reduction in potassium conductance mediated firing rate accomodation that is associated with learning (Moyer *et al.* 1996; Thompson *et al.* 1996; Disterhoft *et al.* 1988). The second possibility arises from the "continuous attractor" concept (Tsodyks and Sejnowski 1995; Samsonovich and McNaughton 1997), in which the coupling of cells with neighboring "place fields" results in a network that may exhibit a continuous random "walk" among neighboring states (rather like Brownian motion in N dimensions) due to the low "energy" barriers between them. Such activity would be analogous to the "delay" activity observed in working memory experiments (e.g. Fuster 1973) in which task related activity persists after the removal of the eliciting cue. In this case, however, the attractor is a continuum of states rather than a fixed point. According to this model, reactivation may reflect not a synaptic bias *per se*, but the fact that the network remains, in a sense, trapped within a set of coupled states, gradually drifting further and further from the recently experienced set, or jumping abruptly to a new one, depending on the "energy landscape" of the synaptic matrix and the "noise" level.

Does affect effect reactivation?

Why are some memories apparently more fully consolidated and apparently more persistent than others? There is an abundance of evidence that the affective value of the experience, whether positive or negative, plays an important role in memory for events that normally depend on an intact hippocampus (e.g. Kesner and Andrus 1982; Kim and Fanselow 1992). There are two possible explanations for such effects, within the framework of the reactivation hypothesis for consolidation. One is that affectively-colored experiences are more robustly reactivated, and hence lead to stronger changes in neocortical horizontal connections. The other is that the reinforcement event induces modulatory signals that act primarily on the plasticity of the neocortical horizontal connections themselves, and that these signals are reactivated in a coherent fashion with the associated neocortical sensory events. Ongoing experiments addressing the effect of both positive and negative reinforcers have thus far failed to reveal any enhancement of the reactivation process (Cowen, Karten, and McNaughton, unpublished observations). We have been able to detect neither an enhancement of the overall reactivation nor a selective enhancement of reactivation of the hippocampal patterns associated directly with the affective stimuli. Although power considerations cannot rule out the existence of a small effect, if present, it does not appear to be of sufficient magnitude to be a plausible explanation for the modulatory effects of affective state on memory. On the other hand, evidence described in a later section does provide some support for the second possibility, that is, that reinforcement signals may be coherently reactivated with the encoded events.

Effects of repetition and memory load on reactivation

As alluded to previously, the number of different states stored during a given encoding phase may adversely affect the apparent retrieval quality, as assessed with current methods. This can be understood in two ways. For activity correlations, the variance of the correlation distribution decreases as the number of different states expressed during the encoding period increases. It tends towards zero as that number approaches all possible states. Because large correlation values disproportionately affect the explained variance measure, the storage and retrieval of small sets of events should be more readily detectable than a large set of events. For population vector-based analyses, the expected overlap with other events increases with the number of events. Thus, in general, both methods are expected to be more accurate if there are fewer "target" patterns. A second consideration is that if the plastic changes underlying the encoding process are not saturated by a single repetition of the event, then a small number of events repeated frequently during a fixed encoding period will lead to more robust reactivation. We recently tested these conjectures by comparing the strength of the EV measure following repeated traversal of a relatively small space (1–2 m of track length) versus an equivalent period of time in which the rats explored a much larger space and hence visited each location rarely, if more than once (Bower *et al.* 2001; Gerrard *et al.* 2001*a*). As expected, in the large space, the distribution of cell pair correlation values was more strongly clustered near zero, and the observed reactivation measure was significantly reduced. The complementary experiment in which space is held constant and the number of repetitions is systematically varied remains to be conducted. At present, it can be concluded that reactivation is reduced following experience in a large environment either because the number of target states is large or because the number of repetitions of each state in the sampling period is low.

Storage and reactivation of memory sequence "snippits"

The population vector and EV methods do not take into consideration information about the temporal order in which events occur. It was pointed out by McNaughton and Morris (1987) that a recurrent version of the Hebb–Marr net is capable of encoding event sequences, provided that the elements of the sequence change relatively rapidly. If not, these nets will either get "stuck" in fixed attractors or exhibit a kind of Brownian motion backwards and forwards within the sequence. It has been speculated elsewhere (Skaggs and McNaughton 1998) that the phenomenon of phase precession described by O'Keefe and Recce (1993) has the consequence of temporally compressing elements of a slowly changing sequence of "place" codes, and might therefore exist expressly for the purpose of sequence encoding. Moreover, during repetitive route following, place fields exhibit the retrograde expansion (Mehta *et al.* 1997) predicted by models in which the recurrent connections develop asymmetry as a consequence of the asymmetric nature of LTP (i.e. presynaptic activity precedes postsynaptic). This expansion is route-specific but not neuron specific and hence is likely to reflect the development of asymmetry in the connections between specific pairs of neurons.

To address the possibility of sequence reactivation, Skaggs and McNaughton (1996) measured the asymmetry of cross-corellograms between pairs of hippocampal neurons during repetitive spatial behavior on a track and during prior and subsequent SWS. During behavior, asymmetric cross corellograms arise because of the partial overlap of place fields that are visited sequentially. There was a significant trend for the asymmetry developed during behavior to be preserved during subsequent SWS, but on a substantially shorter time scale (Fig. 12.7). The reason for this apparent temporal compression is not fully understood; however, there seem to be two possibly related factors. The first is that phase precession leads to temporally asymmetric subpeaks in the cross-corellograms of cells with partially overlapping place fields. These subpeaks are on the time scale of one theta cycle. The second is that, as discussed previously, reactivation during SWS appears to be confined largely to hippocampal SPW events, and these have a similarly brief time course, which would disrupt any long-range sequential correlation structure. A similar preservation of temporal asymmetry, on a compressed time scale can be observed in pairs of simultaneously recorded parietal cortical neurons in rats (Qin *et al.* 1997; Fig. 12.8).

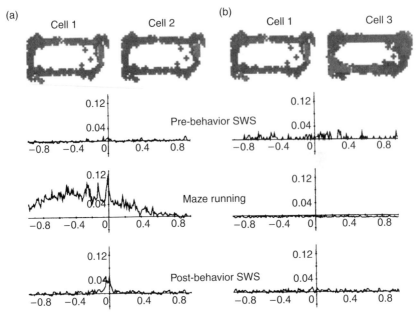

Figure 12.7 An example of preservation of temporal order of firing during SWS related reactivation of hippocampal activation patterns. In this experiment, the rat ran repeatedly around a rectangular track for food reinforcement. Place fields for three cells are illustrated as regions of high firing rate (red) in the upper row. Cells one and two had partly overlapped place fields as indicated also by the broad, asymmetric cross-corellograms during behavior. Note also the asymmetry of the sub-peaks of the cross-correlogram, which is due to the theta phase precession effect. The overall asymmetry is present in the cross-correlogram during SWS after the behavior. Cells one and three had nonoverlapping place fields and were uncorrelated during all three epochs. (See Plate 10.)

Hippocampal readout to neocortex and ventral striatum during LIA

The hypothesis that off-line reactivation, driven by the hippocampus, plays a critical role in memory consolidation leads to two related predictions. First, reactivation should be observed over widespread regions of the neocortex and possibly within some subcortical structures, and second, this reactivation should be coherent both with hippocampal outflow and among the modules that receive this outflow either directly or indirectly. Coherent reactivation between hippocampus and posterior neocortex was observed by Qin *et al.* (1997). Groups of hippocampal and neocortical cells were simultaneously recorded in rats. Correlations were examined among cells within and between areas. All sets of correlations during sleep following a period of spatial behavior were significantly related to those expressed during the behavior, after controlling for the pattern that was present in sleep prior to the behavior. More recently, Hoffman *et al.* (2001) recorded large

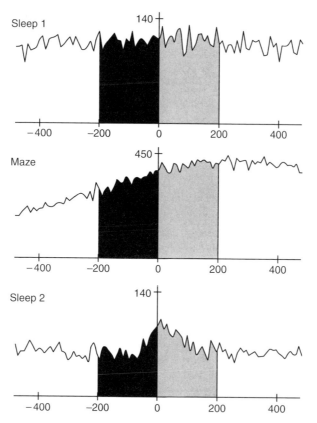

Figure 12.8 An example of preserved but temporally compressed asymmetry in the cross-corellograms for two rat parietal cortical cells (note, these histograms have not been normalized for the total duration of the recording epochs).

ensembles of neurons simultaneously in several neocortical areas in a rhesus monkey. Significant reactivation was observed within and between somatosensory and motor cortex (in opposite hemispheres). Interestingly, however, no reactivation was observed either within dorsal prefrontal cortex or between prefrontal cortex and the other neocortical areas. This negative result is consistent with the hypothesis that the role of the prefrontal system in memory storage may be distinctly different from other areas. Further studies are needed both to confirm the lack of effect and to clarify its significance.

In addition to its widespread direct and indirect output to the neocortex, the hippocampus sends strong projections to two subcortical structures that are important for mnemonic processes: the nucleus accumbens and the amygdala. Reactivation in the amygdala has not yet been studied, but it has been observed in the nucleus accumbens, whose neurons also exhibit modulation during hippocampal sharp waves (Pennartz *et al.* 2001). The importance of the nucleus accumbens in reinforcement-dependent learning, and its close connection with the dopamine systems of the ventral tegmental area, suggests that patterned hippocampal outflow may indeed reactivate not only the sensory patterns associated with a given experience but also the corresponding affective and motor signals. This would provide a basis for the enhanced consolidation of memories associated with strong positive or negative affect.

Overall, it appears that memory trace reactivation is a widespread, although possibly not universal, phenomenon in the brain, and that when and where it occurs it is coherent across diverse structures. It remains for future studies to examine whether and in what manner this reactivation contributes to the establishment of new connections among "lower" brain modules and how the hippocampus acts to integrate and support memories that are distributed across different modules.

The hippocampal–neocortical dialogue

A speculative hypothesis about the nature of the interaction between neocortex and hippocampus during LIA can be proposed on the basis of recent observations on the time course of modulation of neocortical cells relative to the peak of the hippocampal SPW/ripple complex (Battaglia *et al.* 2001). It was observed that for a variable period of a second or more prior to a hippocampal sharp wave, the activity of neocortical cells is significantly attenuated. During the SPW, a (variable) subset of neocortical cells is excited, and then the overall excitability of the neocortex is elevated for a further second or more. Neocortical circuits are known to exhibit slow oscillations (less than 1 Hz) in excitability, that are correlated with high and low states of excitability in subcortical structures such as the striatum. The elevated-activity phase is at least partly an effect of recurrent excitation within neocortical networks (e.g. Sanchez-Vives and McCormick 2000). The observation that hippocampal SPWs are preceded by neocortical quiescence and followed by neocortical activation suggests that the quiescence itself may be a trigger for the hippocampal SPWs and that the SPW, in turn, may trigger a period of cortical processing that substantially outlasts the SPW itself. Judging from the conclusion of Sanchez-Vives and McCormick (2000), the activity during such a period would be sustained by attractor-like dynamics in the neocortex that reflect previously-consolidated memories. It seems plausible to suppose that those previously-consolidated memories may be structurally related to the new memory triggered by the hippocampus. This would provide a possible substrate for incorporation of the new memory into the existing categorical structure of the neocortex, as suggested by Marr (1970) and elaborated by McClelland *et al.* (1995).

Acknowledgments

This work was supported by MH01565, MH46823, NATO Grant CRG972196, and a Human Frontier Science Grant.

References

Ackley, D. H., Hinton, G. E., and Sejnowski, T. J. (1985). A learning algorithm for Boltzmann machines. *Cognitive Science*, **9**, 147–169.

Alvarez, P. and Squire, L. R. (1994). Memory consolidation and the medial temporal lobe: A simple network model. *Proceedings of the National Academy of Science, USA*, **91**, 7041–7045.

Battaglia, F. P., Sutherland, G. R., and McNaughton, B. L. (2001). Widespread modulation of neocortical cell activity during hippocampal sharp waves. *Society for Neuroscience Abstracts*, **27**, 1699.

Bostock, E., Muller, R. U., and Kubie, J. L. (1991). Experience-dependent modifications of hippocampal place cell firing. *Hippocampus*, **1**, 193–206.

Bower, M. R., Euston, D. R., Gebara, N. M., and McNaughton, B. L. (2001). The role of the hippocampus in disambiguating context in a sequence task. *Society for Neuroscience Abstracts*, **27**, 835.

Buzsáki, G. (1986). Hippocampal sharp waves: their origin and significance. *Brain Research*, **398**, 242–252.

Çavus, I. and Teyler, T. (1996). Two forms of long-term potentiation in area CA1 activate different signal transduction cascades. *Journal of Neurophysiology*, **76**, 3038–3047.

Chrobak, J. J. and Buzsáki, G. (1994). Selective activation of deep layer (V-VI) retrohippocampal cortical neurons during hippocampal sharp waves in the behaving rat. *The Journal of Neuroscience*, **14**, 6160–6170.

Corkin, S. (2002). What's new with the amnesic patient H.M.? *Nature Reviews Neuroscience* (in press).

Disterhoft, J. F., Golden, D. T., Read, H. L., Coulter, D. A., and Alkon, D. L. (1988). AHP reductions in rabbit hippocampal neurons during conditioning correlate with acquisition of the learned response. *Brain Research*, **462**, 118–125.

Ekstrom, A. D., Meltzer, J. A., McNaughton, B. L., and Barnes, C. A. (2000). Reactivation of recent hippocampal neural ensemble patterns does not require NMDA receptor dependent encoding. *Society for Neuroscience Abstracts*, **26**, 981.

Fuster, J. M. (1973). Unit activity in prefrontal cortex during delayed-response performance: neuronal correlates of transient memory. *Journal of Neurophysiology*, **36**, 61–78.

Gabriel, M., Foster, K., Orona, E., Saltwick, S. E., and Stanton, M. (1980). Neuronal activity of cingulate cortex, anteroventral thalamus, in hippocampal formation and discriminative conditioning: Encoding and extraction of the significance of conditional stimuli. *Progress in Psychobiology and Physiological Psychology*, **9**, 125–231.

Gerrard, J. L., Bower, M. R., Insel, N., Lipa, P., Barnes, C. A., and McNaughton, B. L. (2001*a*). A long day's journal into night. *Society for Neuroscience Abstracts*, **27**, 1698.

Gerrard, J. L., Kudrimoti, H., McNaughton, B. L., and Barnes, C. A. (2001*b*). Reactivation of hippocampal ensemble activity patterns in the aging rat. *Behavioral Neuroscience*, **115**, 1180–1192.

Gibson, W. G. and Robinson, J. (1992). Statistical analysis of the dynamics of a sparse associative memory. *Neural Networks*, **5**, 645–661.

Hoffman, K. L., Gothard, K. M., Battaglia, F., and McNaughton, B. L. (1998). Self motion updates the hippocampal population code for place in the dark. *Society for Neuroscience Abstracts*, **24**, 932.

Hoffman, K. L., McNaughton, B. L., Lipa, P., Ellmore, T. M., and Stengel, K. (2001). Spontaneous reactivation of recent memory traces in macaque neocortical ensembles. *Society for Neursocience Abstracts*, **27**, 1698.

Kesner, R. P. and Andrus, R. G. (1982). Amygdala stimulation disrupts the magnitude of reinforcement contribution to long-term memory. *Physiological Psychology*, **10**, 55–59.

Kim, J. J. and Fanselow, M. S. (1992). Modality-specific retrograde amnesia of fear. *Science*, **256**, 675–677.

Knierim, J. J., Kudrimoti, H. S., and McNaughton, B. L. (1998). Interactions between idiothetic cues and external landmarks in the control of place cells and head direction cells. *Journal of Neurophysiology*, **79**, 425–466.

Kudrimoti, H. S., Barnes, C. A., and McNaughton, B. L. (1999). Reactivation of hippocampal cell assemblies: Effects of behavioral state, experience, and EEG dynamics. *The Journal of Neuroscience*, **19**, 4090–4101.

Louie, K. and Wilson, M. A. (2001). Temporally structured replay of awake hippocampal ensemble activity during rapid eye movement sleep. *Neuron*, **29**, 145–156.

Markus, E. J., Qin, Y.-L., Leonard, B., Skaggs, W. E., McNaughton, B. L., and Barnes, C. A. (1995). Interactions between location and task affect the spatial and directional firing of hippocampal neurons. *The Journal of Neuroscience*, **15**, 7079–7094.

Marr, D. (1969). A theory of cerebella cortex. *Journal of Physiology*, **202**, 437–470.

Marr, D. (1970). A theory of cerebral neocortex. *Proceedings of the Royal Society of London, B*, **176**, 161–234.

Marr, D. (1971). Simple memory: A theory for arch cortex. *Philosophical Transactions of the Royal Society, B*, **262**, 23–81.

McClelland, J. L., McNaughton, B. L., and O'Reilly, R. C. (1995). Why there are complementary learning systems in the hippocampus and neocortex: Insights from the successes and failures of connectionist models of learning and memory. *Psychological Review*, **102**, 419–457.

McNaughton, B. L. (1982). Long-term synaptic enhancement and short-term potentiation in rat fascia dentata act through different mechanisms. *Journal of Physiology (London)*, **324**, 249–262.

McNaughton, B. L. (1998). The neurophysiology of reminiscence. *Neurobiology of Learning and Memory*, **70**, 252–267.

McNaughton, B. L. and Morris, R. G. M. (1987). Hippocampal synaptic enhancement and information storage within a distributed memory system. *Trends in Neurosciences*, **10**, 408–415.

McNaughton, B. L. and Nadel, L. (1990). Hebb–Marr networks and the neurobiological representation of action in Space. In *Neuroscience and connectionist theory* (eds M. A. Gluck and D. E. Rumelhart), pp. 1–63. Hillsdale: Lawrence Erlbaum Associates, Publishers.

McNaughton, B. L., Douglas, R. M., and Goddard, G. V. (1978). Synaptic enhancement in fascia dentata: Cooperativity among coactive afferents. *Brain Research*, **157**, 277–293.

Mehta, M. R., Barnes, C. A., and **McNaughton, B. L.** (1997). Experience-dependent, asymmetric expansion of hippocampal place fields. *Proceedings of the National Academy of Sciences, USA,* **94,** 8918–8921.

Moyer, J. R. J., Thompson, L. T., and **Disterhoft, J. F.** (1996). Trace eyeblink conditioning increases CA1 excitability in a transient and learning-specific manner. *The Journal of Neuroscience,* **16,** 5536–5546.

Muller, R. U., Kubie, J. L., and **Ranck, J. B., Jr.** (1987). Spatial firing patterns of hippocampal complex-spike cells in a fixed environment. *The Journal of Neuroscience,* **77,** 1935–1950.

Nadel, L., Wilner, J., and **Kurz, E. M.** (1985). Cognitive maps and environmental context. In *Context and learning* (ed. P. D. B. A. Tomie), pp. 385–406. Hillsdale, N. J.: Lawrence Earlbaum.

O'Kane, D. and **Treves, A.** (1992). Why the simplest notion of neocortex as an autoassociative memory would not work. *Network,* **3,** 379–384.

O'Keefe, J. and **Nadel, L.** (1978). In *The hippocampus as a cognitive map.* Oxford, Clarendon Press.

O'Keefe, J. and **Dostrovsky, J.** (1971). The hippocampus as a spatial map. Preliminary evidence from unit activity in the freely-moving rat. *Brain Research,* **34,** 171–175.

O'Keefe, J. and **Recce, M. L.** (1993). Phase relationships between hippocampal place units and the EEG theta rhythm. *Hippocampus,* **3,** 317–330.

Pavlides, C. and **Winson, J.** (1989). Influences of hippocampal place cell firing in the awake state on the activity of these cells during subsequent sleep episodes. *The Journal of Neuroscience,* **9,** 2907–2918.

Pennartz, C. M. A., Geurtsen, A. M. S., Lipa, P., Barnes, C. A., and **McNaughton, B. L.** (2001). Reactivation of neuronal ensembles in the nucleus accumbens during sleep. *Society for Neuroscience Abstracts,* **27,** 500.

Qin, Y.-L., McNaughton, B. L., Skaggs, W. E., and **Barnes, C. A.** (1997). Memory reprocessing in corticocortical and hippocampocortical neuronal ensembles. *Philosophical Transactions of the Royal Society, Series B,* **352,** 1525–1533.

Quirk, G. J., Muller, R. U., and **Kubie, J. L.** (1990). The firing of hippocampal place cells in the dark depends on the rat's recent experience. *The Journal of Neuroscience,* **10,** 2008–2017.

Samsonovich, A. and **McNaughton, B. L.** (1997). Path integration and cognitive mapping in a continuous attractor neural network model. *The Journal of Neuroscience,* **17,** 5900–5920.

Sanchez-Vives, M. V. and **McCormick, D. A.** (2000). Cellular and network mechanisms of rhythmic recurrent activity in neocortex. *Nature Neuroscience,* **3,** 1027–1033.

Sharp, P. E., Blair, H. T., Etkin, D., and **Tzanetos, D. B.** (1995). Influences of vestibular and visual motion information on the spatial firing patterns of hippocampal place cells. *The Journal of Neuroscience,* **15**(1), 173–189.

Shen, B. and **McNaughton, B. L.** (1996). Modeling the spontaneous reactivation of experience-specific hippocampal cell assembles during sleep. *Hippocampus,* **6,** 685–692.

Shen, J., Kudrimoti, H. S., McNaughton, B. L., and **Barnes, C. A.** (1998). Reactivation of neuronal ensembles in hippocampal dentate gyrus during sleep after spatial experience. *Journal of Sleep Research,* **7,** 6–16.

Skaggs, W. E. (1995). Relations between the theta rhythm and activity patterns of hippocampal neurons. Dissertation, University of Arizona, Tucson, Arizona.

Skaggs, W. E. and **McNaughton, B. L.** (1996). Replay of neuronal firing sequences in rat hippocampus during sleep following spatial experience. *Science*, **271**, 1870–1873.

Skaggs, W. E. and **McNaughton, B. L.** (1998). Spatial firing properties of hippocampal CA1 populations in an environment containing two visually identical regions. *The Journal of Neuroscience*, **18**, 8455–8466.

Squire, L. R. and **Zola-Morgan, S.** (1991). The medial temporal lobe memory system. *Science*, **253**, 1380–1386.

Squire, L. R., Cohen, N. J., and **Nadel, L.** (1984). The medial temporal region and memory consolidation: A new hypothesis. In *Memory consolidation* (eds G. Weingartner and E. Parker), pp. 185–210. Hillsdale: Erlbaum.

Staley, K. J., Longacher, M., Bains, J. S., and **Yee, A.** (1998). Presynaptic modulation of CA3 network activity. *Nature Neuroscience*, **1**, 201–209.

Teyler, T. J. and **Discenna, P.** (1986). The hippocampal memory indexing theory. *Behavioral Neuroscience*, **100**, 147–154.

Thompson, L. T., Moyer, J. R. J., and **Disterhoft, J. F.** (1996). Transient changes in excitability of rabbit CA3 neurons with a time course appropriate to support memory consolidation. *Journal of Neurophysiology*, **76**, 1836–1849.

Treves, A. and **Rolls, E. T.** (1991). What determines the capacity of autoassociative memories in the brain? *Network*, **2**, 371–397.

Treves, A. and **Rolls, E. T.** (1992). Computational constraints suggest the need for two distinct input systems to the hippocampal CA3. *Hippocampus*, **2**, 189–200.

Tsodyks, M. and **Sejnowski, T.** (1995). Associative memory and hippocampal place cells. *International Journal of Neural Systems*, **6**(Suppl.), 81–86.

Vanderwolf, C. H., Kramis, R., Gillespie, L. A., and **Bland, B. H.** (1975). Hippocampal rhythmic slow activity and neocortical low-voltage fast activity: Relations to behavior. In *The hippocampus* (eds R. L. Isaacson and K. H. Pribram), Vol. 2, pp. 101–128. New York: Plenum Press.

Wilson, M. A. and **McNaughton, B. L.** (1993). Dynamics of the hippocampal ensemble code for space. *Science*, **261**, 1055–1058.

Wilson, M. A. and **McNaughton, B. L.** (1994). Reactivation of hippocampal ensemble memories during sleep. *Science*, **265**, 676–679.

CHAPTER 13

MAINTENANCE AND MODIFICATION OF FIRING RATES AND SEQUENCES IN THE HIPPOCAMPUS: DOES SLEEP PLAY A ROLE?

GYÖRGY BUZSÁKI, DANIEL CARPI, JOZSEF CSICSVARI, GEORGE DRAGOI, KENNETH HARRIS, DARRELL HENZE, AND HAJIME HIRASE

The means by which large collections of neurons, within and across the vast regions of the brain, can effectively interact is not well understood. Nevertheless, it is clear that these interactions are fundamentally different in states of waking and sleep. The reason for this functional dichotomy is not well understood. It is not impossible that all important actions of the brain are performed in the waking state, leaving no or very little function to sleep. Alternatively, the waking and sleeping brain may cooperate in a meaningful manner. The sleep–wake interaction has some striking characteristics at the hippocampal–neocortical interface and might serve various functional/cognitive/computational processes. Some of these hypothesized processes are maintaining or altering synaptic functions, intrinsic properties of neurons or changing their morphological features. These relatively permanent changes are usually referred to by the term memory representation.

It has been repeatedly claimed that sleep may assist in altering neuronal communication thereby consolidating or erasing information (memories) gathered in the waking brain. This would be a very useful contribution of sleep. After all, we spend one third of our life time in sleep. According to the general two-step framework, initial "encoding" of the events occurs during learning and the encoded events will "consolidate" during sleep. These issues have been recently reviewed by several excellent papers (Guzowski *et al.* 2001; Maquet 2001; Stickgold *et al.* 2001). In most sequential models, however, the nature of sleep critical to memory formation is either not stated or claimed flatly that the rapid eye movement (REM) sleep stage is responsible for benevolent effects of sleep (Karni *et al.* 1994). The idea that REM sleep is the critical ingredient of sleep responsible for memory consolidation likely derives from the association of dreams and REM sleep (Aserinsky 1996). Since dreams may reflect (some) events experienced in the waking state (cf. Winson 1990), it was logical to assume that rehearsal of learned information in dreams could make repeated use of the brain hardware during sleep (Winson 1990; Karni *et al.* 1994; Louie and Wilson 2001).

We have some issues with REM sleep as the critical sleep stage for memory consolidation. First, there is no known mechanism in action during REM sleep that is not present in the "aroused" waking brain. So what special processes are at work in REM sleep that cannot happen in the awake brain? Second, the link between performance gain and REM sleep is very weak (Siegel 2001). Third, chronic elimination of REM sleep and dreams in patients using various antidepressants does not induce memory problems (cf. Vertes and Eastman 2000). Fourth, all animals sleep or rest and learn but only mammals developed REM sleep episodes (Hobson 1995). Finally, if REM sleep can do it all, we are still wasting more than one quarter of our life-time in slow wave sleep (SWS). The contribution of the senior author to the sleep–memory debate was the suggestion that it is SWS that may be critical for consolidating learned information (Buzsáki 1989).

Two-stage model of memory trace formation

The gross EEG states of the hippocampus and associated structures alternate between theta/gamma oscillations and sharp waves (SPW) associated with fast (140–200 Hz) ripples in the CA1 pyramidal layer. Whereas theta oscillations represent a consortium of various structures and intrinsic cellular mechanisms (cf. Bland 1986; Vertes and Kocsis 1997; Buzsáki 2002), SPWs are endogenous to the hippocampus and emerge in the excitatory recurrent circuits of the CA3 region (Buzsáki *et al.* 1983, 1992; Buzsáki 1986; Csicsvari *et al.* 2000). SPWs are transient (40–100 ms) population bursts that involve synchronous discharge of 40,000–80,000 neurons in the CA3–CA1-subicular complex–entorhinal cortex axis (Chrobak and Buzsáki 1994, 1998). SPWs and ripples are present in the hippocampus of all mammals investigated, including humans (Bragin *et al.* 1999). Several features of SPW burst make this network pattern an excellent candidate for inducing neuronal plasticity. First, the time window of the SPW population burst roughly corresponds to the time constant of the NMDA receptor, through which Ca^{2+}, the key ion for the induction of synaptic plasticity, can enter (cf. Kandel 2001). Second, the oscillatory network output (140–200 Hz) is the ideal frequency range for initiating long-term potentiation (LTP; Douglas and Goddard 1975). Third, during the burst there is a 3–5-fold gain of network excitability (Csicsvari *et al.* 1999), creating an ideal condition for synaptic potentiation (Gustafsson and Wigström 1986). SPW burst is an output pattern of the hippocampus, making it possible to transfer information (i.e. neuronal patterns) to neocortical structures (Chrobak and Buzsáki 1994; Siapas and Wilson 1998).

Neuronal activity during sleep can be useful in at least two ways for synaptic plasticity. First, neurons can discharge independently and randomly, thereby erasing synaptic modifications brought about by the awake brain. The expected result is a fresh "tabula rasa" every morning ready to be filled with the excitements of the new day (Crick and Mitchison 1983). Alternatively, neuronal pathways used and modified in the awake

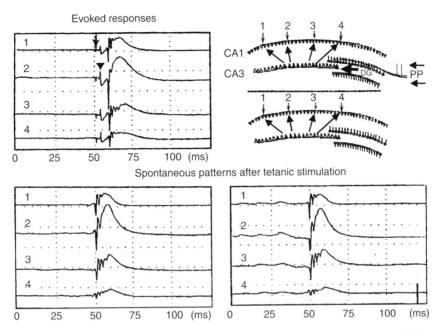

Figure 13.1 Synaptic modification of the CA3 recurrent circuit influences spontaneous population recruitment of neurons. Single pulses of perforant path (PP) stimulation induces a population spike of granule cells (triangle) and trisynaptically evoked population spikes in CA1 (example of a single evoked response in a fimbria-fornix damaged rat). Following tetanic stimulation of PP spontaneous bursts emerge from the CA3 region. Note the similar spatio-temporal distribution of CA1 population spikes in the evoked responses and spontaneous events, indicating similar synaptic routes of recruitment (after Buzsáki 1989).

brain can be replayed repeatedly, perhaps at some altered temporal scale. The repeated activation of the same neurons and same synapses can be useful because some of the underlying molecular processes, for example, synaptic potentiation, are quite protracted (Frey *et al.* 1993). The same principles apply to any sleep patterns, including SPW bursts. In order for the SPW burst to be useful for its desired purpose, it should have a content and the content should be modifiable. The idea that this is a viable mechanism came from a simple experiment, designed to study epileptic patterns rather than memory trace formation *per se* (Fig. 13.1).

In the subcortically deafferented hippocampus, rather stereotypic, large amplitude population bursts occur intermittently (Buzsáki *et al.* 1989). The source and mechanisms of these spontaneous hypersynchronous events are similar to SPWs, except that they are shorter and larger in amplitude. These events display a characteristic waveshape distribution along the septohippocampal axis of the CA1 region, indicating that they are initiated from a localized focus of the CA3 region (Wong and Traub 1983). Importantly, we found that the spatial patterns of these exaggerated SPW burst-like events could be modified. Single pulse stimulation of the perforant path evoked trisynaptic responses with a stereotyped spatial distribution (Fig. 13.1). Tetanic activation of the perforant path leads to the spontaneous occurrence of hypersynchronous population events whose morphology and spatial distribution were identical with the evoked responses, except that they were not preceded by a population discharge of the granule cells (Fig. 13.1). Subsequent tetanization of different subsets of afferents induced different spontaneous population burst patterns.

The simplest interpretation of the above experiment is that tetanic stimulation of the main hippocampal input, the perforant path, changed the synaptic weights within the CA3 recurrent system. Subsets of CA3 neurons with the strongest synaptic connectivity, as a result of afferent activation, became "burst initiators" of subsequently emerging spontaneous population bursts. In essence, cells that were activated by the tetanic input continued to burst together spontaneously. On the bases of these and other related observations it was speculated that similar changes may take place during natural behavior. Specifically, during learning, associated with theta oscillation, task specific activation of the entorhinal input will bring about synaptic changes in the recurrent CA3 system. In the subsequent non-theta state the previously activated neurons are reactivated in a time-compressed manner during SPW bursts. As a result, the behaviorally induced synaptic strengths will be maintained and the "memory representation" in the CA3 region can be transferred to neocortical targets. Details of this two-stage model have been elaborated elsewhere (Buzsáki 1989, 1996, 1998; Chrobak and Buzsáki 1998; Lörincz and Buzsáki 2000). Because SPW bursts occur during immobility, consummatory behaviors, and mostly during SWS, it was inferred that a main function of SWS is consolidation of learned information and the slow transfer of hippocampal content to the neocortex. Some specific predictions of the model are that (i) neurons do not randomly participate in SPW bursts, (ii) synaptic connectivity, firing rates and population patterns in subsequent sleep episodes remain similar unless specifically altered by awake experience, and (iii) SPWs may serve as a mechanism to induce synaptic plasticity. To date, experimental evidence for the model, as discussed below and elsewhere in this book, is still quite slim.

Similarity of long-term firing rates and co-activation in the waking and sleeping brain

The first electrophysiological investigation to examine firing relationship of neuronal patterns in the wake–sleep cycle recorded pairs of CA1 pyramidal neurons during exploration–sleep cycles (Pavlides and Winson 1989). One cell of the pair was a place cell (O'Keefe and Nadel 1978) and the rat was confined physically to the cell's place field to ensure prolonged activation of the neuron. The main finding was that the neuron with sustained activity during exploration continued to fire at a higher rate during subsequent SWS and REM sleep, relative to the control cell. This early experiment was carried out using single wires. Judging from the long bursts of units and the multiple field of most units recorded, isolation of single cells was likely not successful in each case.

Subsequent experiments, using large-scale recordings, did not confirm the suggested correlation between firing rates in the awake and sleeping animal. On the other hand, these studies reported that pyramidal cells with overlapping place fields preserved their pairwise temporal correlations during subsequent sleep but were not correlated with co-activated cell pairs recorded from a sleep episode preceding the awake session (Wilson and McNaughton 1994; Skaggs and McNaughton 1996). Although these physiological experiments were discussed in support of the beneficial role of sleep in learning, it is important to recognize that in the above experiments no learning took place. The rats were exposed to the same environment numerous times prior to the recording session. What was demonstrated is that cells that were co-activated in a 100-ms time windows in the testing apparatus continued to be co-activated in the subsequent sleep period. Surprisingly, the co-activation patterns in the sleep episodes preceding and following the daily routine in the test apparatus were dramatically different (Wilson and McNaughton 1994; Skaggs and McNaughton, 1996). In other words, 24 h after the previous day's experience neuronal activity during sleep did not predict the co-activation of the neurons in a well-learned task. These findings were thus interpreted that no long-term savings are gained by subsequent sleep episodes and co-activation decays with a time constant of approximately 15–30 min. If the effect of awake experience disappears so quickly then what rules apply to firing patterns for the remaining part of sleep? Thus, these physiological observations are in sharp contrast with the beneficial behavioral effects of slow wave sleep in humans where long-term savings have been demonstrated (see Chapters 2 and 3).

The above findings are surprising because if the animal performs the same task repeatedly in an unchanging environment, the sensory and motor-feedback inputs are expected to activate defined subsets of the neuronal populations in the various levels of the neuraxis. For example, the same sets of hippocampal pyramidal cells are re-activated in the same testing apparatus over days or weeks (O'Keefe and Nadel 1978; Thompson and Best 1990). This reactivation may be so because anatomical wiring, synaptic weights and intrinsic properties of the neurons involved do not substantially change over time. If this assumption is correct then the discharge rates and patterns of individual neurons in the presence and absence of external sensory signals (e.g. during sleep) are expected to correlate. Furthermore, if routine, well-learned tasks are performed between sleep episodes, then one might expect that neuronal patterns in those sleep episodes should also be similar. We tested this conjecture by comparing firing rates and co-activation of neurons of neuronal groups in sleep episodes interrupted by performance in a well-trained task, such as food foraging in an open field and running in a wheel.

Discharge frequency of simultaneously recorded pyramidal cells remained remarkably stable across several sleep-wave cycles (up to 10 h tested). Neurons with high firing rates during wheel running (associated with theta oscillation) continued to fire at a high rate while the rat was drinking or staying immobile. Similarly, fast-firing neurons in slow wave sleep sustained their relative high rates during REM sleep (Fig. 13.2; Hirase *et al.* 2001). When firing rates of neuronal populations were compared in two subsequent sleep

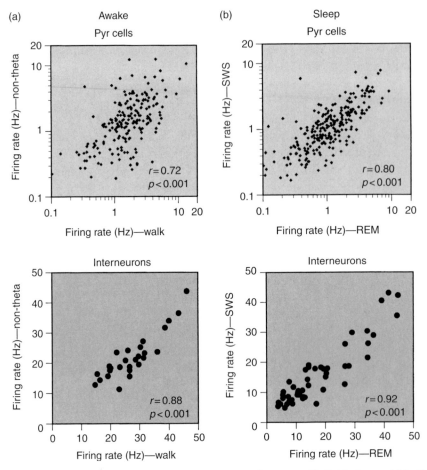

Figure 13.2 Short-term (<30 min) comparison of discharge frequency of individual pyramidal cells and interneurons during different behavioral states. (a) Relationship between firing rates during running in wheel and walking in box (theta behaviors) and drinking/immobility (non-theta). (b) Relationship between firing rates during REM sleep and SWS. The high correlation of firing rates across different stages of sleep indicates that similar cell assemblies are being activated in both SWS and REM sleep (after Hirase *et al.* 2001).

episodes, interrupted by a session in the wheel apparatus or food foraging in an open field, discharge frequencies of individual cells robustly correlated (Fig. 13.3). Similar observations were made on co-activated cell pairs. Neuron pairs with overlapping place fields had higher temporal correlation in the awake rat than pairs with nonoverlapping fields (see also Kudrimoti *et al.* 1999). Confirming previous results (Wilson and McNaughton 1994; Skaggs and McNaughton 1996), the cell pairs with high awake correlation continued to have significantly higher correlation in the subsequent sleep episode than pairs with low awake temporal co-activation. However, this relationship was true also for

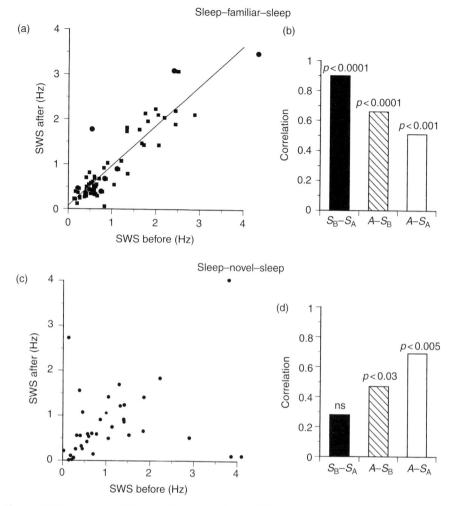

Figure 13.3 Comparison of discharge frequency of pyramidal cells in two successive SWS episodes, interrupted either by a wheel running session (a, Familiar) or novel exploration (c, Novel). "Wheel cells" (filled gray circles) are shown separately in (a), (b), and (d), Mean correlation values for "sleep before" vs "sleep after" (S_B–S_A), "awake" vs "sleep before" (A–S_B) and "awake" vs "sleep after" (A–S_A) sessions in the well-trained running wheel task (b) and in the novel environment (d). Note high and low correlations between successive sleep sessions in the familiar and novel environments, respectively (after Hirase *et al.* 2001).

neuron pairs examined in the preceding sleep episodes. Importantly, co-activation patterns in the sleep episodes preceding and following the awake session strongly correlated. Similar to these observations, Kudrimoti *et al.* (1999) also reported that co-activation patterns during a routine awake behavior could sometimes be predicted from patterns analyzed during the preceding sleep episode.

Altogether the above findings demonstrate that firing patterns observed in a well-learned stereotyped behavioral task are correlated with similar patterns in the sleeping animal. Firing rates correlated not only between awake and SWS states but also between SWS and REM sleep (Pavlides and Winson 1989; Hirase *et al.* 2001). In a recent study, firing patterns of simultaneously recorded pyramidal cells in the awake rat were "replayed" in real time during REM sleep of a subsequent sleep episode (Louie and Wilson 2001). Furthermore, such uncompressed replay of firing patterns was also observed in zebra finches (Dave and Margoliash 2000). The spontaneous activity in the premotor area of the song system during sleep resembled closely the pattern of activity present in the singing bird. Nevertheless, these correlations do not demonstrate that sleep has played any special role in the conservation of firing patterns. One can argue that the correlation of firing rates and pairwise co-activation patterns in the above experiments simply demonstrate the stability of a hard-wired system, rather than learning-based modification of synaptic weights or intrinsic neuronal mechanisms. A possible way to attribute a causal link to the sleep-wake correlations is to perturb them by novel experience.

Experience in a novel environment may alter firing patterns in subsequent sleep

Although a main issue is whether learning can alter synaptic connectivity in such a persistent way that the ensued changes can be detected in subsequent sleep episode(s), to date, very few physiological experiments examined the role of learning on subsequent firing patterns of cell ensembles.

Exposure to a novel situation can result in long-lasting changes in the firing rate distributions of the recorded pyramidal cells. When firing rates of individual neurons in the novel environment and subsequent sleep episode were compared their correlation was stronger than correlation of firing rates between exploration in the novel environment and the preceding sleep episode (Hirase *et al.* 2001). Importantly, firing rates observed in the sleep episodes preceding and following exposure to novelty were poorly correlated (Fig. 13.3). A novel environment had a similar effect on co-activation of neurons pairs as well. Neuron pairs with high awake correlation continued to display high correlation in the subsequent sleep episode. However, some residual correlation was still present between exploration and the preceding sleep session (Kudrimoti *et al.* 1999; Hirase *et al.* 2001), indicating that novelty affects only a part of the neuronal population responsible for the changes observed.

A more direct support for the "replay" of learned neuronal patterns comes from experiments where, instead of pairwise correlations, neuronal sequences were compared. Repeated discharge sequences of neurons across several theta cycles were detected in parallel-recorded spike trains when the rats were exposed to a wheel for the first time. The precise timing of neurons in the awake animal is not surprising given that running in the wheel is rather stereotypic. However, many of the same neuronal sequences were also detected in the subsequent sleep episode (Nadasdy *et al.* 1999). Not only were there significantly more common sequences present during wheel running and subsequent sleep episodes than the number of sequences common in wheel running and preceding sleep but the incidence of sequences in the awake and subsequent sleep episode were also correlated (Fig. 13.4). Although the neurons involved in the sequences were identical, they were "replayed" much faster during sleep than in the waking animal. Most replayed sequences occurred during SPW bursts. In summary, neuronal sequences

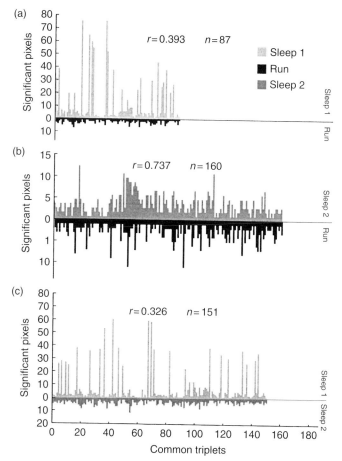

Figure 13.4 Spike sequences during sleep can be influenced by previous novel experience. Histogram of significant triplets common to Sleep 1 and (wheel) Run sessions (a), to Run and Sleep 2 sessions (b) and to Sleep 1 and Sleep 2 sessions (c). A sequence was considered to be "common" if it was significant in both behavior sessions regardless of the interspike intervals (e.g. 4–1–2 at 50, 80, and 5 and 8 ms). Individual triplets are listed on the abscissa. Note that there are almost twice as many triplets common to Run and Sleep 2 sessions than to Sleep 1 and Run session. The r values (Pearson's product moment correlation coefficient) indicate the correlation of the number of common triplets between the respective two sessions (after Nadasdy *et al.* 1999).

during SWS are determined by the dynamics of the SPW process and the synaptic weight changes brought about by previous experience (Kudrimoti *et al.* 1999; Nadasdy *et al.* 1999). In an unchanging environment, discharge sequences of neurons (content of sleep) are expected to remain stable (Lörincz and Buzsáki 2000).

Further support for the ability of novel environment to alter firing patterns comes from experiments in awake animals. When rats were tested repeatedly in the same apparatus the firing patterns of place cells were sometimes substantially reorganized after the animal was exposed to a series of novel environments. The interpretation of the "re-mapping" of neuron discharges in the otherwise familiar environment was that synaptic weights in the CA3 axon collateral system were substantially altered by novelty (McNaughton *et al.* 1996). Similarly, tetanic stimulation-induced LTP of intrahippocampal synapses significantly modified firing rates and maps of hippocampal place cells (Dragoi and Buzsáki 2001).

Taken together, these findings indicate that (i) experience can alter the minute-scale firing rates and patterns of neurons and (ii) the changes are not all or none since some residual correlation is still present between firing patterns of the waking state and the preceding sleep session (Kudrimoti *et al.* 1999; Hirase *et al.* 2001).

Sharp wave burst can modify discharge probability of pyramidal cells

A potential mechanism of modifying firing rates and patterns of neurons is synaptic plasticity (Bliss and Lømo 1973). Although numerous studies have suggested that synaptic strength during theta oscillations can modified (cf. Buzsáki 2002), those experiment used artificial electrical stimulation for both induction and testing of synaptic plasticity. Other studies explicitly suggested that synaptic modification can take place only in the awake but not sleeping animal (Leonard *et al.* 1987). This is unexpected on the basis of the experimental requirements of LTP: proper timing of pre- and postsynaptic activity and strong postsynaptic depolarization with burst of spikes (Levy and Steward 1983; Markram *et al.* 1997). The latter conditions are expected to be present during SPW events, since neurons discharge in sequences and the population burst associated with SPWs in the CA3–CA1-subicular complex–deep layers of the entorhinal cortex can provide a strong depolarization for the participating neurons (Chrobak and Buzsáki 1994).

Some pyramidal cells participate in as many as 40 percent of successive SPWs, whereas the majority discharges less than 10 percent (Ylinen *et al.* 1995). Thus, the question is how the participation probability of a single pyramidal neuron in SPW bursts can be altered. To examine this issue, single neurons or small group of CA1 pyramidal cells were discharged by either direct current injection via an intracellular electrode in anesthetized animals or via extracellular micro-stimulation through a recording tetrode in behaving rats (King *et al.* 1999). Following the pairing between physiological activation of the Schaffer collaterals to CA1 and discharge of the target cells by artificial means, the discharge probability of neurons, associated with the SPW bursts, increased significantly (Fig. 13.5; King *et al.* 1999). These findings suggest that changes in the weights of synaptic afferents by a Hebbian mechanism can be at least one possible mechanism for altering

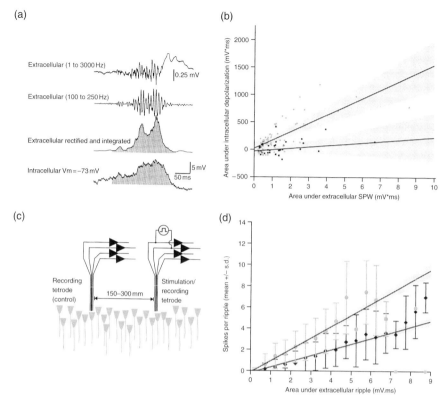

Figure 13.5 Hebbian pairing can increase participation of single pyramidal neurons in SPW events. Upper panels: Integrated ripple (extracellular) activity and the area of the intracellular membrane potential during ripple were correlated (before). During training the extracellular signal was fed back to the impaled neuron so that the cell discharged bursts of action potentials during every SPW burst (50 pairings). Such training increased the response of the neuron to SPW-associated inputs. Bottom panels: Similar experiment in the freely moving rat. First the relationships between ripple, recorded with the control electrode, and integrated multiple unit activity, recorded by both tetrodes, were established. During training units recorded with the training tetrode (stimulation/recording) were consistently discharged by SPW time-locked stimuli. Following training the relative number of spikes associated with SPW/ripple events increased for the activated population (right panel) but not for the control, unstimulated neurons (not shown; after King *et al.* 1999).

firing rates of single neurons. The findings also argue in favor of the possibility that induction of synaptic plasticity may occur also during sleep (but see Leonard *et al.* 1987; Tononi and Cirelli 2001).

Homeostatic maintenance of firing rates

Cortical pyramidal cells fire single spikes and complex spike bursts (Kandel and Spencer 1968; Connors *et al.* 1982; Llinas and Jahnsen 1982; Gray and McCormick 1996).

In hippocampus, pyramidal cells exhibit bursts of 2–6 spikes of decreasing extracellular amplitude at short (≤ 6 ms) intervals (Ranck 1973). Bursts are often assumed to have functions different from single spikes (cf. Lisman 1997). Bursts can have a differential impact "downstream" or can provide a feed-back signal to the synapses that initiated the burst. Burst patterns discharge postsynaptic targets more reliably than the same number of single spikes separated by longer intervals (Miles and Wong 1987; Ali and Thomson 1998; Csicsvari *et al.* 1998) . Due to their prolonged effects, bursts may be able to activate postsynaptic NMDA receptors, in contrast to sparse spikes (Lisman 1997). Nevertheless, the exact downstream role of bursts is not clear. If bursts convey the same information as single spikes, just "stronger," then the behavioral conditions that bring about burst discharges should correspond to the maximum excitation of the bursting neurons (Otto *et al.* 1991; Livingston *et al.* 1996; Lisman 1997). However, the importance of bursts carrying downstream information is not straightforward, since single spikes often carry more information than bursts (Bair *et al.* 1994; Harris *et al.* 2001).

Bursts also play an important role in synaptic plasticity but whether the impact of the burst is downstream or upstream is still debated (Rose and Dunwiddie 1986; Stäubli and Lynch 1987; Huerta and Lisman 1993; Holscher *et al.* 1997). Recent experiments in hippocampal pyramidal neurons indicate that the necessary condition for the induction of LTP is the temporal coordination of presynaptic activity with postsynaptic burst discharge in such a way that presynaptic activity should coincide or precede the burst (Jester *et al.* 1995; Magee and Jonhston 1997; Thomas *et al.* 1998; Pike *et al.* 1999). On the other hand, presynaptic bursting appears neither necessary nor sufficient to induce synaptic plasticity (Paulsen and Sejnowski 2000).

One possible mechanism by which bursts may contribute to synaptic plasticity is through soma-dendritic backpropagation of action potentials. Successfully back-propagating action potentials are much wider in the dendrites than their axonal–somatic counterparts and can trigger Ca^{2+} spikes (Spruston *et al.* 1995; Kamondi *et al.* 1998). In turn, Ca^{2+} spikes lead to burst firing (Wong *et al.* 1979; Traub *et al.* 1994). Both the Ca^{2+} event and the multiple wide dendritic Na^+ spikes can provide the necessary depolarization, with or without activation of N-methyl-D-aspartate (NMDA) receptors, for the induction of synaptic potentiation (Kandel 2001).

If bursts play a critical role in synaptic plasticity, it is important to reveal the conditions that favor their occurrence. In a recent experiment, we examined the occurrence of complex spike bursts in CA1 pyramidal cells on different behaviors. If bursting is produced by strong afferent excitation alone, we hypothesized that the ratio of bursts to single spikes should be largest in the center of the place field (O'Keefe and Nadel 1978) where the strongest depolarization is expected. However, the information about spatial position carried by bursts and single spikes did not show any reliable relationship (Harris *et al.* 2001). Bursts occurred during both theta and non-theta associated behaviors, although the incidence of bursts was significantly higher during non-theta. Coincident bursts of simultaneously recorded neurons were extremely rare and did not appear to be coordinated by any network pattern. The incidence of bursts was similar in animals exposed to a familiar or a novel environment and in the sleep episodes subsequent to familiar environment and novelty (our unpublished findings).

These findings indicate that the occurrence of bursts is not particularly coordinated across different neurons or under the control of particular behaviors. Instead, it is the intrinsic properties of the pyramidal cell and its recent spiking history that appear to determine the incidence of bursts (Harris *et al.* 2001). Examination of the temporal relationship between single spikes and complex spike bursts revealed that the proportion of bursts occurred at times when the neuron discharged at theta (6–8 Hz) frequency. The probability of burst and burst length correlated with the duration of pre-burst neuronal silence. These observations suggested that the ideal condition for burst production is strong dendritic depolarization coupled with a period of non-spiking activity.

Because a main cause of spike backpropagation failure is Na^+ channel inactivation (Spruston *et al.* 1995; Mickus *et al.* 1999), we speculated that the prolonged Na^+ channel inactivation (Henze and Buzsáki 2001) may account for the suppression of burst discharges. Supporting this suggestion, the current-induced burst length, recorded in the soma, correlated with the rising slope of the intracellular action potential (Harris *et al.* 2001). Furthermore, the burst probability and burst length correlated with the extracellular amplitude of the burst-initiator spike, which reflects the magnitude of the slope of the intracellular action potential (Henze *et al.* 2000).

The proposed importance of bursts in synaptic plasticity and the intrinsic regulatory mechanisms of burst discharge in pyramidal neurons provide some interesting possibilities for the regulation of discharge rate in these neurons (Fig. 13.6). Several experiments support the importance of the temporal order of presynaptic and postsynaptic activity in neuronal plasticity (Levy and Steward 1983; Larson and Lynch 1986; Markram *et al.* 1997; Bi and Poo 1998). A weak input, eliciting an excitatory postsynaptic potential (EPSP), followed by a strong, burst inducing input is a necessary and sufficient condition for strengthening the weak input. The shorter the time interval between the weak and strong input, the larger the magnitude of synaptic potentiation. Conversely, reversing the temporal order of the weak and strong can lead to depression of the weak input or depotentiating its previously gained weight increase.

Assuming that the synaptic modification rule also applies to the intact brain, synaptic connections between the same sets of pyramidal neurons would grow *ad infinitum* in a familiar environment with stereotypic behavior. Unless some intrinsic normalizing mechanisms exist to counteract synaptic potentiation (Turrigiano *et al.* 1998), the hippocampal network would eventually become epileptic. According to this conceptual model, strengthening of the weak input will continue as long as the weak input is followed by the burst-inducing input. We propose that bursts may be conceived as a homeostatic mechanism to maintain synaptic strength. Once the weak input becomes suprathreshold, the single spike induced reduction of Na^+ channel availability will reduce burst length or abolish its occurrence altogether. The tighter the temporal relationship between the weak (but now suprathreshold) and strong input, the stronger the "veto effect" of the single spike. Should the strength of the synapse decay with time the weak synaptic input may

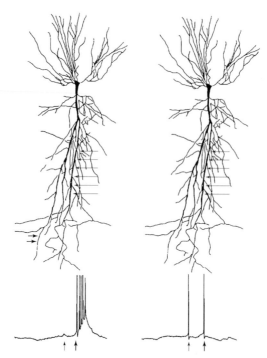

Figure 13.6 Hypothesized effect of activity-dependent burst suppression on synaptic plasticity. A weak input (short arrows) is followed by a strong input (long arrows). If the weak input is subthreshold (left trace), the strong input can trigger a burst, and can lead to strengthening of the weak input (Pike *et al.* 1999; Paulsen and Sejnowski 2000). If the weak input is suprathreshold (right trace), the evoked single spike can inhibit burst response to the same strong input. In effect, the firing of already potentiated afferents reduces the efficacy of the strong input, and inhibits further potentiation. If the efficacy of the weak input decreases below spike threshold, the subsequent burst can again potentiate the weakened synapse (Buzsaki *et al.* 2002).

become subthreshold again. At this point, the strong input becomes instantly effective in inducing a burst, which event will potentiate the weakened synapse. In essence, we propose that the veto effect of single spikes on burst probability is a potential mechanism for maintaining synaptic strength. The suggested homeostatic mechanism is operative in a single cell and depends primarily by the spiking history of the neuron (Henze and Buzsáki 2001). This may explain why bursts in different neurons occur relatively independent from each other and why their occurrence does not require network coordination.

Downstream effects of cortical activity during sleep

Most discussions on sleep concentrate on the influence of subcortical inputs on cortical activity. However, both neocortical and archicortical structures possess strong subcortical outputs (Papez 1937). These subcortical outputs may exert important effects on subcortical nuclei which, in turn, may assist various nonspecific aspects of synaptic plasticity. The main subcortical pathways from the hippocampal formation derive from the principal cells of the hippocampus and subiculum and travel in the fimbria-fornix (Amaral and Witter 1989). Their main targets are the n. accumbens, lateral septum, triangular nucleus, septo-fimbrial nucleus, bed nucleus of stria terminalis and lateral hypothalamus. Many of these targets receive both monosynaptic as well as disynaptic input from the hippocampal formation relayed through the lateral and posterior septum. In contrast to the functional role of the retrohippocampal cortical areas, the possible contribution of the descendent hippocampal outputs to these subcortical areas in memory formation has received scant attention to date. The descending output of the hippocampal formation is known to play an important role in the regulation of endocrine functions (Fischette *et al.* 1980; Seto *et al.* 1983), inhibition of many aspects of the hypothalamic–pituitary axis (Feldman, 1985; Jacobson and Sapolsky 1991) and modulation of circadian rhythms (Yamaoka 1978). Several hormones, whose release is affected by hippocampal activity, have been shown to play a major role in memory consolidation, including corticosteroids, growth hormones, and vasopressin (Kovacs *et al.* 1979; De Wied 1983; McGaugh 1988). For example, it has been demonstrated that post-training intraseptal infusions of both the gamma-amino-butyric-acidergic (GABAergic) agonist muscimol and the antagonist bicuculline can induce dose and time dependent impairments of working/episodic memory as expressed in the rat's performance of a delayed nonmatch-to-sample radial maze task (Chrobak *et al.* 1989). Importantly, many of these effects are exerted in a state-dependent manner. For example, >90 percent of growth hormones are released during stage 4 sleep in humans, a state with highest incidence of SPWs. Because of the

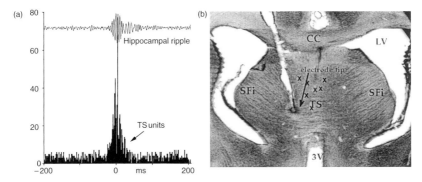

Figure 13.7 Hippocampal excitation of units in the triangular septal nucleus. (a) Relationship between hippocampal ripples, recorded in CA1 pyramidal layer, and unit discharges in the triangular septal nucleus (TS units). Note large increase of TS unit discharges during hippocampal ripples. (b) Tip of the recording tungsten sharp electrode in TS. Recordings sites with similar unit responses during hippocampal ripples in other rats are indicated by X. Sfi, septofimbrial nucleus; CC, corpus callosum; LV, lateral ventricle; 3V, third ventricle.

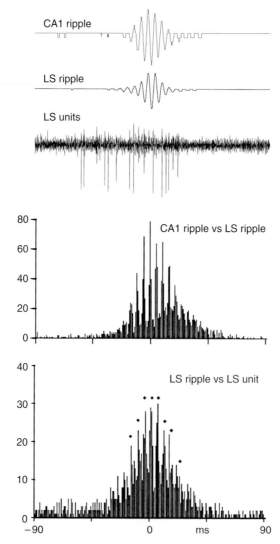

Figure 13.8 Hippocampal excitation of units in the lateral septal nucleus. Hippocampal CA1 ripples (100–300 Hz band-pass), lateral septum field ripple (LS ripple; 100–300 Hz band-pass) and LS unit discharges (600 Hz–6 kHz). Cross-correlation between hippocampal and septal field ripples reveal wave by wave relationship. LS units are modulated by the local (LS) field ripples. Note rhythmic peaks at 5–7 ms intervals (gray diamonds).

protracted nature of memory consolidation, the process can be enhanced or disrupted by various hormonal and neurotransmitter systems related to the internal state of the organism (Walter, 1975; Rigter 1979; Dyball and Patterson 1983; McGaugh 1988; Crowe *et al.* 1990).

We hypothesize that the strong depolarization brought about by SPW activity might be especially effective in the regulation of different autonomic and endocrine functions. As a first step, we examined the neuronal responses of several subcortical targets of the hippocampal formation during SPWs. SPW bursts were associated with several-fold, transient increase of neuronal discharges in the triangular nucleus (Fig. 13.7), septo-fimbrial nucleus, nucleus accumbens, lateral septum, bed nucleus of stria terminalis (Carpi *et al.* 1995). Neurons in the lateral septal nucleus displayed a transient, fast oscillatory rhythm at 140–200 Hz, associated with a field oscillation at the same frequency (Fig. 13.8).

These findings suggest that ascending and descending outputs of the hippocampal formation can exert cooperative influences on the key mechanisms assumed to be involved in memory trace formation. Early steps of the consolidation process may involve transfer of information from the hippocampus to neocortical targets and modification of the synapses involved. The ultimate, long-term modification of the synaptic structure requires several molecular steps (Kandel 2001), many of which can be effectively regulated by circulating hormones.

References

Ali, A. B. and **Thomson, A. M.** (1998). Facilitating pyramid to horizontal oriens—alveus interneurone inputs: dual intracellular recordings in slices of rat hippocampus. *Journal of Physiology*, **507**, 185–199.

Amaral, D. G. and **Witter, M. P.** (1989). The three-dimensional organization of the hippocampal formation: a review of anatomical data. *Neuroscience*, **31**, 571–591.

Aserinsky, E. (1996). The discovery of REM sleep. *Journal of the History of Neuroscience*, **5**, 213–227.

Bair, W., Koch, C., Newsome, W., and **Britten, K.** (1994). Power spectrum analysis of bursting cells in area MT in the behaving monkey. *Journal of Neuroscience*, **14**, 2870–2892.

Bi, G. Q. and **Poo, M. M.** (1998). Synaptic modifications in cultured hippocampal neurons: dependence on spike timing, synaptic strength, and postsynaptic cell type. *Journal of Neuroscience*, **18**, 10464–10472.

Bland, B. H. (1986). Physiology and pharmacology of hippocampal formation theta rhythms. *Progress in Neurobiology*, **26**, 1–54.

Bliss, T. V. and **Lømo, T.** (1973). Long-lasting potentiation of synaptic transmission in the dentate area of the anaesthetized rabbit following stimulation of the perforant path. *Journal of Physiology*, **232**, 331–356.

Bragin, A., Engel, J. Jr, Wilson, C. L., Fried, I., and **Buzsáki, G.** (1999). High-frequency oscillations in human brain. *Hippocampus*, **9**, 137–142.

Buzsáki, G. (1989). Two-stage model of memory trace formation: a role for "noisy" brain states. *Neuroscience*, **31**, 551–570.

Buzsáki, G. (1986). Hippocampal sharp waves: their origin and significance. *Brain Research*, **398**, 242–252.

Buzsáki, G. (1996). The Hippocampo–neocortical dialogue. *Cerebral Cortex*, **6**, 81–92.

Buzsáki, G. (1998). Memory consolidation during sleep: a neurophysiological perspective. *Journal of Sleep Research*, **7**(Suppl.), 17–23.

Buzsáki, G. (2002). Theta oscillations in the hippocampus. *Neuron* **33**, 325–340.

Buzsáki, G., Ponomareff, G. L., Bayardo, F., Ruiz, R., and **Gage, F. H.** (1989). Neuronal activity in the subcortically denervated hippocampus: a chronic model for epilepsy. *Neuroscience*, **28**, 527–538.

Buzsáki, G., Bragin, A., Chrobak, J. J., Nadasdy, Z., Sik, A., and **Ylinen, A.** (1994). Oscillatory and intermittent synchrony in the hippocampus: Relevance for memory trace formation. In: *Temporal coding in the brain* (eds G. Buzsàki, R. R. Llinás, W. Singer, A. Berthoz, and Y. Christen) pp. 145–172. Springer-Verlag, Berlin.

Buzsáki, G., Csiesvari, J., Dragoi, G., Harris, K. D., Henze, D. A., and **Hirase, H.** (2002). Homeostatic maintenance of neuronal excitability by burst discharges in vivo. *Cerebral Cortex* **12**, 893–899.

Buzsáki, G., Horvath, Z., Urioste, R., Hetke, J., and **Wise, K.** (1992). High-frequency network oscillation in the hippocampus. *Science*, **256**, 1025–1027.

Buzsáki, G., Leung, L. W., and **Vanderwolf, C. H.** (1983). Cellular bases of hippocampal EEG in the behaving rat. *Brain Research*, **287**, 139–171.

Carpi, D., Sik, A., and **Buzsáki, G.** (1995). Activity of nucleus triangularis septi (TS) neurons to theta and sharp waves in the behaving rat. *Society for Neuroscience Abstracts*, Vol. 21, pp. 473.14.

Chrobak, J. J., Stackman, R. W., and **Walsh, T. J.** (1989). Intraseptal administration of muscimol produces dose-dependent memory impairments in the rat. *Behavioral Neural Biology*, **52**, 357–369.

Chrobak, J. J. and **Buzsáki, G.** (1994). Selective activation of deep layer (V–VI) retrohippocampal cortical neurons during hippocampal sharp waves in the behaving rat. *Journal of Neuroscience*, **14**, 6160–6170.

Chrobak, J. J. and **Buzsáki, G.** (1998). Operational dynamics in the hippocampal–entorhinal axis. *Neuroscience and Biobehavioral Review*, **22**, 303–310.

Connors, B. W., Gutnick, M. J., and **Prince, D. A.** (1982). Electrophysiological properties of neocortical neurons *in vitro*. *Journal of Neurophysiology*, **48**, 1302–1320.

Csicsvari, J., Hirase, H., Mamiya, A., and **Buzsáki, G.** (2000). Ensemble patterns of hippocampal CA3–CA1 neurons during sharp wave-associated population events. *Neuron*, **28**, 585–594.

Crick, F. and **Mitchison, G.** (1983). The function of dream sleep. *Nature*, **304**, 111–114.

Crowe, S. F., Ng, K. T., and **Gibbs, M. E.** (1990). Memory consolidation of weak training experiences by hormonal treatments. *Pharmacology, Biochemistry and Behavior*, **37**, 729–734.

Cullinan, W. E., Herman, J. P., and **Watson, S. J.** (1993). Ventral subicular interaction with the hypothalamic paraventricular nucleus: evidence for a relay in the bed nucleus of the stria terminalis. *Journal of Comparative Neurology*, **332**, 1–20.

Dave, A. S. and **Margoliash, D.** (2000). Song replay during sleep and computational rules for sensorimotor vocal learning. *Science*, **290**, 812–816.

De Wied, D. (1983). Central actions of neurohypophysial hormones. *Progress in Brain Research*, **60**, 155–167.

Dragoi, G. and **Buzsáki, G.** (2001). Influence of long term potentiation on the stability of hippocampal place field cells. *Society of Neuroscience Abstracts*, **27**, 537.5.

Douglas, R. M. and **Goddard, G. V.** (1975). Long-term potentiation of the perforant path-granule cell synapse in the rat hippocampus. *Brain Research*, **86**, 205–215.

Dyball, R. E. and **Paterson, A. T.** (1983). Neurohypophysial hormones and brain function: the neurophysiological effects of oxytocin and vasopressin. *Pharmacology and Therapeutics*, **20**, 419–436.

Feldman, S. (1985). Neural pathways mediating adrenocortical responses. *Federal Proceedings*, **44**, 169–175.

Fischette, C. T., Komisaruk, B. R., Edinger, H. M., Feder, H. H., and **Siegel, A.** (1980). Differential fornix ablations and the circadian rhythmicity of adrenal corticosteroid secretion. *Brain Research*, **195**, 373–387.

Frey, U., Huang, Y. Y., and **Kandel, E. R.** (1993). Effects of cAMP simulate a late stage of LTP in hippocampal CA1 neurons. *Science*, **260**, 1661–4166.

Gray, C. M. and **McCormick, D. A.** (1996). Chattering cells: superficial pyramidal neurons contributing to the generation of synchronous in the visual cortex. *Science*, **274**, 109–113.

Gustafsson, B. and **Wigström, H.** (1986). Hippocampal long-lasting potentiation produced by pairing single volleys and brief conditioning tetani evoked in separate afferents. *Journal of Neuroscience*, **6**, 1575–1582.

Guzowski, J. F., McNaughton, B. L., Barnes, C. A., and **Worley, P. F.** (2001). Imaging neural activity with temporal and cellular resolution using FISH. *Current Opinion in Neurobiology*, **11**, 579–584.

Harris, K. D., Hirase, H., Leinekugel, X., Henze, D. A., and **Buzsáki, G.** (2001). Temporal interaction between single spikes and complex spike bursts in hippocampal pyramidal cells. *Neuron*, **32**, 141–149.

Hebb, D. (1949). *Organization of behavior*. Wiley, New York.

Henze, D. A. and **Buzsáki, G.** (2001). Action potential threshold of hippocampal pyramidal cells *in vivo* is increased by recent spiking activity. *Neuroscience*, **105**, 121–130.

Henze, D. A., Borhegyi, Z., Csicsvari, J., Mamiya, A., Harris, K. D., and **Buzsáki, G.** (2000). Intracellular features predicted by extracellular recordings in the hippocampus *in vivo*. *Journal of Neurophysiology*, **84**, 390–400.

Hirase, H., Leinekugel, X., Czurkó, A., Csicsvari, J., and **Buzsáki, G.** (2001). Firing rates of hippocampal neurons are preserved during subsequent sleep episodes and modified by novel awake experience. *Proceedings of the National Academy Sciences, USA*, **98**, 9386–9390.

Hobson, J. A. (1995). *Sleep*. Scientific American Library. W. H. Freeman and Co., New York, NY.

Holscher, C., Anwyl, R., and **Rowan, M. J.** (1997). Stimulation on the positive phase of hippocampal theta rhythm induces long-term potentiation that can Be depotentiated by stimulation on the negative phase in area CA1 *in vivo*. *Journal of Neuroscience*, **17**, 6470–6477.

Huerta, P. T. and Lisman, J. E. (1993). Heightened synaptic plasticity of hippocampal CA1 neurons during a cholinergically induced rhythmic state. *Nature*, **364**, 723–725.

Jacobson, L. and Sapolsky, R. (1991). The role of the hippocampus in feedback regulation of the hypothalamic–pituitary–adrenocortical axis. *Endocrine Reviews*, **12**, 118–134.

Jakab, R. L. and Leranth, C. (1995). Septum. In *The rat nervous system* (ed. P. George), pp. 405–442. Academic Press, Sydney.

Jester, J. M., Campbell, L. W., and Sejnowski, T. J. (1995). Associative EPSP—spike potentiation induced by pairing orthodromic and antidromic stimulation in rat hippocampal slices. *Journal of Physiology*, **484**, 689–705.

Kamondi, A., Acsady, L., Wang, X. J., and Buzsáki, G. (1998). Theta oscillations in somata and dendrites of hippocampal pyramidal cells *in vivo*: activity-dependent phase-precession of action potentials. *Hippocampus*, **8**, 244–261.

Kandel, E. R. (2001). The molecular biology of memory storage: a dialogue between genes and synapses. *Science*, **294**(5544), 1030–1038.

Kandel, E. R. and Spencer, W. A. (1968). Cellular neurophysiological approaches in the study of learning. *Physiological Reviews*, **48**, 65–134.

Karni, A., Tanne, D., Rubenstein, B. S., Askenasy, J. J., and Sagi, D. (1994). Dependence on REM sleep of overnight improvement of a perceptual skill. *Science*, **265**, 679–682.

King, C., Henze, D. A., Leinekugel, X., and Buzsáki, G. (1999). Hebbian modification of a hippocampal population pattern in the rat. *Journal of Physiology*, **521**, 159–167.

Kovacs, G. L., Bohus, B., and Versteeg, D. H. (1979). The effects of vasopressin on memory processes: the role of noradrenergic neurotransmission *Neuroscience*, **4**, 1529–1537

Kudrimoti, H. S., Barnes, C. A., and McNaughton, B. L. (1999). Reactivation of hippocampal cell assemblies: effects of behavioral state, experience, and EEG dynamics. *Journal of Neuroscience*, **19**, 4090–4101.

Larson, J. and Lynch, G. (1986). Induction of synaptic potentiation in hippocampus by patterned stimulation involves two events. *Science*, **232**, 985–988.

Leonard, B. J., McNaughton, B. L., and Barnes, C. A. (1987). Suppression of hippocampal synaptic plasticity during slow-wave sleep. *Brain Research*, **425**, 174–177.

Levy, W. B. and Steward, O. (1983). Temporal contiguity requirements for long-term associative potentiation/depression in the hippocampus. *Neuroscience*, **8**, 791–797.

Lisman, J. E. (1997). Bursts as a unit of neural information: making unreliable synapses reliable. *Trends in Neuroscience*, **20**, 38–43.

Livingstone, M. S., Freeman, D. C., and Hubel, D. H. (1996). Visual responses in V1 of freely viewing monkeys. *Cold Spring Harbor Symposia on Quantitative Biology*, **61**, 27–37.

Llinas, R. and Jahnsen, H. (1982). Electrophysiology of mammalian thalamic neurones *in vitro*. *Nature*, **297**, 406–408.

Louie, K. and Wilson, M. A. (2001). Temporally structured replay of awake hippocampal ensemble activity during rapid eye movement sleep. *Neuron*, **29**, 145–156.

Lörincz, A. and **Buzsáki, G.** (2000). Two-phase computational model training long-term memories in the entorhinal–hippocampal region. *Annals of the New York Academy of Sciences*, **911**, 83–111.

Magee, J. C. and **Johnston, D.** (1997). A synaptically controlled, associative signal for Hebbian plasticity in hippocampal neurons. *Science*, **275**, 209–213.

Maquet, P. (2001). The role of sleep in learning and memory. *Science*, **294**, 1048–1052.

Markram, H., Lubke, J., Frotscher, M., and **Sakmann, B.** (1997). Regulation of synaptic efficacy by coincidence of postsynaptic APs and EPSPs. *Science*, **275**, 213–215.

McGaugh (1988). Involvement of hormonal and neuromodulatory system in the regulation of memory storage. *Annual Review of Neuroscience*, **12**, 255–287.

McNaughton, B. L., Barnes, C. A., Gerrard, J. L., Gothard, K., Jung, M. W., Knierim, J. J., Kudrimoti, H., Qin, Y., Skaggs, W. E., Suster, M., and **Weaver, K. L.** (1996). Deciphering the hippocampal polyglot: the hippocampus as a path integration system. *Journal of Experimental Biology*, **199**, 173–185.

Mickus, T., Jung, H., and **Spruston, N.** (1999). Properties of slow, cumulative sodium channel inactivation in rat hippocampal CA1 pyramidal neurons. *Biophysical Journal*, **76**, 846–860.

Miles, R. and **Wong, R. K.** (1987). Latent synaptic pathways revealed after tetanic stimulation in the hippocampus *Nature*, **329**, 724–726.

Nadasdy, Z., Hirase, H., Czurko, A., Csicsvari, J., and **Buzsáki, G.** (1999). Replay and time compression of recurring spike sequences in the hippocampus. *Journal of Neuroscience*, **19**, 9497–9507, 1999.

O'Donnell, P. and **Grace, A. A.** (1995). Synaptic interactions among excitatory afferents to nucleus accumbens neurons: hippocampal gating of prefrontal cortical input. *Journal of Neuroscience*, **15**, 3622–3639.

O'Keefe, J. and **Nadel, L.** (1978). *The Hippocampus as a cognitive map*. Clarendon Press, Oxford.

Otto, T., Eichenbaum, H., Wiener, S. I., and **Wible, C. G.** (1991). Learning-related patterns of CA1 spike trains parallel stimulation parameters optimal for inducing hippocampal long-term potentiation. *Hippocampus*, **1**, 181–192.

Papez, J. W. (1937). A proposed mechanism of emotion. *Archives of Neurology and Psychiatry*, **38**, 725–743.

Paulsen, O. and **Sejnowski, T. J.** (2000). Natural patterns of activity and long-term synaptic plasticity. *Current Opinion in Neurobiology*, **10**, 172–179.

Pavlides, C. and **Winson, J.** (1989). Influences of hippocampal place cell firing in the awake state on the activity of these cells during subsequent sleep episodes. *Journal of Neuroscience*, **9**, 2907–2918.

Pike, F. G., Meredith, R. M., Olding, A. W., and **Paulsen, O.** (1999). Rapid report: postsynaptic bursting is essential for 'Hebbian' induction of associative long-term potentiation at excitatory synapses in rat hippocampus. *Journal of Physiology, London*, **518**, 571–576.

Ranck, J. B., Jr. (1973). Studies on single neurons in dorsal hippocampal formation and septum in unrestrained rats. I. Behavioral correlates and firing repertoires. *Experimental Neurology*, **41**, 461–531.

Rigter, H. and Van Riezen, H. (1979). Pituitary hormones and amnesia. *Current Developments in Psychopharmacology*, **5**, 67–124.

Rose, G. M. and Dunwiddie, T. V. (1986). Induction of hippocampal long-term potentiation using physiologically patterned stimulation. *Neuroscience Letters*, **69**, 244–248.

Seto, K., Saito, H., Otsuka, K., and Kawakami, M. (1983). Influence of electrical stimulation of the limbic structure on insulin level in rabbit's plasma. *Experimental and Clinical Endocrinology*, **81**, 347–349.

Siapas, A. G. and Wilson, M. A. (1988). Coordinated interactions between hippocampal ripples and cortical spindles during slow-wave sleep. *Neuron*, **21**, 1123–1128.

Siegel, J. M. (2001). The REM sleep-memory consolidation hypothesis. *Science*, **294**, 1058–1063. Review.

Skaggs, W. E. and McNaughton, B. L. (1996). Replay of neuronal firing sequences in rat hippocampus during sleep following spatial experience. *Science*, **271**, 1870–1873.

Spruston, N., Schiller, Y., Stuart, G., and Sakmann, B. (1995). Activity-dependent action potential invasion and calcium influx into hippocampal CA1 dendrites. *Science*, **268**, 297–300.

Staubli, U. and Lynch, G. (1987). Stable hippocampal long-term potentiation elicited by 'theta' pattern stimulation. *Brain Research*, **435**, 227–234.

Stickgold, R., Hobson, J. A., Fosse, R., and Fosse, M. (2001). Sleep, learning, and dreams: off-line memory reprocessing. *Science*, **294**, 1052–1057.

Thomas, M. J., Watabe, A. M., Moody, T. D., Makhinson, M., and O'Dell, T. J. (1998). Post-synaptic complex spike bursting enables the induction of LTP by theta frequency synaptic stimulation. *Journal of Neuroscience*, **18**, 7118–7126.

Thompson, L. T. and Best, P. J. (1990). Long-term stability of the place-field activity of single units recorded from the dorsal hippocampus of freely behaving rats. *Brain Research*, **509**, 299–308.

Tononi, G. and Cirelli, C. (2001). Modulation of brain gene expression during sleep and wakefulness: a review of recent findings. *Neuropsychopharmacology*, **25**, S28–S35.

Traub, R. D., Jefferys, J. G., Miles, R., Whittington, M. A., and Toth, K. (1994). A branching dendritic model of a rodent CA3 pyramidal neurone. *Journal of Physiology London*, **481**, 79–95.

Turrigiano, G. G., Leslie, K. R., Desai, N. S., Rutherford, L. C., and Nelson, S. B. (1998). Activity-dependent scaling of quantal amplitude in neocortical neurons. *Nature*, **391**, 892–896.

Vertes, R. P. and Eastman, K. E. (2000). The case against memory consolidation in REM sleep. *Behavioral Brain Science*, **23**, 867–876.

Vertes, R. P. and Kocsis, B. (1997). Brainstem–diencephalo-septohippocampal systems controlling the theta rhythm of the hippocampus. *Neuroscience*, **81**, 893–926.

Walter, R., Hoffman, P. L., Flexner, J. B., and Flexner, L. B. (1975). Neurohypophyseal hormones, analogs, and fragments: their effect on puromycin–induced amnesia. *Proceedings of National Academy of Sciences, USA*, **72**, 4180–4184.

Wilson, M. A. and McNaughton, B. L. (1994). Reactivation of hippocampal ensemble memories during sleep. *Science*, **265**, 676–682.

Winson, J. (1990). The meaning of dreams. *Scientific American*, **263**, 86–96.

Wong, R. K. and **Traub, R. D.** (1983). Synchronized burst discharge in disinhibited hippocampal slice. I. Initiation in CA2–CA3 region. *Journal of Neurophysiology*, **49**, 442–458.

Wong, R. K., Prince, D. A., and **Basbaum, A. I.** (1979). Intradendritic recordings from hippocampal neurons. *Proceedings of the National Academy of Sciences, USA*, **76**, 986–990.

Yamaoka, S. (1978). Participation of limbic-hypothalamic structures in the circadian rhythm of slow wave sleep and paradoxical sleep in the rat. *Brain Research*, 255–268.

Ylinen, A., Bragin, A., Nadasdy, Z., Jando, G., Szabo, I., Sik, A., and **Buzsáki, G.** (1995). Sharp wave-associated high-frequency oscillation (200 Hz) in the intact hippocampus: network and intracellular mechanisms. *Journal of Neuroscience*, **15**, 30–46.

CHAPTER 14

NEURONAL PLASTICITY DURING SLEEP OSCILLATIONS IN CORTICOTHALAMIC SYSTEMS

MIRCEA STERIADE AND IGOR TIMOFEEV

Background

This chapter postulates that, far from being epiphenomena with little or no functional significance, spontaneously occurring brain rhythms during slow wave sleep (SWS) produce plastic changes in thalamic and neocortical neurons. Plasticity can be defined as an alteration in neuronal responsiveness and in the strength of connections among neurons, which depends on the history of a given neuronal circuit, a mechanism through which information is stored. Such changes may occur at different sites in the brain. Here, the emphasis is placed on corticothalamic networks.

Although earlier hypotheses assumed that SWS is associated with global cortical inhibition (Pavlov 1923) that produces an "abject annihilation of consciousness" (Eccles 1961), recent intracellular recordings during natural states of vigilance of behaving cats demonstrate that neocortical neurons display a rich spontaneous activity during SWS (Steriade *et al.* 2001; Timofeev *et al.* 2001) (Fig. 14.1(a)), despite the fact that, simultaneously, the thalamus undergoes a global inhibition that prevents the transfer of signals from the external world to the neocortex (Steriade 2001*a*). This suggests that, during SWS, corticocortical operations are preserved and may lead to reorganization and specification of neuronal circuits in cortex and target structures (Steriade *et al.* 1993*a*). Our view is corroborated by studies using indicators of neuronal activities during SWS in humans, revealing more marked changes in those neocortical areas that are implicated in memory tasks and decision-making during wakefulness (Maquet *et al.* 1997).

In this chapter, we discuss the role played by augmenting responses elicited by stimuli at 10 Hz, which are the experimental model of sleep spindles, in producing plastic changes in neuronal properties through the rhythmic repetition of spike-bursts and spike-trains fired by thalamic and cortical neurons. Thalamically generated spindles (7–14 Hz) represent an electrographic landmark of early SWS stages. They also follow the depolarizing phase of the cortically generated slow oscillation (0.5–1 Hz), which is a pervasive brain rhythm during SWS in both animals and humans (Steriade *et al.* 1993*c*;

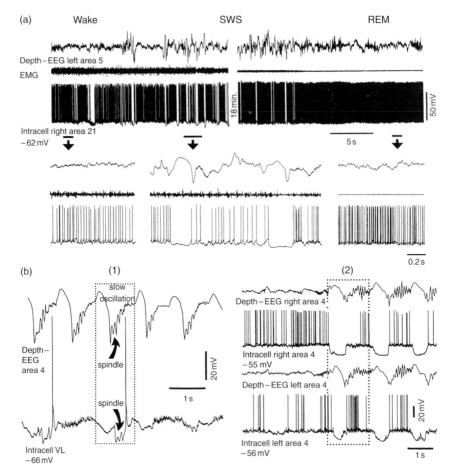

Figure 14.1 Changes in membrane potential and firing patterns during natural wake and sleep states and coalescence of different sleep oscillations into complex wave patterns. (a) Chronically implanted cat. Regular-spiking neuron from posterior association suprasylvian area 21 was intracellularly recorded (together with electromyogram (EMG) and electroencephalogram (EEG) from area 5) during transition from wake to SWS and, further, to REM sleep (there is a non-depicted period of 18 min during SWS). Periods marked by horizontal bars are expanded below (arrows). Note tonic firing during both waking and REM sleep, and cyclic hyperpolarizations associated with depth-positive EEG field potentials during SWS. (b) Cats under ketamine–xylazine anesthesia. (1) intracellular recording of thalamocortical (TC) neuron from ventrolateral (VL) nucleus, together with EEG waves from the depth of cortical area 4 where VL nucleus projects. The excitatory component (depth-negative, downward deflection) of the slow cortical oscillation (0.9 Hz) is followed by a sequence of spindle waves at ∼10 Hz (arrows), generated in the thalamus. This combination gives rise to what are called K-complexes in human sleep. One typical cycle of these two combined rhythms (slow oscillation and spindles) is indicated by the dotted box; note that the hyperpolarizing IPSPs building up spindles may lead to a postinhibitory rebound. (2) dual simultaneous intracellular recordings from cortical neurons (right and left areas 4) show that EEG synchronization is concomitant with simultaneous hyperpolarizations in neocortical neurons. EEG activated pattern at left, and occurrence of EEG synchronization. Only when both cells simultaneously displayed large hyperpolarizations, was the EEG fully synchronized with the patterns of slow oscillation and brief spindle sequences (modified from Steriade *et al.* 2001 (a); Timofeev and Steriade 1997 (b1); Contreras and Steriade 1995 (b2)).

Achermann and Borbély 1997; Amzica and Steriade 1997) and has the virtue of grouping other SWS rhythms, such as spindles and delta (Steriade *et al.* 1993*d*). The synchronous firing of cortical neurons during the slow oscillation triggers the thalamic neuronal equipment that generates spindles, thalamic reticular (RE), and thalamocortical (TC) neurons. The coalescence of the slow oscillation and a brief sequence of spindle waves (Fig. 14.1(b2)) forms the K-complex during SWS in both experimental animals and humans.

The mechanisms of augmenting responses, which have been introduced as a model of naturally occurring spindles (Morison and Dempsey 1943), have been revealed intracellularly in cortical slices maintained *in vitro* (Castro-Alamancos and Connors 1996), in simplified preparations and intact neuronal networks *in vivo* (Steriade and Timofeev 1997; Timofeev and Steriade 1998; Steriade *et al.* 1998*c*), and *in computo* (Bazhenov *et al.* 1998*a,b*).

Plasticity during and outlasting augmenting responses

Intrathalamic augmenting responses

There are two types of intrathalamic augmenting responses recorded from TC neurons in decorticated animals (Steriade and Timofeev 1997). One of them is based on the progressive depolarization of these neurons in response to thalamic stimuli at 10 Hz, is thus termed *high-threshold* (HT) (Fig. 14.2(a)), and may be ascribed to a high-threshold Ca^{2+} conductance (Hernández-Cruz and Pape 1989; Kammermeier and Jones 1997). The other type of intrathalamic augmentation is termed *low-threshold* (LT) because it develops from progressively growing LT responses (Deschênes *et al.* 1984; Jahnsen and Llinás 1984) resulting from the increase in Cl^--dependent inhibitory postsynaptic potentials (IPSPs) during successive stimuli at 10 Hz (Fig. 14.2(b)).

These two (HT and LT) types of augmenting responses in TC neurons are due to opposite changes produced in gamma-amino-butyric-acidergic (GABAergic) RE neurons by intrathalamic stimulation at different intensities (Timofeev and Steriade 1998; Fig. 14.3). Decremental responses elicited in RE neurons by low-intensity thalamic stimuli are due to intra-RE inhibitory processes, through dendrodendritic and recurrent collateral axonal contacts (Deschênes *et al.* 1985; Yen *et al.* 1985; Liu *et al.* 1995) that mediate $GABA_{A-B}$ IPSPs (Ulrich and Huguenard 1996; Sanchez-Vives and McCormick 1997). The decremental responses in RE neurons would produce a progressive release from inhibition in target TC neurons, with the consequence of developing HT augmenting responses in TC neurons. By contrast, the incremental responses in RE neurons, obtained with higher-intensity stimuli, would produce a progressive hyperpolarization in TC neurons, with the consequence of de-inactivating the Ca^{2+}-mediated LT conductance and increasing postinhibitory rebound spike-bursts.

Thalamic plasticity occurs during augmenting responses and consists of progressive diminution in IPSPs and increased number of action potentials in HT spike-bursts elicited by thalamic volleys (Steriade and Timofeev 1997). The depolarization area

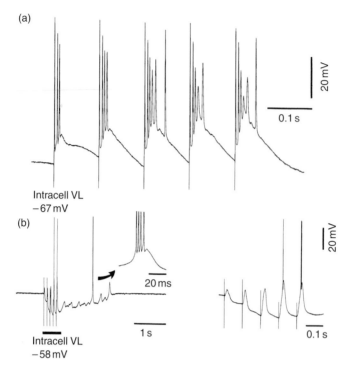

Figure 14.2 Short-term plasticity in the thalamus of decorticated cats. Ketamine–xylazine anesthesia. (a) Intrathalamic augmenting responses of high-threshold (HT) type. Intracellular recording of thalamocortical (TC) neuron from the ventrolateral (VL) nucleus shows HT augmenting responses of VL neuron to local VL stimulation (5 pulses at 10 Hz), occurring at a progressively depolarized level. Responses consisted of an early antidromic action potential, followed by orthodromic spikes displaying progressive augmentation and spike inactivation. (b) Low-threshold (LT) augmenting responses of TC neurons from VL nucleus, developing from progressive increase in IPSP-rebound sequences and followed by a self-sustained spindle. Arrow indicates expanded spike-burst (action potentials truncated). The part marked by horizontal bar and indicating augmenting responses is expanded at right (modified from Steriade and Timofeev 1997).

(mV × ms) increases during successive HT augmenting responses. In responses elicited by pulse-trains at 10 Hz, there is a dramatic increase in the depolarization area from the first to the fifth response in the first and second pulse-trains, with progressive increases during subsequent pulse-trains (Fig. 14.4).

Thalamocortical augmenting responses

Dual simultaneous intracellular recordings from TC and cortical neurons during thalamically evoked augmenting responses revealed a selective enhancement of the secondary depolarization in cortical neurons, from the second and following stimuli in pulse-trains at 10 Hz, which is initiated at 7–16 ms and is associated with diminished amplitude of

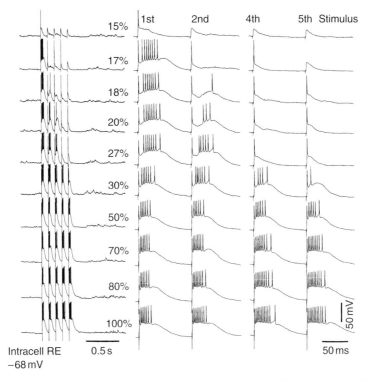

Figure 14.3 Intensity-dependency of decremental and incremental intracellular responses of rostral thalamic reticular (RE) neuron to repetitive (10 Hz) stimulation of ventrolateral (VL) nucleus. Decorticated cat under ketamine–xylazine anesthesia. Left: lower speed; responses to all the five stimuli in a pulse-train at 10 Hz. Middle and right, higher speed; responses to first and second and fourth and fifth stimuli, respectively. Decremental responses were observed with stimuli at 15–30% of maximal intensity. Incremental responses occurred at high intensities (70–100%). At half intensity (50%) there was virtually no change in the number of spikes evoked by the five stimuli in the pulse-train (from Timofeev and Steriade 1998).

the early excitatory post synaptic potential (EPSP) (Steriade *et al.* 1998*c*). This is the essential feature of augmenting responses in the intact brain.

   The decreased amplitude of the primary EPSP during augmenting responses might be partially due to the shunting action of cortically generated IPSPs. However, other factors are more likely involved in the decreased amplitude of cortical primary EPSP. Stimulation at dorsal thalamic sites simultaneously excites, in addition to TC axons and perikarya, corticothalamic and/or prethalamic axons. The second and following stimuli in the pulse-train at 10 Hz reach TC neurons in a hyperpolarized state, which prevents TC neurons to reach firing threshold when driven by corticothalamic and/or prethalamic axons. The absence of short-latency firing of TC neurons largely contributes to the diminished amplitude of the primary EPSP in cortical neurons. By contrast, the EPSPs that occur at a hyperpolarized level of TC neurons are able to activate LTSs crowned by

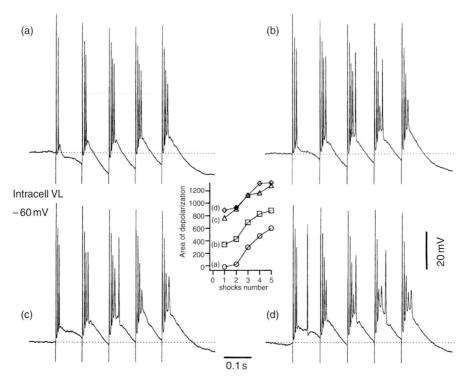

Figure 14.4 Short-term plasticity from repetitive intrathalamic augmenting responses of the high-threshold type. Intracellular recording of VL neuron in cat with ipsilateral hemidecorticaion and callosal cut. Ketamine–xylazine anesthesia. Progressive and persistent increase in the area of depolarization by repeating the pulse-trains. Pulse-trains consisting of five stimuli at 10 Hz were applied to the VL every 2 s. The VL cell was recorded under +0.5 nA (−60 mV); at rest, the membrane potential was −72 mV. Responses to four pulse-trains (a–d) are illustrated; (a) and (b) were separated by 2 s; (c) and (d) were also separated by 2 s and followed 14 s after (b). The responses to 5-shock train consisted of an early antidromic spike, followed by orthodromic spikes displaying progressive augmentation and spike inactivation. Note that, with repetition of pulse-trains, IPSPs elicited by preceding stimuli in the train were progressively reduced until their complete obliteration and spike-bursts contained more action potentials with spike inactivation. The graph depicts the increased area of depolarization from the first to the fifth responses in each pulse-train as well as from pulse-train (a) to pulse-trains (b) and (d) (from Steriade and Timofeev 1997).

fast Na$^+$ spikes, which mediate the secondary depolarization (will longer latency) during augmenting responses of cortical neurons.

Thus, at least two, nonexclusive factors account for the increased amplitude of the cortical secondary depolarizing component during augmentation. (i) The postinhibitory spike-bursts during the LT augmenting responses in TC neurons precede by ~3 ms the augmented depolarization in cortical neurons (Fig. 14.5(b3)). (ii) Progressively stronger volleys from TC neurons during LT-type augmenting responses can

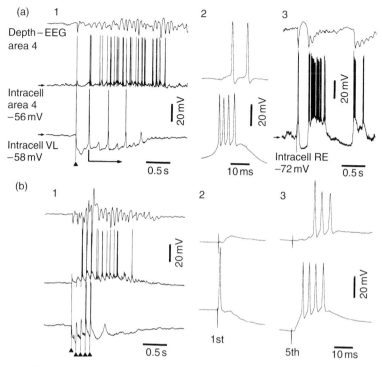

Figure 14.5 Self-sustained oscillatory activity (∼10 Hz) in cortical neuron after augmenting responses is accompanied by sustained hyperpolarization in simultaneous recorded TC neuron. Cat under barbiturate anesthesia. Dual intracellular recording of cortical neuron from area 4 and TC neuron from ventrolateral (VL) nucleus (a1–2) and (b), and intracellular recording from RE neuron in the peri-VL district (a3). (a1) single stimulus (arrowhead) to thalamic VL nucleus produces, after the initial excitation and a period of inhibition in both neurons, a series of oscillatory waves in cortex, whereas the VL neuron remained hyperpolarized and displayed occasional LTSs and burst discharges (the first spike-burst is expanded (a2). (a3) same VL stimulus produces rhythmic spike-bursts in RE neuron. (b) pulse-train (5 stimuli at 10 Hz) applied to VL nucleus produced augmenting responses in cortical neuron, whereas simultaneously recorded VL neuron displayed hyperpolarization (same neurons as in a1–2). First and fifth responses are expanded (b2) and (b3), respectively). Note persistent oscillatory activity at 10 Hz in cortical neuron, after cessation of thalamic stimulation (from Steriade and Timofeev 2001).

activate local-circuit inhibitory neurons in cortex, hyperpolarize pyramidal neurons, and de-inactivate Ca^{2+}-dependent LT currents in these neurons (Kawaguchi 1993; de la Peña and Geijo-Barrientos 1996), thus generating augmented waves. During spindle oscillations too, rhythmic spike-bursts from TC neurons produce inhibitory effects on cortical pyramidal neurons, as demonstrated by the transformation of reversed IPSPs, recorded with Cl^--filled micropipettes, into robust bursts resembling paroxysmal depolarizations during seizures (Contreras *et al.* 1997).

Simultaneous intracellular recordings from cortical and TC neurons demonstrate that the former display post-augmenting oscillatory activities in the same frequency range as that of evoked augmenting responses, whereas the latter remained hyperpolarized because of the pressure from the GABAergic RE neurons (Steriade *et al.* 1998*c*). These data show that intracortical circuits have a major influence on the incoming inputs from TC neurons and can amplify oscillatory activity arising in the thalamus. Figure 14.5(a1–2) shows that, with single thalamic stimuli, the initial response in TC neurons is followed by a biphasic, $GABA_{A-B}$ IPSP and a sequence of hyperpolarizations in the frequency range of spindles, which favor the occurrence of spike-bursts crowning low-threshold spikes (LTSs). The prolonged inhibition of TC neurons is probably generated by RE neurons that fire repeated spike-bursts in response to a single stimulus to the dorsal thalamus (panel (a3) in Fig. 14.5). Simultaneously, the intracellularly recorded cortical neuron displays a depolarizing plateau giving rise to trains of action potentials that are associated with self-sustained oscillations in cortical electroencephalogram (EEG). Similarly, opposing activity patterns in TC and cortical neurons are seen with pulse-trains of five stimuli at 10 Hz (Fig. 14.5(b)).

Thus, although cortical potentials are directly produced by thalamofugal volleys (see subthreshold EPSPs and full-blown action potentials in cortical neuron, following the action potentials in TC neuron, in Fig. 14.5(b3)), the cortex uses its own machinery to elaborate oscillatory responses that outlast thalamic stimuli, despite the fact that, simultaneously, TC neurons remain under a prolonged hyperpolarization. This activity pattern, which implicates intracortical activity that may amplify corticipetal volleys arising in the thalamus and may even be independent on thalamic activity, corroborates data on the active role of cortical circuitry in the genesis of spindles (Kandel and Buzsáki 1997).

To sum up, although TC neurons have a high propensity to fire spike-bursts and trigger incremental responses in target neocortical neurons, the latter have the ability to maintain and develop self-sustained oscillations. This is an autonomous, intracortically generated activity, within the frequency range of the previous stimulus-evoked responses, since TC neurons continue to remain hyperpolarized following augmenting responses because of the inhibitory pressure from GABAergic RE neurons.

Intracortical augmenting responses

Compared with augmenting responses elicited in cortical neurons by thalamic stimuli, corticocortical augmenting responses are less ample and the progressive growing amplitude of successive responses is much less evident (Steriade *et al.* 1998*c*). The difference is accounted for by the complete absence of, or reduction in spike-bursts size arising in TC neurons when intracortical stimulation is used.

Some features of augmenting responses elicited in isolated cortical slabs (Timofeev *et al.* 2002) are similar to those found in corticocortical augmenting responses recorded in intact cortex (Steriade *et al.* 1998*c*), but augmenting potentials within the slab can only be evoked by using relatively high-intensity stimuli, which suggests that they occur as a network-related phenomenon requiring a sufficient number of activated cortical neurons and axons.

Despite the fact that intracortical augmenting responses are less ample than in the presence of the thalamus, plastic changes occur in cortex and they are independent of thalamic events. Rhythmic repetition of pulse-trains at 10 Hz changes the response pattern of cortical neurons within isolated slabs *in vivo* (Timofeev *et al.* 2002). These alterations in neuronal responsiveness during augmenting responses elicited in isolated cortical slabs are mediated by synaptic and intrinsic factors. The synaptic factors are demonstrated by the requirement of setting into action an increased neuronal population for the elaboration of incremental responses. To test the role of intrinsic factors in the generation of short- or medium-range enhancement of excitability, the paradigm of cellular conditioning (Baranyi *et al.* 1991) or a modification of it can be used. Association, at appropriate time-intervals, between electrical stimuli within the cortical slab that elicit subthreshold synaptic depolarizations with direct depolarizations induced by current pulses can lead to suprathreshold synaptic depolarizations after a variable number of conditioning-testing stimuli (Fig. 14.6). Low-intensity, extracellular electrical stimulation within isolated cortical slabs elicits active periods (200–300 ms) that are not associated with action potentials. The association of extracellular electrical stimuli with depolarizing current steps induces, after a repetition of 20–50 such combined stimuli, a state in which extracellular stimuli, with the same intensity as when they were subthreshold, elicit active periods with action potentials. This increased excitability can last for 3–4 min and thus indicates that synaptic responses associated with firing of postsynaptic response may induce a mid-term increase in excitability of cortical neurons (Cissé *et al.* 2001).

It was postulated that the hippocampus orchestrates neocortical memory retrieval during consolidation, and simultaneous recordings from neurons in the hippocampus and neocortex showed that memory trace reactivation is coherent at these two levels, leading to the suggestion that the initiation site of the reactivation process is area CA3 (Buzsáki 1989, 1998; Siapas and Wilson 1998; Kudrimoti *et al.* 1999; Sutherland and McNaughton 2000). Although in the intact brain the hippocampal–neocortical dialog is obviously important in the consolidation of memory traces, the experimental results from isolated neocortical slabs (Timofeev *et al.* 2002) and from the intact cortex in athalamic animals (Steriade *et al.* 1993*d*; see below, Fig. 14.10) show that neocortical networks alone are capable of neuronal plasticity, even if at a more rudimentary level.

Prethalamic stimuli do not produce augmenting responses

As mentioned above, dorsal thalamic stimulation activates axons from a series of ascending and descending systems. We tested the possibility that fibers from ascending systems, arising in brainstem and related structures, also produce augmenting responses, and we recorded TC neurons while stimulating at 10 Hz cerebellothalamic axons in brachium conjunctivum (BC). TC neurons responded to BC stimuli with short-latency (1.2 ms)

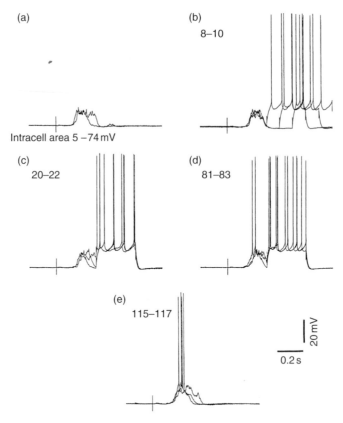

Figure 14.6 Intracellular conditioning in cortical slab from area 5. Cat under ketamine–xylazine anesthesia. (a) Stimulus within the slab evoked a long-latency, subthreshold depolarizing event. This was the conditioned (C) stimulus. (b) Depolarizing current pulses (unconditioned, U, stimulus) followed the C stimulus at three time-intervals (trials 8–10). (c) Trials 20–22 with C immediately followed by U stimulus. (d) Beginning of development from subthreshold to suprathreshold C responses (trials 81–83). (e and c) Stimulus alone elicited suprathreshold responses in all trials (115–117). The extinction procedure is not depicted here (unpublished experiment by I Timofeev and M Steriade).

EPSPs, which gave rise to action potentials at more depolarized levels, but did not evoke augmenting responses with rhythmic stimuli at 10 Hz (Fig. 14.7).

Corticothalamic augmenting responses and their consequences

As shown above, plasticity may occur within the thalamus of decorticated animals or within the isolated neocortex, and thus can be investigated in both simplified *in vivo* preparations and even in slices maintained *in vitro*. However, the full development of mechanisms leading to the coalescence of different SWS oscillatory types and to the storage of information requires preserved connectivity between the cortex and thalamus,

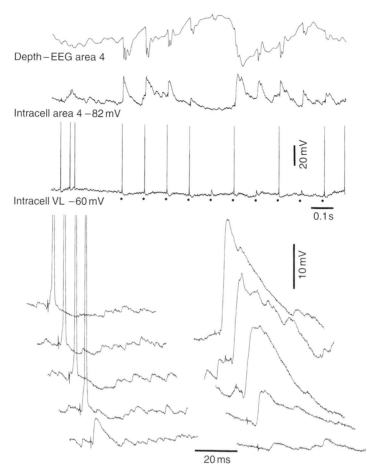

Figure 14.7 Stimulation of cerebellothalamic projection pathway (brachium conjunctivum, BC) does not elicit augmenting responses in thalamocortical systems. Cat under ketamine–xylazine anesthesia. Simultaneous recording of depth negative EEG together with intracellular recordings from a cortical cell (area 4) and a TC cell from VL nucleus. Stimuli in the pulse-train at 10 Hz indicated by dots. Expansion of the early parts of responses to the first five stimuli of VL cell (bottom left) and cortical cell (bottom right) is shown. BC stimulation revealed a monosynaptic EPSP in the TC cell leading to spikes. Hyperpolarization during depth-positivity of EEG prevented the cortical cell from firing and the cell had a small amplitude EPSP. The responsiveness of TC and cortical cells was affected by the slow oscillation but did not increment during the train of stimuli at 10 Hz (from Bazhenov *et al.* 1998*b*).

under the control of generalized modulatory systems. The differences between the results obtained in simplified preparations and in the intact brain are reported elsewhere (Steriade 2001*b*).

Repeated spike-bursts evoked by volleys applied to corticothalamic pathways or resulting from spontaneous oscillations may lead to self-sustained activity patterns, resembling

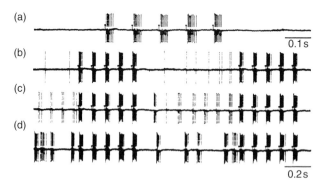

Figure 14.8 Development from corticothalamic augmenting responses to self-sustained activity. Brainstem-transected cat. Cortically evoked spike-bursts in thalamic VL neuron (a). Motor cortex stimulation was applied with pulse-trains at 10 Hz delivered every 1.3 s. In (a), the pattern of cortically evoked responses at the onset of rhythmic pulse-trains (faster speed than in (b)–(d)). (b)–(d) responses at later stages of stimulation. Stimuli are marked by dots. In (b)–(d) stimuli and evoked spike-bursts are aligned. Note progressive appearance of spontaneous spike-bursts resembling the evoked ones, as a form of "memory" in the corticothalamic circuit (from Steriade 1991).

those evoked in the late stages of stimulation (Fig. 14.8). Such changes are due to resonant activities in closed loops, as in "memory" processes (Steriade 1991).

One of the mechanisms implicated in neuronal plasticity as a result of rhythmic spike-bursts during augmenting responses associated with large depolarization area may be the Ca^{2+} entry in TC and cortical neurons (Steriade *et al.* 1993b; Berridge 2000; Sejnowski and Destexhe 2000). There are several mechanisms that may underlie increased responsiveness promoted by sleep spindles, the oscillation that we mimicked by augmenting responses. During the depolarizing phases of sleep oscillations or as an effect of repeated pulse-trains leading to augmenting responses, neuronal firing results in local increase in the $[K^+]_o$, which enhances neuronal excitability, thus providing conditions for amplification of responses that may remain effective up to 15 min (see Fig. 14.9 in Timofeev *et al.* 2002). The increased $[Ca^{2+}]_i$ in association with concurrent synaptic inputs may activate protein kinase A (PKA) and/or ras/mitogen-activated protein kinase (Abel *et al.* 1997; Dolmetsch *et al.* 2001) that seem to be involved in memory consolidation.

Development from self-sustained normal oscillations to paroxysmal states

Plasticity processes are regarded as beneficial for the storage of information, but they can eventually lead, with prolonged stimuli, to self-sustained discharges of the epileptic type. This was demonstrated in many central structures. Self-sustained after-discharges are gradually generated from incremental responses in amygdalo–hippocampal circuits and the waveform as well as frequency of potentials during the self-sustained after-discharge are nearly identical to those of responses during the final period of stimulation

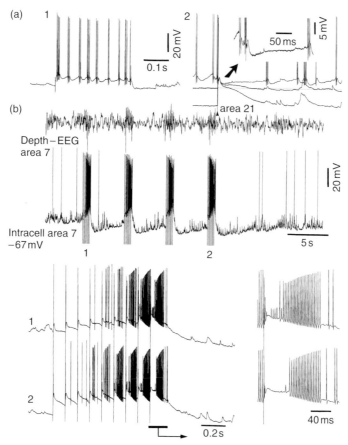

Figure 14.9 Progressively growing depolarization during cortically evoked augmenting responses in cortical FRB neuron from cat suprasylvian area 7. Barbiturate anesthesia. Close intracortical stimulation, in adjacent area 21. (a1) identification of FRB neuron by depolarizing current step (0.5 nA). (a2) synaptic responses of this neuron to single stimulus to area 21 are dominated by IPSPs. The three V_m levels are under +1 nA, at rest (−67 mV), and under −1 nA. *B*, responses of this FRB neuron to four pulse-trains, each consisting of 9 pulses at 10 Hz applied to area 21. Responses to pulse-trains 1 and 2 (last) are expanded below, and responses to the last stimulus in these pulse-trains are further expanded at right (arrow). The neuron persistently depolarized during stimulation. At depolarized levels of the V_m, IPSPs evoked by area 21 stimuli (see a2) shunted the early occurring spikes. The latency and duration of the spike shunting (lasting for 20–50 ms and seen in the expanded traces at bottom right) is consistent with the latency and duration of the early IPSP observed in the upper right panel (a2) (unpublished experiment by Timofeev and Steriade).

(Steriade 1964). In behaving monkeys, augmenting responses led to self-sustained seizure consisting of spike-wave (SW) complexes at ∼3 Hz that were confined to neocortex as they were recorded from the cortical depth, without any reflection at the surface (Steriade 1974). These data suggested that at least some types of SW seizures are cortically generated. Indeed, we demonstrated more recently that complex seizures, resembling the electrographic pattern of Lennox–Gastaut syndrome and consisting of SW complexes at 2–3 Hz interspersed with fast runs at 10–15 Hz, (i) are initiated in neocortex (Steriade *et al.* 1998*a*); (ii) spread to the thalamus only after 5–7 s (Neckelmann *et al.* 1998); and (iii) are associated with steady hyperpolarization and phasic IPSPs in TC neurons, generated by GABAergic RE neurons that faithfully follow each paroxysmal depolarizing shift in neocortical neurons (Steriade and Contreras 1995; Timofeev *et al.* 1998).

In some cases, enhanced neuronal excitability following augmenting responses is so powerful that it reaches a level close to that underlying paroxysmal activity. Figure 14.9 shows such an enhancement in which the potentiation of responsiveness in a fast-rhythmic-bursting (FRB) cortical neuron, which resulted at the end of pulse-trains at 10 Hz, took the pattern of a paroxysmal response. Compared to regular-spiking and intrinsically-bursting neurons, deeply lying FRB neurons, some of them with thalamic projections (Steriade *et al.* 1998*b*), display a much higher propensity to produce powerful spike-bursts during augmenting responses, in which the primary and secondary depolarizations coalesce and result in an increased number of action potentials (Steriade *et al.* 1998*c*; Steriade and Timofeev 2001). Their projections to the thalamus, and in particular to rostral intralaminar nuclei that return their axons to widespread cortical areas (Jones 1985), can bring into action cortical areas that are distant to the initial source of corticothalamic drive, and thus increase the synchronization process.

After complete hemithalamectomy (Fig. 14.10(b)), ipsilateral cortical association neurons display augmenting responses to 10-Hz stimulation of homotopic points in the contralateral cortex. Repetition of pulse-trains lead to a progressive depolarization of membrane potential, increase in the depolarization area of responses, and increased number of action potentials in response to testing stimuli (Steriade *et al.* 1993*c*). These progressive changes in membrane potential and synaptic properties are especially pronounced in intrinsically-bursting cells that can be recorded not only in deep layers, as conventionally assumed, but also more superficially, in layer III of cat association cortex that receives callosal inputs (Fig. 14.10(a)). After protracted callosal volleys, leading to progressive increase in membrane depolarization and greater number of action potentials in spike-bursts during augmenting responses, cortical neurons reach the status of self-sustained seizure, with spike-bursts at ~8–10 Hz, a frequency range similar to that of evoked responses during the last period of cortical stimulation (Fig. 14.10(a)).

The changes in responsiveness of cortical neurons, which lead to self-sustained oscillations of the paroxysmal type, are already initiated during rhythmic stimulation with pulse-trains at 10 Hz. Such changes consist of the appearance of "spontaneous" depolarizing events, occurring between pulse-trains and having the same frequency as that used in these pulse-trains. That plastic changes in cortex are independent of thalamic events is shown not only by dual intracellular recordings demonstrating progressive

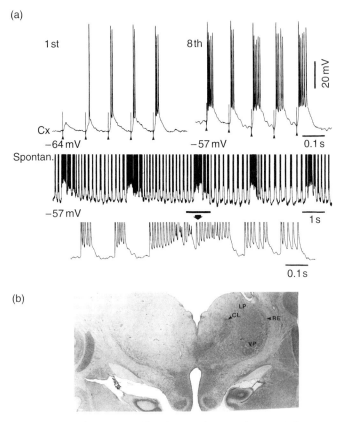

Figure 14.10 Changes in membrane potential and responsiveness of neocortical neuron after repetitive callosal volleys in a thalamically lesioned cat (see bottom panel with kainic thalamic lesion, ipsilateral to the recorded cortical neuron). Intracellular recording from intrinsically-bursting neuron recorded at 1.5-mm depth in area 7. Urethane anesthesia. (a) Responses to repetitive stimulation (5-shock trains at 10 Hz, repeated every 3 s) of the contralateral area 7. The intracortical augmenting responses to the first and eighth trains are illustrated. Note depolarization by about 7 mV and increased number of action potentials within bursts after repetitive stimulation. Below, self-sustained, paroxysmal activity following repeated stimulation, as shown in the top panel. This activity consisted of rhythmic spike-bursts at ~8–10 Hz, interspersed with longer bursts at a slower frequency (~0.4 Hz). (b) Excitotoxic, kainate-induced lesion of the ipsilateral thalamus. Abbreviations: CL, LP, RE, and VP, centrolateral, lateroposterior, reticular and ventroposterior thalamic nuclei (modified from Steriade *et al.* 1993*d*).

depolarization, enhanced responsiveness, and self-sustained oscillations of neocortical neurons, concomitant with the hyperpolarization of TC neurons, but also by evidence of plasticity leading to paroxysmal activity in isolated cortical slabs *in vivo* (Fig. 14.11).

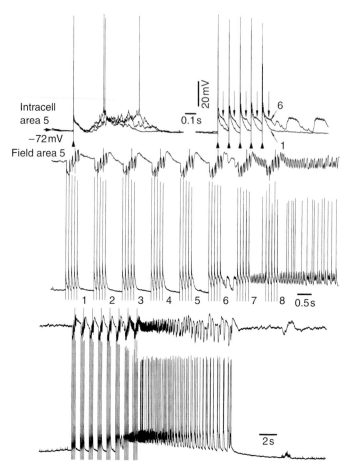

Figure 14.11 Repeated pulse-trains at 10 Hz may lead to self-sustained paroxysm. Intracellular recording from a neuron in cortical suprasylvian slab of cat under ketamine–xylazine anesthesia. Upper left displays responses to single stimuli applied within the slab. Upper right displays superimposed responses to the first and sixth trains in a series of 5-stimuli pulse-trains at 10 Hz, delivered every second. Note the increased responses to the sixth pulse-train, especially in the late component of the response (marked by arrows). The whole period of stimulation is shown in the middle panel. This increased responsiveness on repeated 10-Hz pulse-trains led to the electrical seizure shown at bottom (from Timofeev *et al.* 2002).

Concluding remarks

The above data show that naturally occurring SWS oscillations and their experimental models, such as augmenting responses that mimic sleep spindles, produce progressive depolarization in the membrane potential of neocortical neurons, their increased responsiveness that may be short- or medium-range (up to 15 min), self-sustained oscillations with the same waveform and frequencies as those of evoked responses in prior stages of stimulation, and may develop into paroxysmal activity. Although the full development of these alterations is best seen with intact corticothalamic loops, plastic changes in neuronal responsiveness are also seen in the absence of thalamus and, at a more rudimentary level, in isolated neocortical slabs *in vivo*. Together with intracellular recordings in naturally sleeping animals, showing high discharge rates in SWS (Steriade *et al.* 2001; Timofeev *et al.* 2001), these results suggest that neocortical neurons are the sites of processes leading to consolidation of memory traces during SWS. It was suggested that both SWS and REM sleep are implicated in the process of network reorganization and memory consolidation, in the sense that early SWS stages favor retention of declarative memories, whereas sleep during late night, when episodes of REM sleep prevail, favors the retention of nondeclarative memories (Plihal and Born 1997). The role of REM sleep was challenged on the basis of a series of arguments, among them the stress induced in experiments with REM sleep deprivation (see Vertes and Eastman 2000; Siegel 2001). The role of SWS in memory consolidation is substantiated by results using ocular dominance plasticity during the critical period in cats (Frank *et al.* 2001) and by potentiation of discrimination tasks in humans if the training period is followed by sleep, the enhancement correlating more closely to SWS (Gais *et al.* 2000; Stickgold *et al.* 2000; see also Maquet 2001).

Acknowledgments

This work was made possible by grants from the Medical Research Council of Canada (presently, Canadian Institutes for Health Research), Human Frontier Science Program, National Institute of Health of the USA, and Fonds de la recherché en santé du Québec. We thank P. Giguère for technical assistance.

References

Abel, T., Nguyen, P. V., Barad, M., Deuel, T. A., Kandel, E. R., and **Bourtchouladze, R.** (1997). Genetic demonstration of a role for PKA in the late phase of LTP and in hippocampus-based long-term memory. *Cell*, **88**, 615–626.

Achermann, P. and **Borbély, A.** (1997). Low-frequency (<1 Hz) oscillations in the human sleep EEG. *Neuroscience*, **81**, 213–222.

Amzica, F. and **Steriade, M.** (1997). The K-complex: its slow (<1 Hz) rhythmicity and relation to delta waves. *Neurology*, **49**, 952–959.

Baranyi, A., Szente, M. B., and **Woody, C. D.** (1991). Properties of associative long-lasting potentiation induced by cellular conditioning in the motor cortex of conscious cats. *Neuroscience*, **42**, 321–334.

Bazhenov, M., Timofeev, I., Steriade, M., and **Sejnowski, T. J.** (1998*a*). Cellular and network models for intrathalamic augmenting responses during 10-Hz stimulation. *Journal of Neurophysiology*, **79**, 2730–2748.

Bazhenov, M., Timofeev, I., Steriade, M., and Sejnowski, T. J. (1998b). Computational models of thalamocortical augmenting responses. *Journal of Neuroscience*, **18**, 6444–6465.

Berridge, M. J. (2000). Calcium signaling systems in neurons: synaptic plasticity and sleep. In *The regulation of sleep* (eds A. A. Borbély, O. Hayaishi, T. J. Sejnowski, and J. S. Altman), pp. 65–75. Human Frontier Science Program, Strasbourg.

Buzsáki, G. (1989). Two-stage model of memory trace formation: a role for "noisy" brain states. *Neuroscience*, **31**, 551–570.

Buzsáki, G. (1998). Memory consolidation during sleep: a neurophysiological perspective. *Journal of Sleep Research*, **7**(Suppl. 1), 17–23.

Castro-Alamancos, M. A. and Connors, B. W. (1996). Cellular mechanisms of the augmenting response: short-term plasticity in a thalamocortical pathway. *Journal of Neuroscience*, **16**, 7742–7756.

Cissé, Y., Timofeev, I., Grenier, F., and Steriade, M. (2001). Intracellular pairing with synaptic activation leads to neocortical plasticity. *Society for Neuroscience Abstracts*, **27**, 366.

Contreras, D. and Steriade, M. (1995). Cellular basis of EEG slow rhythms: a study of dynamic corticothalamic relationships. *Journal of Neuroscience*, **15**, 604–622.

Contreras, D., Destexhe, A., and Steriade, M. (1997). Intracellular and computational characterization of the intracortical inhibitory control of synchronized thalamic inputs *in vivo*. *Journal of Neurophysiology*, **78**, 335–350.

Deschênes, M., Paradis, M., Roy, J. P., and Steriade, M. (1984). Electrophysiology of neurons of lateral thalamic nuclei in cat: resting properties and burst discharges. *Journal of Neurophysiology*, **51**, 1196–1219.

Deschênes, M., Madariaga-Domich, A., and Steriade, M. (1985). Dendrodendritic synapses in cat reticularis thalami nucleus, a structural basis for thalamic spindle synchronization. *Brain Research*, **334**, 169–171.

Dolmetsch, R. E., Pajvani, U., Fife, K., Spotts, J. M., and Greenberg, M. E. (2001). Signaling to the nucleus by an L-type calcium channel-calmodulin complex through the MPA kinase pathway. *Science*, **294**, 333–339.

Eccles, J. C. (1961). Chairman's opening remarks. In *The nature of sleep* (eds G. E. W. Wolstenholme and M. O'Connor), pp. 1–3. Churchill, London.

Frank, M. G., Issa, N. P., and Stryker, M. P. (2001). Sleep enhances plasticity in the developing visual cortex. *Neuron*, **30**, 275–287.

Gais, S., Plihal, W., Wagner, U., and Born, J. (2000). Early sleep triggers memory for early visual discrimination skills. *Nature Neuroscience*, **3**, 1335–1339.

Hernández-Cruz, A. and Pape, H. C. (1989). Identification of two calcium currents in acutely dissociated neurons from the rat lateral geniculate nucleus. *Journal of Neurophysiology*, **61**, 1270–1283.

Jahnsen, H. and Llinás, R. (1984). Ionic basis for electroresponsiveness and oscillatory properties of guinea-pig thalamic neurones *in vitro*. *Journal of Physiology London*, **349**, 227–247.

Jones, E. G. (1985). *The thalamus*. Plenum, New York.

Kammermeier, P. J. and **Jones, S. W.** (1997). High-voltage-activated calcium currents in neurons acutely isolated from the ventrobasal nucleus of the rat thalamus. *Journal of Neurophysiology*, **77**, 465–475.

Kandel, A. and **Buzsáki, G.** (1997). Cellular-synaptic generation of sleep spindles, spike-and-wave discharges, and evoked thalamocortical responses in the neocortex of rat. *Journal of Neuroscience*, **17**, 6783–6797.

Kawaguchi, Y. (1993). Groupings of nonpyramidal and pyramidal cells with specific physiological and morphological characteristics in rat frontal cortex. *Journal of Neurophysiology*, **69**, 416–431.

Kudrimoti, H. S., Barnes, C. A., and **McNaughton, B. L.** (1999). Reactivation of hippocampal cell assemblies: effects of behavioral state, experience, and EEG dynamics. *Journal of Neuroscience*, **19**, 4090–4101.

Liu, X. B., Warren, R. A., and **Jones, E. G.** (1995). Synaptic distribution of afferents from reticular nucleus in ventroposterior nucleus of cat thalamus. *Journal of Comparative Neurology*, **352**, 187–202.

Maquet, P. (2001). The role of sleep in learning and memory. *Science*, **294**, 1048–1052.

Maquet, P., Degueldre, C., Delfiore, G., Aerts, J., Péters, J. P., Luxen, A., and **Franck, G.** (1997). Functional neuroanatomy of human slow wave sleep. *Journal of Neuroscience*, **17**, 2807–2812.

Morison, R. S. and **Dempsey, E. W.** (1943). Mechanisms of thalamocortical augmentation and repetition. *American Journal of Physiology*, **138**, 297–308.

Neckelmann, D., Amzica, F., and **Steriade, M.** (1998). Spike-wave complexes and fast components of cortically generated seizures. III. Synchronizing mechanisms. *Journal of Neurophysiology*, **80**, 1480–1494.

Pavlov, I. P. (1923). "Innere Hemmung" der bedingten Reflexe und der Schlaf—ein und derselbe Prozess. *Skandinavisches Archiv für Physiologie*, **44**, 42–58.

de la Peña, E. and **Geijo-Barrientos, E.** (1996). Laminar localization, morphology, and physiological properties of pyramidal neurons that have low-threshold calcium current in the guinea-pig medial frontal cortex. *Journal of Neuroscience*, **16**, 5301–5311.

Plihal, W. and **Born, J.** (1997). Effects of early and late nocturnal sleep on declarative and procedural memory. *Journal of Cognitive Neuroscience*, **9**, 534–547.

Sanchez-Vives, M. V. and **McCormick, D. A.** (1997). Inhibitory interactions between perigeniculate GABAergic neurons. *Journal of Neuroscience*, **17**, 8894–8908.

Sejnowski, T. J. and **Destexhe, A.** (2000). Why do we sleep? *Brain Research*, **886**, 208–223.

Siapas, A. G. and **Wilson, M. A.** (1998). Coordinated interactions between hippocampal ripples and cortical spindles during slow-wave sleep. *Neuron*, **21**, 1123–1128.

Siegel, J. M. (2001). The REM sleep—memory consolidation hypothesis. *Science*, **294**, 1058–1063.

Steriade, M. (1964). Development of evoked responses into self-sustained activity within amygdalo-hippocampal circuits. *Electroencephalography and Clinical Neurophysiology*, **16**, 221–236.

Steriade, M. (1974). Interneuronal epileptic discharges related to spike-and-wave cortical seizures in behaving monkeys. *Electroencephalography and Clinical Neurophysiology*, **37**, 247–263.

Steriade, M. (1991). Alertness, quiet sleep, dreaming. In *Cerebral cortex, Vol. 9, Normal and altered states of function* (eds A. Peters and E. G. Jones), pp. 279–357. Plenum, New York.

Steriade, M. (2001*a*). Impact of network activities on neuronal properties in corticothalamic systems. *Journal of Neurophysiology*, **86**, 1–39.

Steriade, M. (2001*b*). *The intact and sliced brain*. The MIT Press, Cambridge (MA).

Steriade, M. and Contreras, D. (1995). Relations between cortical and thalamic cellular events during transition from sleep pattern to paroxysmal activity. *Journal of Neuroscience*, **15**, 623–642.

Steriade, M. and Timofeev, I. (1997). Short-term plasticity during intrathalamic augmenting responses in decorticated cats. *Journal of Neuroscience*, **17**, 3778–3795.

Steriade, M. and Timofeev, I. (2001). Corticothalamic operations through prevalent inhibition of thalamocortical neurons. *Thalamus and Related Systems*, **1**, 225–236.

Steriade, M., Contreras, D., Curró Dossi, R., and Nuñez, A. (1993*a*). The slow (<1 Hz) oscillation in reticular thalamic and thalamocortical neurons: scenario of sleep rhythm generation in interacting thalamic and neocortical networks. *Journal of Neuroscience*, **13**, 3284–3299.

Steriade, M., McCormick, D. A., and Sejnowski, T. J. (1993*b*). Thalamocortical oscillation in the sleeping and aroused brain. *Science*, **262**, 679–685.

Steriade, M., Nuñez, A., and Amzica, F. (1993*c*). A novel slow (<1 Hz) oscillation of neocortical neurons *in vivo*: depolarizing and hyperpolarizing components. *Journal of Neuroscience*, **13**, 3252–3265.

Steriade, M., Nuñez, A., and Amzica, F. (1993*d*). Intracellular analysis of relations between the slow (<1 Hz) neocortical oscillation and other sleep rhythms. *Journal of Neuroscience*, **13**, 3266–3283.

Steriade M., Amzica, F., Neckelmann, D., and Timofeev, I. (1998*a*). Spike-wave complexes and fast runs of cortically generated seizures. II. Extra- and intracellular patterns. *Journal of Neurophysiology*, **80**, 1456–1479.

Steriade, M., Timofeev, I., Dürmüller, N., and Grenier, F. (1998*b*). Dynamic properties of corticothalamic neurons and local cortical interneurons generating fast rhythmic (30–40 Hz) spike bursts. *Journal of Neurophysiology*, **79**, 483–490.

Steriade, M., Timofeev, I., Grenier, F., and Dürmüller, N. (1998*c*). Role of thalamic and cortical neurons in augmenting responses: dual intracellular recordings *in vivo*. *Journal of Neuroscience*, **18**, 6425–6443.

Steriade, M., Timofeev, I., and Grenier, F. (2001). Natural waking and sleep states: a view from inside neocortical neurons. *Journal of Neurophysiology*, **85**, 1969–1985.

Stickgold, R., Whitbee, D., Schirmer, B., Patel, V., and Hobson, J. A. (2000). Visual discrimination improvement. A multi-step process occurring during sleep. *Journal of Cognition Neuroscience*, **12**, 246–254.

Sutherland, G. R. and McNaughton, B. (2000). Memory traces reactivation in hippocampal and neocortical neuronal ensembles. *Current Opinion in Neurobiology*, **10**, 180–186.

Timofeev, I. and **Steriade, M.** (1997). Fast (mainly 30–100 Hz) oscillations in the cat cerebellothalamic pathway and their synchronization with cortical potentials. *Journal of Physiology (London)*, **504**, 153–168.

Timofeev, I. and **Steriade, M.** (1998). Cellular mechanisms underlying intrathalamic augmenting responses of reticular and relay neurons. *Journal of Neurophysiology*, **79**, 2716–2729.

Timofeev, I., Grenier, F., and **Steriade, M.** (1998). Spike-wave complexes and fast runs of cortically generated seizures. IV. Paroxysmal fast runs in cortical and thalamic neurons. *Journal of Neurophysiology*, **80**, 1495–1513.

Timofeev, I., Grenier, F., and **Steriade, M.** (2001). Disfacilitation and active inhibition in the neocortex during the natural sleep-wake cycle: an intracellular study. *Proceedings of the National Academy of Sciences, USA*, **98**, 1924–1929.

Timofeev, I., Grenier, F., Bazhenov, M., Houweling, A., Sejnowski, T. J., and **Steriade, M.** (2002). Short- and medium-term plasticity associated with augmenting responses in cortical slabs and spindles in intact cortex of cats *in vivo. Journal of Physiology (London)*, **542**, 583–598.

Ulrich, D. and **Huguenard, J. R.** (1996). GABA$_B$ receptor-mediated responses in GABAergic projection neurones of rat nucleus reticularis thalami *in vitro. Journal of Physiology London*, **493**, 845–854.

Vertes, R. P. and **Eastman, K. E.** (2000). The case against memory consolidation in REM sleep. *Behavioral Brain Science*, **23**, 867–876.

Yen, C. T., Conley, M., Hendry, S. H. C., and **Jones, E. G.** (1985). The morphology of physiologically identified GABAergic neurons in the somatic sensory part of the thalamic reticular nucleus in the cat. *Journal of Neuroscience*, **5**, 2254–2268.

CELLULAR LEVEL

Consolidation of the memory trace is known to rely on gene expression and protein synthesis (McGaugh 2000). Therefore, the description of the effects of sleep on recent memory traces would not be complete without the characterization of the molecular processes taking place at the cellular level during this state. Unfortunately, the latter endeavor is still in its early stages. While there are now several reports on gene expression during wakefulness and sleep (Tononi and Cirelli 2001), only a handful of studies have tried to specify activity-dependent gene expression during sleep.

Hellman and Abel (University of Pennsylvania) set the stage to this section in describing the framework within which cognitive neurosciences consider memory processes. They stress the existence of multiple memory systems, the prevalent role of the hippocampal formation in explicit memory and the important phenomenon of temporally graded retrograde amnesia after hippocampal lesions. They then turn to the description of the molecular processes underlying memory consolidation. They provide some clues on how sleep could influence these processes. They emphasize the modulatory context set by acetylcholine during REM sleep and the role of adenosine in synaptic plasticity. They finish by describing the role of NMDA receptors in memory consolidation and its possible relation to the replay of firing patterns within the rat hippocampus during post-exposure sleep.

Within this general framework, the chapter by Pavlides (The Rockefeller University, New York) and Ribeiro (Duke University Medical Center, Durham) focus on the modulation by previous waking experience of the expression of immediate early gene *zif-268* in rat hippocampus and neocortex during sleep. For the first time, they provide evidence at the cellular level, for the re-expression *zif-268* during REM sleep, after exposure to various kinds of experiences during wakefulness. These observations are particularly important, given the role of *zif-268* in neural plasticity. The parallel between these cellular processes and the reactivations of hippocampal firing patterns during post-training REM sleep is striking. These data further support the potential role played by the reactivation of memory processes during post-training sleep.

The last chapter, by Krueger *et al.* (Washington State University, Pullman), is particularly important in understanding two intricate-sleep functions. Sleep is modulated by the activity performed during previous waking periods. For didactic purposes, the activity-dependent processes can be viewed as either use-dependent or experience-dependent. The former are intimately linked to the neuronal workload during the preceding waking period. They are related to the restorative function of sleep and probably have a limited time course. The latter are tightly related to memory processes and entail the expansion of the behavioral repertoire after the exposure to a new environment. In contrast to restoration, consolidation might go on long after the last training session has ended.

Here, Krueger *et al.* show that various compounds (such as NO and various hormones, and cytokines) share three main functional features. They are released in response to neural activity; they are somnogenic and they trigger a cascade of events involved in neural plasticity. After reviewing the somnogenic factors which are released in an activity-dependent manner, they focus on two examples, more closely related to neural plasticity. First, the expression of nerve growth factor (NGF), a neurotrophin involved in neural plasticity, is modulated by sleep/sleep deprivation only in neurones with an elevated activity during previous waking periods. Second, they concentrate on metalloproteinase-9 which is involved in the interaction between neurones and extracellular matrix, a critical feature in neural plasticity. It is shown that sleep deprivation modifies the cerebral expression of the metalloproteinase-9 induced by spatial learning. These studies open the way to the study of sleep-related activity-dependent molecular processes.

References

McGaugh, J. L. (2000). Memory—a century of consolidation. *Science*, **287**, 248–251.

Tononi, G. and Cirelli, C. (2001). Modulation of brain gene expression during sleep and wakefulness: a review of recent findings. *Neuropsychopharmacology*, **25**, S28–S35.

CHAPTER 15

MOLECULAR MECHANISMS OF MEMORY CONSOLIDATION

KEVIN M. HELLMAN AND TED ABEL

The recall of memories during dreams has suggested that memory is consolidated during sleep. Indeed, memory even appears to be replayed in rodents during sleep (Nadasdy *et al.* 1999; Louie and Wilson 2001), and sleep is necessary for consolidation of certain memory tasks (Smith *et al.* 1998; Stickgold *et al.* 2000; Graves *et al.* 2001*b*). Recent research at the molecular, pharmacological, behavioral, and genetic levels has defined molecular mechanisms that mediate the consolidation of memory (Abel and Lattal 2001). Interestingly, the specific molecular mechanisms that mediate certain forms of memory storage are regulated by sleep systems, suggesting that sleep and memory consolidation may involve similar molecular mechanisms. To establish a relationship between sleep and memory consolidation, it is crucial to understand the biochemical signaling pathways underlying these processes. In this chapter, we will discuss these processes, focusing on REM sleep and the potential role of acetylcholine, NREM sleep, and hippocampal sharp waves, and glutamate, as well as the role of intracellular signaling mechanisms in memory consolidation.

Memory consists of several stages including learning (acquisition), consolidation, and retrieval (Abel and Lattal 2001) (Fig. 15.1). Our discussions here will focus on the process of memory consolidation (McGaugh 2000), which occurs in the period following learning, rather than on learning itself. This period of memory consolidation represents a time during which memories are labile and can be either weakened or strengthened by experience, by neural activity or by specific neurotransmitters, as might occur during different stages of sleep. This chapter will focus on the hippocampus for several reasons. First, the hippocampus is known to play a role in the consolidation of memory for specific tasks such as spatial learning in rodents (Riedel *et al.* 1999), and this consolidation is known to be sensitive to sleep deprivation (Smith and Rose 1996). Second, neurons within the hippocampus undergo dramatic changes in firing rates during the sleep/wake cycle, generating an 8 Hz (theta) rhythm during rapid-eye movement (REM) sleep and exploratory behavior (Buzsáki *et al.* 1983) and sharp waves accompanied by 200 Hz bursts during non-rapid eye movement (NREM) sleep (Buzsáki 1986). These observations suggest that memory traces within the hippocampus may be altered by sleep states. In particular, REM sleep may create a specific chemical and physiological environment within the hippocampus that promotes memory

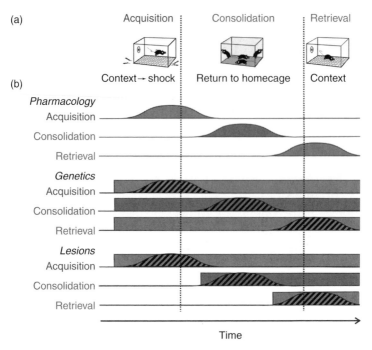

Figure 15.1 Three stages of memory. Three different stages of memory in contextual fear conditioning (a) have been examined using pharmacology, genetics, and lesions. During acquisition, learning occurs and memory is initially established. After acquisition, the memory is stabilized during consolidation. During retrieval, the memory is expressed as altered behavior, in this case, freezing in response to exposure to the context. (b) Pharmacological approaches can be best used to discretely alter a single stage without affecting the two other stages because of their temporal resolution. Lesion studies have allowed for the identification of specific brain regions involved in memory and genetic studies have identified the molecular components of memory storage. The development of reversible lesion and genetic approaches (hatched shading) has enabled these techniques to be used to study selectively each stage in memory storage (reproduced with permission from Abel and Lattal 2001). (See Plate 12.)

consolidation (Graves *et al.* 2001*b*). Third, the study of synaptic plasticity in the hippocampus has helped identify several components of the molecular cascade responsible for memory storage (Abel and Lattal 2001) (Fig. 15.2). This molecular machinery includes the *N*-methyl-*D*-aspartate (NMDA) glutamate receptor as well as intracellular signal transduction cascades such as the cyclic AMP/protein kinase A/cyclic AMP response binding protein (cAMP/PKA/CREB) pathway (Abel and Lattal 2001). Recent work at the genetic and pharmacological levels has suggested that some of the same molecular pathways that play a role in memory storage also regulate sleep/wake states in rodents and rest/activity states in *Drosophila* (Hendricks *et al.* 2001; Graves *et al.* 2001*a,b*). Thus, the hippocampus represents an ideal brain region in which to explore the molecular mechanisms of memory consolidation and their relationship to sleep.

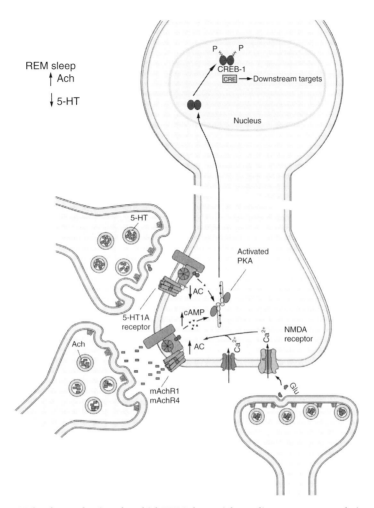

Figure 15.2 Molecular mechanisms by which REM sleep might mediate memory consolation within the hippocampus. During REM sleep increased levels of acetylcholine and decreased levels of serotonin can trigger a molecular cascade via G-protein-coupled receptors. Subsequent changes in the second messenger cAMP, the activation of PKA and CREB could enhance memory consolidation (reproduced with permission from Graves *et al.* 2001*b*). (See Plate 13.)

The idea that memory is consolidated from a labile state to a more permanent state following training has its origins in studies of human subjects in the late nineteenth century. Müller and Pilzecker (1900) found that recent memory is sensitive to retroactive interference by performing a series of human experiments in which subjects were required to memorize word lists. When subjects were required to learn additional material soon after the initial learning, memory for the initial material deteriorated. When the learning of this additional material was delayed, however, no retroactive interference was observed. Ribot (1901) found strong evidence for this hypothesis in his experience with patients with neurological diseases. He found that patients with amnesia had much more complete memories of childhood than adulthood. This led him to postulate that older memories are more resistant to organic damage because it takes time for new memories to become more permanent.

The hippocampus and anterograde amnesia

Humans with memory disturbances have provided an important foundation for memory consolidation research. The well-known case, a patient H. M., underwent an operation at age 27 to remove both hippocampi and surrounding structures in the temporal lobe in an effort to ameliorate his temporal lobe epilepsy. Although the operation was successful at reducing his seizures, H. M. completely lost the ability to remember facts and events for more than a couple of minutes (see Milner *et al.* 1998 for review). The patient H. M. was able to remember and repeat a sequence of digits for several minutes, but once distracted he immediately forgot. On the other hand, H. M. was able to learn and remember new motor tasks including difficult mechanical puzzles. When a puzzle was subsequently presented to him, he reported that he had never seen such a puzzle before in his life. Nevertheless, his performance at solving puzzles greatly improved compared to his original performance. H. M. was always able to remember childhood events, but was never able to remember events that occurred after his operation. This evidence suggests that H. M. had impaired memory consolidation and not just a general impairment in learning or cognition. Moreover, this evidence suggests that the hippocampus plays an important role in memory consolidation for specific kinds of tasks, namely the conscious recollection of facts and events.

The patient H. M.'s anterograde amnesia (inability to remember new things), however, may not be explained by hippocampal impairments alone because subsequent magnetic resonance imaging revealed that the hippocampus was not the only region damaged during his operation (Corkin *et al.* 1997). Importantly, selective hippocampal lesions in other patients produced memory impairments similar to those of H. M. In a patient R. B., a bilateral lesion in area CA1 of the hippocampus was found after he demonstrated severe anterograde amnesia (Zola-Morgan *et al.* 1986). Likewise, a patient E. P., who suffered selective bilateral damage to the hippocampus after a viral infection, exhibited anterograde amnesia for names, objects, and locations (Stefanacci *et al.* 2000). Primate studies have confirmed that lesions of the hippocampus will produce anterograde amnesia (see Zola-Morgan and Squire 2001 for review). Furthermore, lesioning the temporal lobe structures adjacent to the hippocampus (the perirhinal cortex and parahippocampal gyrus) in monkeys produces profound memory impairments (Zola-Morgan *et al.* 1989). In fact, the severe impairments in humans such as H. M.'s may be due to lesions in the perirhinal cortex and parahippocampal gyrus as well as the hippocampus.

In rodents, hippocampal lesions can also produce anterograde amnesia in two behavioral tasks: contextual fear conditioning and the hidden platform or spatial version of the Morris water maze (Morris *et al.* 1982; Phillips and LeDoux 1992; Kim *et al.* 1993). Fear conditioning is a form of associative learning in which rodents are trained to associate a neutral stimulus (such as a specific context) with an aversive stimulus (such as a mild foot shock) (LeDoux 2000; Maren 2001). In contextual fear conditioning, rodents are trained to associate a specific cage with a shock (Fig. 15.3). Rodents display their fear by freezing upon exposure to the training context during a subsequent retrieval test. The advantage of this task is that it can be learned in a single trial that enables acquisition, consolidation, and retrieval to be studied independently (Fig. 15.1). In the hidden platform or spatial version of the Morris water maze, the goal is for the rodent to find a submerged platform in a pool of opaque water (Morris *et al.* 1982) (Fig. 15.4). Each day, the rodent is placed into the pool at a random position along the edge of the pool and explores the pool until it learns to use spatial clues in the room to locate the platform. Measuring how long it takes the rodent to get to the platform tests its performance; a probe trial verifies that it is using spatial clues. During probe trials, the hidden platform is removed and the path used is recorded with a video camera.

Genetic alterations specific to the hippocampus also create anterograde amnesia. Tsien *et al.* (1996) created mice lacking the NMDA-R1 glutamate receptor in only a subregion (area CA1) of the hippocampus. Mice lacking NMDA-R1 receptors in area CA1 are impaired at both contextual fear conditioning and spatial learning in the Morris water maze (Tsien *et al.* 1996; Rampon *et al.* 2000). Furthermore, these mice do not display NMDA receptor dependent forms of synaptic plasticity in area CA1 (Tsien *et al.* 1996). Together these results support the hypothesis that synaptic plasticity and NMDA receptors in the hippocampus may be necessary for contextual and spatial learning in rodents.

Rodents with hippocampal lesions or without hippocampal NMDA-R1 receptors, however, were able to learn a visible platform version of the Morris water maze (Morris *et al.* 1982; Tsien *et al.* 1996). In this version of the Morris water maze, a visual cue is used to assess the ability of a rodent to find the platform relative to the cue instead of a specific hidden location. This task, in which the platform is marked with a visible cue and the position of the platform moves from trial to trial, is a form of procedural learning that is sensitive to lesions of the striatum (Packard and McGaugh 1992). This version of the water maze also provides a way to measure swimming ability, visual acuity, and motivation to escape the water, thus controlling for potential performance effects of genetic, or pharmacological, or lesion manipulations.

Multiple memory systems

The accumulation of evidence that lesions of specific brain regions produce selective memory impairments has suggested that different brain systems are responsible for memory storage for different tasks (Squire *et al.* 2001; Fig. 15.5). Long-term memory has been subdivided by cognitive neuroscientists into categories based on the information learned: explicit and implicit memory (Fig. 15.5). Explicit memory is the conscious memory of facts and events such as names, or the knowledge of whether one ate breakfast that particular morning. The hippocampal and medial

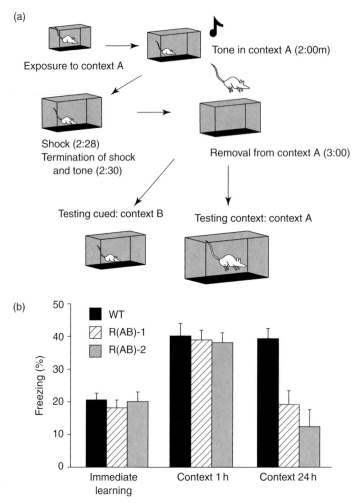

Figure 15.3 Fear conditioning. The procedure for fear conditioning is shown schematically in (a). Rodents are placed into the training context for 2 min. After this period, a 30-s tone is played that concludes with a 2-s foot shock. After another 30-s context exposure, the mouse is removed. In this training procedure, both the context and the tone are conditioned stimuli and the foot shock serves as an unconditioned stimulus. Upon return to the chamber, the mouse will exhibit freezing as an indication of fear that results from the memory of being shocked in the context. Exposure to the tone in a novel context will also produce freezing behavior. The percentage of the time spent freezing in wild type (WT) and two lines of R(AB) transgenic mice is shown in panel (b). R(AB) transgenic mice express an inhibitor of PKA in neurons within the hippocampus, and these mutant mice exhibit long-term memory deficits in contextual fear conditioning. Transgenic R(AB) mice with an impairment in long-term memory display normal levels of freezing immediately after fear conditioning and 1 h later—but reduced levels of freezing when retested 24 h later. Cued fear conditioning is not impaired in R(AB) transgenics (modified with permission from Abel *et al.* 1997).

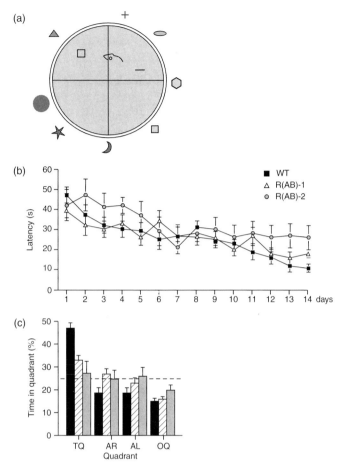

Figure 15.4 Spatial learning in the Morris water maze. In the spatial version of the Morris water maze, a mouse swims to find a platform hidden underneath the surface of opaque water (a). The mouse uses spatial clues within the room to find the platform. It is possible to determine the strategy used by the mouse to find the hidden platform with probe trials. During probe trials, the hidden platform is removed and the path used by the mouse to search for the hidden platform is recorded with a video camera and subsequently analyzed. R(AB) transgenic mice exhibit spatial learning deficits (b and c). Initially, wild type (WT) mice and R(AB) transgenic mice have similar latencies to find the platform. However, after 14 days after training WT mice remember the location of the platform much better than mutant mice (b). During a probe trial on the day after the end of training (c), WT mice spend more time than R(AB) mice in the quadrant of the pool in which the platform was located during training (training quadrant, TQ) and not in the adjacent right (AR), adjacent left (AL), or opposite quadrant (OQ) ((a) modified with permission Kandel *et al.* 2001; (b) and (c) from Abel *et al.* 1997). (See Plate 14.)

temporal lobe system plays a critical role in explicit memory, as described above for H. M. Implicit memory involves unconscious learning, which is often procedural in nature. For example, learned motor skills and emotional associations could be considered implicit memory. In terms of brain regions, the striatum and cerebellum

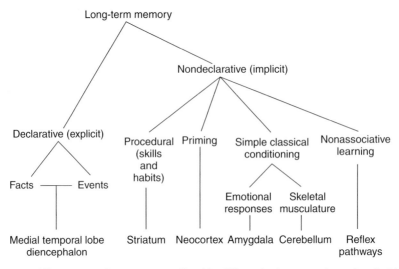

Figure 15.5 Different types of memory are mediated by different brain systems (reproduced with permission from Milner *et al.* 1998).

are important for learned motor skills (Saint-Cyr *et al.* 1988), whereas the amygdala is important for emotional learning such as fear conditioning (Bechara *et al.* 1995; LeDoux 2000).

The understanding of how multiple memory systems work has permitted sophist-icated interpretation of behavioral experiments in humans and experimental animals. Because a task, such as the water maze or fear conditioning, can be configured in different ways to recruit distinct neural systems, it is possible to design "dissoci-ation" experiments in which lesions to one brain region result in impairments in only one variation of the task (e.g. McDonald and White 1993; Bechara *et al.* 1995). Because each variation of the task has similar sensory, motor, attention, motiva-tion and performance requirements, dissociation experiments allow the investigator to more directly identify effects on learning and memory. These types of experiments are also critically important for the studies of the effects of manipulations such as sleep deprivation, pharmacological treatments, or genetic alterations on learning and memory.

The hippocampus and retrograde amnesia

Despite the differential role of distinct brain regions in explicit and implicit memory, both types of memory undergo consolidation in the period following training (McGaugh 2000). Disruption of this process of consolidation produces retrograde amnesia. Although our discussion thus far has focused on anterograde impairments in hippo-campal lesioned patients, damage to the hippocampus also produces a time-limited *retrograde* amnesia in human studies (Squire *et al.* 2001). Events preceding the lesions were difficult for patients to remember, but events that occurred many years prior to the lesions were easily remembered in patients with hippocampal damage. Some patients with temporal lobe epilepsy also display temporally graded retrograde amnesia similar to patients with hippocampal lesions (Seidenberg *et al.* 2002). This human evidence supports the idea that the hippocampus makes information learned between 1 day and up to 20 years more permanent (Squire *et al.* 2001).

Animal studies also provide strong support for the hypothesis that the hippocampus is crucial for memory consolidation. The time-limited retrograde amnesia that follows hippocampal lesions has been demonstrated in a striking fashion using contextual fear conditioning (Kim and Fanselow 1992; Anagnostaras *et al.* 1999). Using a powerful within-subjects experimental design, the Fanselow lab has shown that memory for a recently trained context is impaired by hippocampal lesion, whereas memory for a remotely trained context is unaffected (Anagnostaras *et al.* 1999). Monkeys with hippocampal lesions have better recognition of objects learned months prior compared to objects learned two weeks before the hippocampal lesion (Zola-Morgan and Squire 1990).

Hippocampal inactivation produces retrograde amnesia for spatial learning suggesting that the hippocampus also plays a critical role in the consolidation of spatial learning (Riedel *et al.* 1999). The injection of the reversible AMPA receptor antagonist LY326325 into the hippocampus has the effect of inactivating the entire hippocampus. Inactivation of the hippocampus by AMPA receptor blockade for several days following training in the spatial version of the Morris water maze impaired spatial memory measured 16 days after training. By contrast, a single day of hippocampal inactivation did not impair memory consolidation. This inactivation procedure does not permanently destroy the hippocampus, because when mice treated with the AMPA receptor antagonist for several days were given the opportunity to learn the spatial version of the Morris water maze without inactivation, they were able to learn the task successfully. These results strongly suggest that the hippocampus is necessary for the consolidation of spatial memory that occurs in the days following training.

The time-limited nature of the retrograde amnesia following hippocampal lesions implies that the destruction of the hippocampus does not destroy all long-term memories. Therefore, the hippocampus is likely to be a locus where consolidation occurs, with permanent memory storage elsewhere. Metabolic imaging studies support the hypothesis that the hippocampus mediates the transfer of information to cortex for permanent storage (Bontempi *et al.* 1999). Mice trained in a radial maze task display elevated levels of metabolic activity within the hippocampus immediately after training. With longer retention intervals, metabolic activity after testing in the hippocampus decreases, whereas the amount of activity in frontal and temporal cortex increases. This suggests that the circuitry involved in solving this maze task shifts from the hippocampus to the cortex over the period of consolidation as long-term memory is established.

Sleep and memory consolidation for hippocampus-dependent tasks

Our discussion above suggests that the hippocampus is important for the consolidation of certain forms of memory storage. What mechanisms might mediate this process as well as the subsequent stable storage of memory elsewhere in another brain region such as the cortex? Much work has focused on the role that synaptic plasticity may play in acquisition (Martin *et al.* 2000; Abel and Lattal 2001), but what accounts for the longer-term forms of modulation that occur during consolidation? As discussed in this volume, sleep is ideally suited for modulating hippocampal function during memory consolidation (e.g. see Graves *et al.* 2001*b*). During different sleep/wake states, the hippocampus exhibits distinct patterns of neuronal activity (Buzsáki *et al.* 1983). Further, the alterations in the levels of specific neurotransmitters that occur in different sleep/wake states can modulate the "broadcasting" of information from the hippocampus to the cortex (Stickgold *et al.* 2001).

Two broad approaches have been taken to explore the role of sleep in memory consolidation for hippocampus-dependent tasks (reviewed in Graves *et al.* 2001*b*). One approach has been to perturb sleep/wake states following training by sleep deprivation, by administration of pharmacological reagents that alter sleep, or by stimulation of brain regions during specific stages of sleep. A second approach has been to record sleep/wake states after training in an attempt to correlate these changes with memory consolidation.

One of the major challenges in investigating the role of sleep in memory consolidation is the design of appropriate experiments that control for "nonspecific" behavioral effects of sleep deprivation (such as stress) and for the effects of learning on sleep/wake states that may not be specific to the learning *per se* but result from the stimuli and handling that occur during training. Like the studies of the role of the hippocampus in memory storage, the examination of the role of sleep in memory consolidation benefits most from "dissociation" experiments. Smith and Rose (1996, 1997; described in Chapter 6 of this book) have taken this approach using different versions of the Morris water maze to examine the role of sleep in memory storage. REM sleep increases in rats after training for the hidden platform (spatial) version of the Morris water maze, but not following training for the visible platform version. In parallel, REM sleep deprivation, given during a specific time following training, impaired memory for the hidden platform version of the Morris water maze without altering memory for the visible platform version. Because the hidden platform version of the Morris water maze is a spatial task that is dependent on hippocampal function, whereas the visible platform task is a procedural task that is dependent on striatal functioning, these results argue for a specific role of REM sleep in memory consolidation during a specific time window following hippocampus-dependent learning. Further, because the two versions of the water maze used in this study have similar sensory, motor, and motivational requirements, these experiments control for the "nonspecific" effects of swimming and handling on sleep/wake states. Recent work (Graves *et al.* 2000) suggests that total sleep deprivation in the first 5 h immediately following fear conditioning training, selectively impairs memory consolidation for contextual fear conditioning without altering cued fear conditioning, thus supporting the idea that sleep is particularly important for the consolidation of memory storage for hippocampus-dependent tasks.

Given these findings, what are the cellular and molecular processes by which the sleep/wake states alter hippocampal function? In the remainder of this chapter, we will discuss these processes, focusing on REM sleep and the potential role of acetylcholine (Ach), NREM sleep and sharp waves, the potential role of glutamate and the role of intracellular signaling mechanisms in memory consolidation. Our hope is that this molecular and cellular approach will provide a unique avenue by which to explore the functions of sleep in memory storage.

Acetylcholine, REM sleep, and memory consolidation

During NREM and REM sleep, there are dramatic changes in the levels of modulatory neurotransmitters throughout the brain, including the hippocampus. During NREM sleep, levels of norepinephrine, serotonin, and Ach all decline as compared to waking (Segal and Bloom 1974; McCormick 1992; Aston-Jones *et al.* 2001). During REM sleep, levels of norepinephrine and serotonin continue to drop to near zero, but levels of Ach increase to levels comparable to that observed during waking (McCormick 1992). Given the finding of Smith and Rose (1997) that REM sleep may play a critical role in memory consolidation for hippocampus-dependent tasks, it is appropriate to focus our attention initially on the role of Ach in the hippocampus in memory consolidation.

Many studies have explored the role of the cholinergic system in learning and memory, particularly for hippocampus-dependent tasks. Learning increases the level of Ach in the hippocampus (Fadda *et al.* 1996; Nail-Boucherie *et al.* 2000). When rats are placed into a maze, there is an increase in Ach levels in the hippocampus for a period of 10 min. When maze learning is reinforced with food, Ach levels are higher and last throughout the entire learning period. Furthermore, Ach levels are elevated during the period between learning trials outside of the maze. Contextual fear conditioning elevates levels of hippocampal Ach (Nail-Boucherie *et al.* 2000), and rodents trained for contextual fear conditioning display higher levels of Ach when re-exposed to the conditioning chamber (Nail-Boucherie *et al.* 2000).

During REM sleep as well as during exploration, the cholinergic projections via the fimbria/fornix from the medial septum and diagonal band drive theta (~8 Hz) oscillations in the hippocampus (Vanderwolf 1969; Buzsáki 2002). O'Keefe and Dostrovsky (1971) discovered that individual hippocampal cells encoding location fire during theta activity. To confirm that activity during sleep represents activity from prior wakefulness, electrophysiologists have made recordings of hippocampal neural activity as animals are exposed to novel spatial contexts and during subsequent sleep episodes (see Chapters 12, 13, and 16). Pavlides and Winson (1989) first noted that hippocampal place cells that were active after a spatial experience were also active during the subsequent sleep period. These correlations occur during REM sleep and are in phase with the theta oscillation (Poe *et al.* 2000). Neurons encoding a novel location will fire in phase with the theta oscillation producing synchronized depolarization, and such depolarization synchronized with the theta oscillation is known to promote synaptic plasticity (Huerta and Lisman 1993). Louie and Wilson (2001) also found that hippocampal unit activity during wakefulness was replayed during REM sleep. Thus, increased levels of Ach could facilitate memory consolidation and synaptic plasticity in the hippocampus during such "replays" during REM sleep.

Cholinergic receptors are divided into two broad categories, nicotinic and muscarinic, based on the agonists that selectively activate each class of receptor (Nestler *et al.* 2001). Nicotinic receptors are ligand-gated ion channels that allow the passage of potassium and sodium (and to a lesser extent calcium) when the receptor is occupied by two molecules of Ach. Muscarinic receptors are G-protein-coupled receptors that can modulate intracellular signaling pathways as well as the activity of ion channels. Carbachol, a muscarinic agonist, when injected into the medial pontine reticular formation, has the ability to induce a state remarkably similar to REM sleep (Baghdoyan *et al.* 1989). Within the hippocampus, carbachol induces theta oscillations and modulates synaptic plasticity (Huerta and Lisman 1993). Neuromodulators such as Ach may not only modify synaptic transmission within the hippocampus itself, but they may also alter communication between the hippocampus and other brain regions (Hasslemo 1995, 1999). In this context, the low levels of Ach during NREM sleep may be as important as the high levels that occur during REM sleep and waking (Hasslemo 1999).

Much of the work examining the role of cholinergic mechanisms in memory consolidation has focused on muscarinic receptors in part because of the effects of carbachol on hippocampal synaptic transmission. Systemic post-training injections of muscarinic antagonists block memory consolidation for one-trial inhibitory (passive) avoidance (Roldan *et al.* 1997). Muscarinic antagonists are effective at blocking consolidation when given immediately post-training or at 6 h post-training (Doyle *et al.* 1993). This task also exhibits sensitivity to post-training REM sleep deprivation (Smith 1995). Further, post-training administration of the muscarinic agonist oxotremorine enhances the consolidation of inhibitory avoidance learning (Castellano *et al.* 1999). One drawback of these studies in the context of our current discussion, however, is that drugs were not administered to the hippocampus and the behavioral experiments do not distinguish between the hippocampus and other brain regions such as the amygdala. Intrahippocampal injection of oxotremorine, a cholinergic muscarinic agonist, also enhances consolidation of memory for a brightness discrimination task when administered post-training (Grecksch *et al.* 1978), but little is known about the role of specific brain systems and the role of sleep/wake states in memory consolidation for this task. In spatial learning in the water maze, scopolamine infused into the hippocampus blocks acquisition, but not consolidation (Riekkeinen and Riekkeinen 1997). Similarly, systemic injection of the cholinergic antagonist atropine post-training does not impair consolidation of spatial learning (Hagan *et al.* 1986). Consolidation of spatial reference memory in the radial arm maze, however, is sensitive to scopolamine, a muscarinic antagonist, administered 30 min–3 h following training (Toumane and Durkin 1993).

Cholinergic agonists and antagonists have a measurable effect on memory consolidation of contextual fear conditioning. When administered systemically, pre-training, but not immediate post-training, injections of scopolamine blocked contextual fear conditioning (Anagnostaras *et al.* 1995, 1999). Intrahippocampal injections of scopolamine prior to training block acquisition of contextual fear conditioning (Gale *et al.* 2001). Muscarinic receptors may also play a role in the consolidation of contextual fear conditioning. Using systemic administration, Rudy (1996) found that scopolamine impaired consolidation of both context and tone fear conditioning when administered 3 h after training. Wallenstein and Vago (2001) demonstrated that the cholinergic system within the hippocampus is important for both acquisition and consolidation of fear conditioning. Scopolamine directly injected into the hippocampus impairs contextual fear conditioning, but not cued conditioning when either administered prior to training, or up to 48 h after training. Consistent with a role for muscarinic Ach receptors in memory storage for contextual fear conditioning, knockout mice lacking the M1 muscarinic receptor have been reported to have contextual fear conditioning deficits (Anagnostaras *et al.* 2000; Miyakawa *et al.* 2001).

Human and animal studies have also revealed cognitive effects of nicotine (Rezvani and Levin 2001), suggesting that this type of Ach receptor may play a role in memory storage. Nicotine enhances acquisition in the spatial version of the Morris water maze (Socci *et al.* 1995) and passive avoidance (Brioni and Arneric 1993). Further, nicotine enhances synaptic transmission by increasing calcium influx (Gray *et al.* 1996) and nicotine induces long-term potentiation (LTP) in the hippocampus (Hamid *et al.* 1997). Thus, nicotinic cholinergic receptors may also play a role in memory consolidation, perhaps even interacting with muscarinic mechanisms because nicotine can act to facilitate the release of Ach (Levin and Rose 1991). Such ideas, however, remain speculative and require further experimental investigation.

Nevertheless, it remains to be discovered whether cholinergic activity within the hippocampus during REM sleep plays a role in memory consolidation. Graves *et al.* hypothesized that cholinergic activity during REM sleep promotes both theta activity and leads to the molecular cascade responsible for memory consolidation via muscarinic receptors (Graves *et al.* 2001*b*; Fig. 15.2). What is clearly needed is the study of a task sensitive to REM sleep deprivation combined with selective pharmacological or genetic manipulation of cholinergic action in a spatially and temporally restricted fashion.

Adenosine and memory consolidation

Adenosine is a neurotransmitter that has been the focus of many studies in sleep/wake regulation because of its potential role as a chemical mediator of the sleep-inducing effects of prolonged wakefulness and sleep deprivation (Porkka-Heiskanen *et al.* 1997; Dunwiddie and Masino 2001). Caffeine, an adenosine receptor antagonist, promotes wakefulness and appears to increase arousal and attention (Fredholm *et al.* 1999). In addition, pharmacological studies have demonstrated that adenosine receptor antagonists other than caffeine reduce sleep (Lin *et al.* 1997) and that adenosine receptor agonists promote sleep (Portas *et al.* 1997). Levels of adenosine increase in the basal forebrain with extended wakefulness and dissipate with subsequent sleep (Porkka-Heiskanen *et al.* 1997). Adenosine may function by inhibiting neuronal activity in the cholinergic nuclei responsible for the regulation of arousal (Rainnie *et al.* 1994). In addition to changes in regions of the central nervous system that regulate sleep, levels of adenosine have been found to increase in the hippocampus during a rodent's active period (Huston *et al.* 1996). This observation raises the possibility that adenosine may modulate hippocampal function at different points in the sleep/wake cycle as well as at different times in the circadian cycle. Further, adenosine levels are known to increase with sleep deprivation (Basheer *et al.* 2000) and thus, sleep deprivation may exert its effects in part by altering adenosine levels.

Adenosine can have an inhibitory (Dunwiddie and Masino 2001) or excitatory (Sebastiao and Ribeiro 1996) effect on neuronal activity, depending on the type of receptor activated. Adenosine is not stored in synaptic vesicles, nor is it released in a calcium-dependent fashion. Rather, adenosine is made in the extracellular space from adenine nucleotides and released from intracellular stores by facilitated diffusion transporters (Dunwiddie and Masino 2001). Once present extracellularly, adenosine can act on four different G-protein receptor subtypes that inhibit or activate adenylyl cyclase that alter potassium or calcium channel function or activate phospholipase C (Dunwiddie and Masino 2001). Importantly, these intracellular signaling pathways regulated by adenosine have been implicated in synaptic plasticity and memory storage (Abel and Lattal 2001) (Fig. 15.6). Indeed, adenosine modulates synaptic transmission, depotentiation and LTP in the hippocampus, although the nature of this effect depends on the particular receptor type activated. A_1 receptor antagonists facilitate LTP, so endogenous adenosine may act to suppress synaptic plasticity (de Medonça and Ribeiro 2001). A_2 receptor activation enhances synaptic transmission and A_1 receptor activation exerts an opposite effect (Kessey and Mogul 1998; Fujii *et al.* 2000). In the case of A_2 receptors, the blockade of LTP by A_2 receptor antagonists can be reversed by treatment with a membrane permeable analog of cAMP, suggesting that A_2 receptors act via this intracellular signaling pathway to modulate hippocampal synaptic transmission (Kessey and Mogul 1998).

Adenosine receptor agonists and antagonists appear to alter learning and memory in rodents (de Medonça and Ribeiro 2001). In terms of memory consolidation, caffeine administered post-training improves memory for a step-through inhibitory avoidance task in mice. This effect appears to be via the action of caffeine acting on A_{2a} receptors because the selective A_{2a} receptor antagonist SCH58261 has an effect similar to caffeine (Kopf *et al.* 1999).

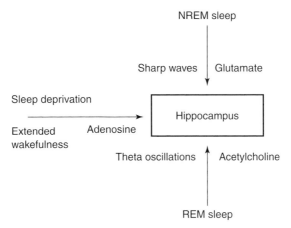

Figure 15.6 Neurochemical mechanisms by which sleep/wake states and sleep deprivation might modulate memory consolidation. During REM sleep, increased levels of Ach in the hippocampus trigger the molecular cascade that stabilizes previously acquired memories. During NREM sleep, sharp waves cause rapid and repeated glutamate receptor activation within the hippocampus, which is known to cause changes in synaptic strength. During sleep deprivation, high levels of adenosine may inhibit the molecular cascades necessary for long-term memory consolidation.

From the perspective of sleep/wake regulation, researchers have focused on the role of adenosine as a sleep-promoting substance whose levels increase with extended wakefulness and sleep deprivation. Our discussion here suggests that changes in adenosine levels across the sleep/wake and circadian cycle or sleep deprivation have the potential to modulate memory consolidation, although the exact mechanisms and brain systems affected have not been precisely defined. Given the importance of the cAMP signaling pathway for memory consolidation, it is intriguing to speculate that adenosine acting through this pathway may enable the sleep/wake cycle to modulate memory storage.

NMDA receptors and memory consolidation

Our discussion thus far has focused on the role of the hippocampus in memory consolidation, and the possible role of sleep/wake states and the neuromodulatory compounds Ach and adenosine in this process. For the remainder of this chapter we will focus on experiments that explore the molecular and cellular mechanisms of memory consolidation and attempt to understand how sleep/wake states might regulate these processes.

Much work on the cellular and molecular mechanisms of memory storage for hippocampus-dependent tasks has focused on the role of LTP, an activity-dependent form of synaptic plasticity, in acquisition (Miller and Mayford 1999; Martin *et al.* 2000; Abel and Lattal 2001). LTP has been especially well-characterized in hippocampal area CA1 at the synapse between the Schaffer collateral axons from CA3 pyramidal cells onto

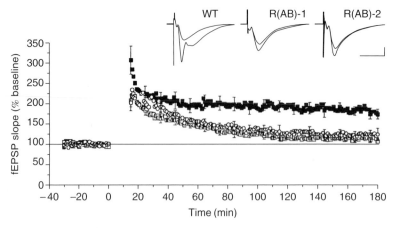

Figure 15.7 R(AB) transgenic mice exhibit impaired long-lasting LTP. LTP was examined in hippocampal slices from R(AB) transgenic and wild type mice by recording extracellularly from hippocampal area CA1 while stimulating CA3 axons. After repeated tetanic stimulation, the field potentials measured in CA1 increase in slope and amplitude. R(AB) mice with reduced neuronal PKA activity are unable to maintain long-lasting forms of LTP. Representative field potentials before and 180 min after LTP induction are shown above. Scale bars: 2 mV, 10 ms (modified with permission from Abel *et al.* 1997).

CA1 neurons (Fig. 15.7). In hippocampal area CA1, the induction of many forms of LTP is critically dependent on the NMDA receptor. In parallel, pharmacological or genetic inhibition of hippocampal NMDA receptors impairs the acquisition of hippocampus-dependent tasks such as spatial learning or contextual fear conditioning (see Martin *et al.* 2000 and Izquierdo and McGaugh 2000 for review). NMDA receptors have a special role in memory because of their voltage-sensitive and ligand-dependent properties. These properties of the NMDA receptor allow for coincidence detection during memory acquisition, a property that may be especially important for associative learning as well as spatial learning.

Do NMDA receptors play a role in the consolidation of hippocampus-dependent tasks? Could LTP mediate consolidation as well as acquisition? How would sleep/wake states interact with this process? Although many experiments have demonstrated that NMDA receptors are important for acquisition, very few studies have successfully demonstrated a role for NMDA receptors in memory consolidation. In the case of step-down inhibitory avoidance, NMDA receptor blockade immediately after training impairs consolidation (Izquierdo *et al.* 1992), and recent reports suggest that agmatine, an endogenous polyamine and noncompetitive NMDA receptor antagonist, impairs consolidation of contextual fear conditioning (Stewart and McKay 2000).

Recent studies using a regulatable transgenic mouse model support the role of NMDA receptors in the hippocampus during memory consolidation (Shimizu *et al.* 2000). Although other genetic studies have indicated that NMDA receptors are required for acquisition of contextual fear conditioning and the Morris water maze and for LTP

(Tsien *et al.* 1996; Rampon *et al.* 2000), previous experiments did not examine what happens when NMDA receptors are intact during acquisition but lacking during consolidation. To control the expression of NMDA receptors both spatially and temporally, Shimizu *et al.* (2000) deleted the existing NMDA-NR1 receptor gene in hippocampal area CA1 and used the tetracycline-regulated system in combination with Cre recombinase to restore expression of the NMDA receptor in that area. In this temporally regulated system NMDA receptor expression in area CA1 is turned off, when doxycycline (a tetracycline analog with a high blood–brain barrier permeability) is put in the food or drinking water. In the absence of doxycycline, NMDA receptors are expressed in area CA1. In these transgenic mice, NMDA currents and LTP were abolished by doxycycline after 3–5 days of treatment. Furthermore, the doxycycline treatment eradicated NMDA expression as assayed by immunohistochemistry.

Although lesion studies have indicated that hippocampal function is required for consolidation, Shimizu *et al.* (2000) provided the first evidence that NMDA receptors in the hippocampus are also needed for consolidation using this regulated approach. When

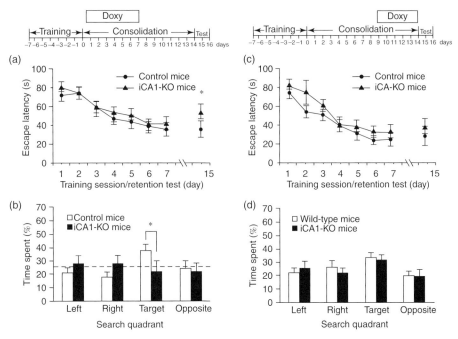

Figure 15.8 NMDA receptors and the consolidation of spatial memory. During the first week after training the inducible reduction in NMDA receptor expression in the hippocampus of CA1 NMDA-KO mice is induced by doxycycline (doxy) treatment and produces impairments in spatial memory in the Morris water maze as revealed by latency to reach the platform in a retention test (a) and spatial reference for the target quadrant in a probe trial (b) Impairments are not observed when NMDA receptor expression is reduced from days 9 to 14 after training (c) and (d) (reproduced with permission from Shimizu *et al.* 2000).

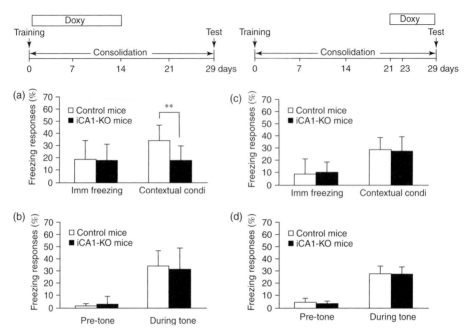

Figure 15.9 NMDA receptors and the consolidation of contextual fear conditioning. The induced loss of NMDA receptor expression in the hippocampus produces impairments in contextual fear conditioning when it occurs during the first two weeks after training (a). Conditioning to the tone conditioning (b) is not altered by this treatment. When NMDA receptor expression is reduced the week before testing, no impairment was seen in either contextual fear conditioning (c) or tone conditioning (d) (reproduced with permission from Shimizu *et al.* 2000).

doxycycline was used to eliminate NMDA receptor expression in the hippocampus after training for one week, mice displayed impaired long-term memory for spatial learning in the Morris water maze (Fig. 15.8). In this study, mice were tested 15 and 16 days after training and presumably NMDA receptors had returned before testing. Furthermore, when doxycycline was administered on the ninth day after training until testing, no significant memory impairments were seen. These results suggest that NMDA receptors in the hippocampus are needed for consolidation during the first week after training. A similar paradigm was used to demonstrate that NMDA receptors are needed for consolidation of contextual fear conditioning (Fig. 15.9). When doxycycline was given to these mice for two weeks after training, impairments in contextual fear conditioning but not tone conditioning were observed in a test 29 days after training. In contrast, when doxycycline was given to mice one week before the retrieval test, no impairment was seen in either contextual or tone fear conditioning.

Based on this data, Shimizu *et al.* (2000) suggest that during the week after training NMDA receptors in the hippocampus are involved in the consolidation of both spatial and contextual memory. The relatively slow time course of action of doxycycline in this regulated genetic system makes it difficult to define more precisely the exact time window during which NMDA receptors are required for consolidation. It is important to note, however, that the findings from this genetic approach have not been supported by pharmacological studies in which NMDA receptor blockade is maintained over several days during the consolidation of spatial learning (Day and Morris 2001). Future genetic and pharmacological experiments are clearly needed to investigate this intriguing idea that NMDA receptors in the hippocampus may play a role in memory consolidation.

How might NMDA receptor activation within the hippocampus after training mediate memory consolidation? One possibility is that NMDA receptors become activated during basal synaptic transmission after training, as has been suggested to occur under certain circumstances in other brain systems (Li *et al.* 1996; Partridge *et al.* 2000). Another possibility is that NMDA-receptor-dependent plasticity during consolidation might lead to the gradual strengthening of synaptic connections within the hippocampus, within the cortex or in hippocampal–cortical connections. During NREM sleep, electrophysiological phenomena such as sharp waves create an environment suitable for synaptic plasticity, which may be responsible for memory consolidation in the hippocampus (Buzsáki 1986; King *et al.* 1999; Kudrimoti *et al.* 1999; Nadasdy *et al.* 1999). Thus, the repeated excitation often used to induce LTP occurs in the hippocampus during NREM sleep. In addition, during NREM sleep, the hippocampus appears to "replay" firing patterns that occurred during wakefulness (Nadasdy *et al.* 1999). Sharp waves in the hippocampus during NREM sleep are synchronized with spindle oscillations in the cortex, and this may serve to broadcast information to the cortex (Siapas and Wilson 1998). These simultaneous oscillations spatially and temporally regulate depolarization of neurons in the cortex and hippocampus. The physiological literature thus supports the idea that these electrical events in the hippocampus during NREM sleep may mediate memory consolidation. Furthermore, the recall of spatial memory in human subjects is superior after sleep dominated by NREM sleep (Plihal and Born 1999) suggesting that NREM sleep facilitates the consolidation of explicit or declarative memory in humans.

The intracellular mechanisms of memory consolidation and sleep

As discussed above, many of the neurotransmitter systems that mediate memory consolidation and sleep/wake regulation alter the levels of intracellular second messengers, which in turn activate a variety of signaling cascades. In terms of long-term memory storage and memory consolidation, the ultimate result of these signaling pathways is the induction of new gene expression and the synthesis of new proteins leading to long-lasting changes in neuronal function.

Behavioral studies in organisms ranging from *Aplysia* to *Drosophila* to rodents have supported the idea of protein synthesis in memory consolidation (see Milner *et al.* 1998 for review). Anisomycin, a protein synthesis inhibitor, interferes with memory consolidation and selectively blocks long-term memory storage (Abel and Kandel 1998). In fear conditioning, anisomycin reduces long-term memory for the context when administered

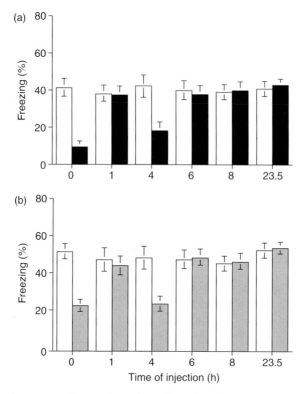

Figure 15.10 The time course of PKA and protein synthesis dependent processes in memory consolidation. The effects of (a) anisomycin, a protein synthesis inhibitor, and (b) Rp-cAMPs, a PKA inhibitor, administered at different time points after contextual fear conditioning in Bourtchouladze *et al.* 1998. The significant effect on memory consolidation when these drugs are administered immediately after training and 4 h later is suggestive of two waves of memory consolidation (reproduced with permission from Bourtchouladze *et al.* 1998).

immediately after training or 4 h after training (Bourtchouladze *et al.* 1998) (Fig. 15.10). No effect is seen when administered during the first, sixth, eighth, or twenty-fourth hour after training. Proteins crucial to the consolidation of contextual fear conditioning are thus apparently synthesized in two "waves," one immediately after training and one 4 h later. In terms of synaptic plasticity, long-lasting forms of LTP within the hippocampus are sensitive to disruption by the inhibition of protein synthesis (reviewed in Huang *et al.* 1996) and the inhibition of RNA synthesis (Nguyen *et al.* 1994). Shorter-lasting forms of LTP, however, do not require protein synthesis. Disrupting protein synthesis will also disrupt sleep. Multiple studies have shown that protein synthesis inhibitors including anisomycin dramatically reduce REM sleep—and possibly increase NREM sleep (Gutwein *et al.* 1980). Drucker-Colin *et al.* (1979) found that phasic REM was reduced in cats administered protein synthesis inhibitors.

Are these effects of protein synthesis inhibition on sleep related to the effects on memory consolidation? Sleep-deprivation studies demonstrating the importance of REM sleep as well as the effects of anisomycin on REM sleep, suggest two hypotheses: either REM sleep leads to the protein synthesis necessary for memory consolidation, or protein synthesis affects REM sleep and memory consolidation via independent pathways. Gutwein *et al.* (1980) supports the hypothesis that anisomycin disrupts memory consolidation by disrupting REM sleep by comparing the time course of the effect of anisomycin on memory impairment and REM sleep. Their results show that the time course for impairments in inhibitory avoidance and REM sleep deprivation caused by anisomycin is similar for several dosages. Thus, the disruption of protein synthesis may reduce the levels of crucial proteins that may interfere with REM sleep and memory consolidation.

The mechanisms of how anisomycin affects sleep remain to be investigated; however, the protein synthesis cascade involved in memory consolidation has been a major focus in memory research. The cAMP/PKA pathway appears to play a critical role in initiating the molecular events that lead to the activation of transcription and new protein synthesis during long-term memory storage (Abel *et al.* 1997). Studies characterizing the role of cAMP in learning and memory either have measured levels of cAMP after learning tasks or used drugs that interfered with cAMP signaling. In step-down inhibitory avoidance, a hippocampus-dependent task, levels of cAMP in the hippocampus increase 30 and 180 min after training (Bernabeu *et al.* 1996). In this particular task, levels of PKA activity remain elevated for over 6 h (Bernabeu *et al.* 1997). Levels of cAMP may increase as a result of the activation of G-protein-coupled receptors or as the result of calcium influx via NMDA receptors or voltage-gated calcium channels. Pharmacology experiments support the hypothesis that increased levels of cAMP lead to memory consolidation. Stimulators of PKA activity improve memory when administered 3 or 6 h after inhibitory avoidance training (Bernabeu *et al.* 1997; Bevilaqua *et al.* 1997). In fact, drugs that reduce cAMP levels and PKA activity impair memory for this task when injected directly into the hippocampus, and drugs that increase cAMP levels and PKA activity enhance memory (Bevilaqua *et al.* 1997). Effects of altering levels of cAMP are also seen in contextual fear conditioning. Rolipram, a phosphodiesterase inhibitor that increases cAMP levels, improves long-term memory, but not short-term memory for contextual fear conditioning (Barad *et al.* 1998).

A downstream target of cAMP, PKA also plays a role in consolidation. cAMP binds to the regulatory subunits of PKA in order to activate it. Transgenic mice expressing a dominant negative form of the regulatory subunit of PKA (R(AB)) in the hippocampus have reduced PKA activity levels (Abel *et al.* 1997). In these mice, the CaMKIIα promoter was used to limit expression postnatally to neurons in forebrain to reduce the possibility of developmental defects. R(AB) transgenic mice exhibit deficits in hippocampus-dependent tasks including spatial learning in the Morris water maze (Fig. 15.4). In fear conditioning, R(AB) transgenic mice exhibit selective deficits in long-term memory for contextual fear conditioning, suggesting that PKA plays a critically important role in the hippocampus in memory consolidation (Fig. 15.3). Electrophysiologically, R(AB) transgenic mice have impairments in long-term forms of LTP, while short-term forms of LTP and basal synaptic transmission are not altered (Abel *et al.* 1997; Woo *et al.* 2000) (Fig. 15.7). In addition, *in vivo* electrophysiology has revealed that long-term, but not short-term, instabilities in hippocampal place fields are seen in R(AB) mice (Rotenberg *et al.* 2000). When mice are exposed to a novel environment, initial place cell activity is similar in R(AB) and control mice. One hour after exposure to the novel environment, stable place cell fields were still seen in R(AB) and control mice. After 24 h, R(AB) place cell fields shifted to new locations within the environment, although control mice continued to demonstrate place cell organization similar to the original context.

Pharmacological experiments have defined a role for PKA in memory consolidation. Rp-cAMPS (a cAMP analog that blocks PKA activity) impairs long-term fear conditioning memory when injected immediately after training or 4 h after training (Bourtchouladze *et al.* 1998; Fig. 15.10). This same time window after fear conditioning is also sensitive to anisomycin, strongly suggesting that cAMP leads to protein synthesis immediately after and 4 h after fear conditioning. Therefore, the cAMP/PKA pathway is important for memory consolidation.

During sleep, cAMP may also play a role as a regulatory molecule. Levels of cAMP in the brainstem are regulated by sleep, temperature, ultradian and circadian cycles. Sleep deprivation decreases levels of cAMP, and recovery sleep increases levels of cAMP in the preoptic region, but not the cortex (Perez *et al.* 1982). During the normal sleep/wake cycle, levels of cAMP also decrease in the preoptic region during wakefulness, but increase after sleep (Perez *et al.* 1982). Rolipram, which increases the availability of cAMP, also increases wakefulness for 1 h immediately after injection (Lelkes *et al.* 1998). Capece and Lydic (1997) found that cAMP in the medial pontine reticular formation modulates carbachol-induced REM sleep in cats. Compounds that increase cAMP levels injected into this brain structure similarly reduced levels of carbachol-induced REM sleep, but had no apparent effect on spontaneous REM sleep. Although carbachol-induced REM sleep has many of the features of spontaneous REM sleep, they operate through slightly different mechanisms. However, the additional REM sleep seen after learning tasks might be similar to carbachol-induced REM sleep.

Additional experiments must be done to determine if cAMP plays a role simultaneously in both REM sleep and memory consolidation. As discussed above, neurotransmitter systems that promote wakefulness and memory consolidation both elevate levels of cAMP. Studies of sleep/wake states in R(AB) transgenic mice as well as other genetically modified mice may help researchers understand the relationship between sleep and memory consolidation in specific brain regions.

Gene expression is induced by PKA signaling by phosphorylating the cAMP-response element binding protein (CREB), an inducible transcription factor that plays a role in long-term memory storage in a number of organisms (Silva *et al.* 1998). Thirty minutes after training, fear conditioned mice have higher levels of phosphorylated CREB in hippocampal areas CA3 and CA1 than unpaired controls and naïve animals, and levels of a CRE-driven reporter gene are increased in the hippocampus following contextual fear conditioning (Impey *et al.* 1998). Recent work using regulated transgenic systems has revealed that CREB within the hippocampal area CA1 is important for long-term memory (Pittenger *et al.* 2002).

The relationship between CREB and sleep is apparent in several organisms. In rodents, Cirelli *et al.* (1996) has shown CREB phosphorylation levels in the cortex are higher during waking than sleep. Sleep deprivation increases CREB phosphorylation in cortex suggesting that wakefulness, whether during the normal sleep/wake cycle or not, induces CREB phosphorylation. The locus coeruleus, the noradrenergic nucleus, is essential for increasing CREB phosphorylation in cortex during wakefulness (Cirelli *et al.* 1996). Mice lacking the alpha and delta isoforms of CREB exhibit decreased wakefulness and increased NREM sleep, supporting the hypothesis that CREB is important for maintaining wakefulness (Graves *et al.* 2001*a*). Whether these alterations in sleep/wake state in CREB mutant mice explain the memory impairments observed in these mice (Bourtchouladze *et al.* 1994; Kogan *et al.* 1997; Gaas *et al.* 1998; Graves *et al.* 2002) will require further research.

Conclusion

We have described in this chapter how neuromodulators and electrophysiological phenomena in the hippocampus during NREM and REM sleep affect intracellular signaling pathways that are known to mediate memory consolidation. The hippocampus appears to be a locus for consolidation during sleep, because it is required for the consolidation of spatial learning and contextual fear conditioning and these tasks require sleep for consolidation. During this period of sleep, replay of activity occurs in the hippocampus in oscillations that have the ability to alter synaptic plasticity, perhaps via molecular cascades involved in LTP (Abel and Lattal 2001). Nevertheless, future experiments are required to identify how the hippocampus consolidates memory at a molecular level during sleep. Behavioral experiments are required to identify the effects of NREM sleep deprivation on memory consolidation and its molecular machinery in the hippocampus. Pharmacological manipulations can be used to discover how Ach and adenosine influence memory consolidation in the hippocampus during sleep. Most importantly, characterization of genetically engineered mice, especially those using spatially and temporally restricted systems, will help identify genes involved in both sleep and memory consolidation within the hippocampus.

Acknowledgments

Our research is supported by grants from the Merck Foundation, the National Institutes of Health, the University of Pennsylvania Research Foundation, the Packard Foundation and the Whitehall Foundation to T. Abel, and by a National Institutes of Health National Research Service Award fellowship to K. M. Hellman. We thank Noreen O'Connor-Abel for her comments.

References

Abel, T. and **Kandel, E.** (1998). Positive and negative mechanisms that mediate long-term memory storage. *Brain Research Brain Research Reviews*, **26**, 360–378.

Abel, T. and **Lattal, K. M.** (2001). Molecular mechanisms of memory acquisition, consolidation and retrieval. *Current Opinion in Neurobiology*, **11**, 180–187.

Abel, T., Nguyen, P. V., Barad, M., Deuel, T. A., Kandel, E. R., and **Bourtchouladze, R.** (1997). Genetic demonstration of a role for PKA in the late phase of LTP and in hippocampus-based long-term memory. *Cell*, **88**, 615–626.

Anagnostaras, S. G., Maren, S., and **Fanselow, M. S.** (1995). Scopolamine selectively disrupts the acquisition of contextual fear conditioning in rats. *Neurobiology of Learning and Memory*, **64**, 191–194.

Anagnostaras, S. G., Maren, S., and **Fanselow, M. S.** (1999). Temporally graded retrograde amnesia of contextual fear after hippocampal damage in rats: within-subjects examination. *Journal of Neuroscience*, **19**, 1106–1114.

Anagnostaras, S. G., Murphy, G. G., Hamilton, S. E., Nathanson, N. M., and **Silva, A. J.** (2000). Learning and memory in cholinergic muscarinic M1 receptor knockout mice. *Society for Neuroscience*, **26**, 1809.

Aston-Jones, G., Chen, S., Zhu, Y., and **Oshinsky, M. L.** (2001). A neural circuit for circadian regulation of arousal. *Nature Neuroscience*, **4**, 732–738.

Baghdoyan, H. A., Lydic, R., Callaway, C. W., and **Hobson, J. A.** (1989). The carbachol-induced enhancement of desynchronized sleep signs is dose dependent and antagonized by centrally administered atropine. *Neuropsychopharmacology*, **2**, 67–79.

Barad, M., Bourtchouladze, R., Winder, D. G., Golan, H., and **Kandel, E.** (1998). Rolipram, a type IV-specific phosphodiesterase inhibitor, facilitates the establishment of long-lasting long-term potentiation and improves memory. *Proceedings of the National Academy of Sciences, USA*, **95**, 15020–15025.

Basheer, R., Porkka-Heiskanen, T., Strecker, R. E., Thakkar, M. M., and **McCarley, R. W.** (2000). Adenosine as a biological signal mediating sleepiness following prolonged wakefulness. *Biological Signals Receptors*, **9**, 319–327.

Bechara, A., Tranel, D., Damasio, H., Adolphs, R., Rockland, C., and **Damasio, A. R.** (1995). Double dissociation of conditioning and declarative knowledge relative to the amygdala and hippocampus in humans. *Science*, **269**, 1115–1118.

Bernabeu, R., Bevilaqua, L., Ardenghi, P., Bromberg, E., Schmitz, P., Bianchin, M., Izquierdo, I., and **Medina, J. H.** (1997). Involvement of hippocampal cAMP/cAMP-dependent protein kinase signaling pathways in a late memory consolidation phase of aversively motivated learning in rats. *Proceedings of the National Academy of Sciences, USA*, **94**, 7041–7046.

Bernabeu, R., Schmitz, P., Faillace, M. P., Izquierdo, I., and **Medina, J. H.** (1996). Hippocampal cGMP and cAMP are differentially involved in memory processing of inhibitory avoidance learning. *Neuroreport*, **7**, 585–588.

Bevilaqua, L., Ardenghi, P., Schroder, N., Bromberg, E., Schmitz, P. K., Schaeffer, E., Quevedo, J., Bianchin, M., Walz, R., Medina, J. H., and **Izquierdo, I.** (1997). Drugs acting upon the cyclic adenosine monophosphate/protein kinase A signalling pathway modulate memory consolidation when given late after training into rat hippocampus but not amygdala. *Behavioral Pharmacology*, **8**, 331–338.

Bontempi, B., Laurent-Demir, C., Destrade, C., and Jaffard, R. (1999). Time-dependent reorganization of brain circuitry underlying long-term memory storage. *Nature*, **400**, 671–675.

Bourtchouladze, R., Abel, T., Berman, N., Gordon, R., Lapidus, K., and Kandel, E. R. (1998). Different training procedures recruit either one or two critical periods for contextual memory consolidation, each of which requires protein synthesis and PKA. *Learning and Memory*, **5**, 365–374.

Bourtchouladze, R., Frenguelli, B., Blendy, J. A., Cioffi, D., Schutz, G., and Silva, A. J. (1994). Deficient long-term memory in mice with a targeted mutation of the cAMP-responsive element-binding protein. *Cell*, **79**, 59–68.

Brioni, J. D. and Arneric, S. P. (1993). Nicotinic receptor agonists facilitate retention of avoidance training: participation of dopaminergic mechanisms. *Behavioral Neural Biology*, **59**, 57–62.

Buzsáki, G. (1986). Hippocampal sharp waves: their origin and significance. *Brain Research*, **398**, 242–252.

Buzsáki, G. (2002). Theta oscillations in the hippocampus. *Neuron*, **33**, 325–340.

Buzsáki, G., Leung, L. W., and Vanderwolf, C. H. (1983). Cellular bases of hippocampal EEG in the behaving rat. *Brain Research*, **287**, 139–171.

Capece, M. L. and Lydic, R. (1997). cAMP and protein kinase A modulate cholinergic rapid eye movement sleep generation. *American Journal of Physiology*, **273**, R1430–R1440.

Castellano, C., Cabib, S., Puglisi-Allegra, S., Gasbarri, A., Sulli, A., Pacitti, C., Introini-Collison, I. B., and McGaugh, J. L. (1999). Strain-dependent involvement of D1 and D2 dopamine receptors in muscarinic cholinergic influences on memory storage. *Behavioral Brain Research*, **98**, 17–26.

Cirelli, C., Pompeiano, M., and Tononi, G. (1996). Neuronal gene expression in the waking state: a role for the locus coeruleus. *Science*, **274**, 1211–1215.

Corkin, S., Amaral, D. G., Gonzalez, R. G., Johnson, K. A., and Hyman, B. T. (1997). H. M.'s medial temporal lobe lesion: findings from magnetic resonance imaging. *Journal of Neuroscience*, **17**, 3964–3979.

Day, M. and Morris, R. G. (2001). Memory consolidation and NMDA receptors: discrepancy between genetic and pharmacological approaches. *Science*, **293**, 755.

de Medonça, A. and Ribeiro, J. A. (2001). Adenosine and synaptic plasticity. *Drug Development Research*, **52**, 283–290.

Doyle, E., Regan, C. M., and Shiotani, T. (1993). Nefiracetam (DM-9384) preserves hippocampal neural cell adhesion molecule-mediated memory consolidation processes during scopolamine disruption of passive avoidance training in the rat. *Journal of Neurochemistry*, **61**, 266–272.

Drucker-Colin, R., Zamora, J., Bernal-Pedraza, J., and Sosa, B. (1979). Modification of REM sleep and associated phasic activities by protein synthesis inhibitors. *Experimental Neurology*, **63**, 458–467.

Dunwiddie, T. V. and Masino, S. A. (2001). The role and regulation of adenosine in the central nervous system. *Annual Review of Neuroscience*, 24, 31–55.

Fadda, F., Melis, F., and Stancampiano, R. (1996). Increased hippocampal acetylcholine release during a working memory task. *European Journal of Pharmacology*, 307, R1–R2.

Fredholm, B. B., Battig, K., Holmen, J., Nehlig, A., and Zvartau, E. E. (1999). Actions of caffeine in the brain with special references to factors that contribute to its widespread use. *Pharmacological Reviews*, 51, 83–133.

Fujii, S., Kato, H., Ito, K., Itoh, S., Yamazaki, Y., Sasaki, H., and Kuroda, Y. (2000). Effects of A1 and A2 adenosine receptor antagonists on the induction and reversal of long-term potentiation in guinea pig hippocampal slices of CA1 neurons. *Cellulary and Molecular Neurobiology*, 20, 331–350.

Gaas, P., Wolfer, D. P., Balschun, D., Rudolph, D., Frey, U., Lipp, H., and Schutz, G. (1998). Deficits in memory tasks of mice with CREB mutations depend on gene dosage. *Learning and Memory*, 5, 274–288.

Gale, G. D., Anagnostaras, S. G., and Fanselow, M. S. (2001). Cholinergic modulation of pavlovian fear conditioning: effects of intrahippocampal scopolamine infusion. *Hippocampus*, 11, 371–376.

Graves, L., Blendy, J., Pack, A., and Abel, T. (2001a). Increased NREM in mutant mice lacking CREB. *Sleep*, 24, A422.

Graves, L., Pack, A., and Abel, T. (2001b). Sleep and memory: a molecular perspective. *Trends in Neuroscience*, 24, 237–243.

Graves, L. A., Dalvi, A., Lucki, I., Blendy, J. A., and Abel, T. (2002). Behavioral analysis of CREB mutation on a B6/129 F1 hybrid background. *Hippocampus*, 12, 18–26.

Graves, L. A., Heller, E., Pack, A., and Abel, T. (2000). The role of sleep in hippocampus-dependent long-term memory. *Sleep*, 23, A393.

Gray, R., Rajan, A. S., Radcliffe, K. A., Yakehiro, M., and Dani, J. A. (1996). Hippocampal synaptic transmission enhanced by low concentrations of nicotine. *Nature*, 383, 713–716.

Grecksch, G., Ott, T., and Matthies, H. (1978). Influence of post-training intrahippocampally applied oxotremorine on the consolidation of a brightness discrimination. *Pharmacology, Biochemistry, and Behavior*, 8, 215–218.

Gutwein, B. M., Shiromani, P. J., and Fishbein, W. (1980). Paradoxical sleep and memory: long-term disruptive effects of Anisomycin. *Pharmacology, Biochemistry, and Behavior*, 12, 377–384.

Hagan, J. J., Tweedie, F., and Morris, R. G. (1986). Lack of task specificity and absence of posttraining effects of atropine on learning. *Behavioral Neuroscience*, 100, 483–493.

Hamid, S., Dawe, G. S., Gray, J. A., and Stephenson, J. D. (1997). Nicotine induces long-lasting potentiation in the dentate gyrus of nicotine-primed rats. *Neuroscience Research*, 29, 81–85.

Hasslemo, M. E. (1995). Neuromodulation and cortical function: modeling the physiological basis of behavior. *Behavioral Brain Research*, 67, 1–27.

Hasslemo, M. E. (1999). Neuromodulation: acetylcholine and memory consolidation. *Trends in Cognitive Sciences*, 3, 351–359.

Hendricks, J. C., Williams, J. A., Panckeri, K., Kirk, D., Tello, M., Yin, J. C., and Sehgal, A. (2001). A non-circadian role for cAMP signaling and CREB activity in Drosophila rest homeostasis. *Nature Neuroscience*, **4**, 1108–1115.

Huang, Y. Y., Nguyen, P. V., Abel, T., and Kandel, E. (1996). Long-lasting forms of synaptic potentiation in the mammalian hippocampus. *Learning Memory*, **3**, 74–85.

Huerta, P. T. and Lisman, J. E. (1993). Heightened synaptic plasticity of hippocampal CA1 neurons during a cholinergically induced rhythmic state. *Nature*, **364**, 723–725.

Huston, J. P., Haas, H. L., Boix, F., Pfister, M., Decking, U., Schrader, J., and Schwarting, R. K. W. (1996). Extracellular adenosine levels in neostriatum and hippocampus during rest and activity periods of rats. *Neuroscience*, **73**, 99–107.

Impey, S., Smith, D. M., Obrietan, K., Donahue, R., Wade, C., and Storm, D. R. (1998). Stimulation of cAMP response elements (CRE)-mediated transcription during contextual learning. *Nature Neuroscience*, **7**, 595–601.

Izquierdo, I., da Cunha, C., Rosat, R., Jerusalinsky, D., Ferreira, M. B., and Medina, J. H. (1992). Neurotransmitter receptors involved in post-training memory processing by the amygdala, medial septum, and hippocampus of the rat. *Behavioral and Neural Biology*, **58**, 16–26.

Izquierdo, I. and McGaugh, J. L. (2000). Behavioral pharmacology and its contribution to the molecular basis of memory consolidation. *Behavioral Pharmacology*, **11**, 517–534.

Kessey, K. and Mogul, D. J. (1998). Adenosine A2 receptors modulate hippocampal synaptic transmission via a cyclic-AMP-dependent pathway. *Neuroscience*, **84**, 59–69.

Kim, J. J. and Fanselow, M. S. (1992). Modality-specific retrograde amnesia of fear. *Science*, **256**, 675–677.

Kim, J. J., Rison, R. A., and Fanselow, M. S. (1993). Effects of amygdala, hippocampus, and periaqueductal gray lesions on short- and long-term contextual fear. *Behavioral Neuroscience*, **107**, 1093–1098.

King, C., Henze, D. A., Leinekuge, I. X., and Buzsáki, G. (1999). Hebbian modification of a hippocampal population pattern in the rat. *Journal of Physiology*, **521**, 159–167.

Kogan, J. H., Frankland, P. W., Blendy, J. A., Coblentz, J., Marowitz, Z., Schutz, G., and Silva, A. J. (1997). Spaced training induces long-term memory in CREB mutant mice. *Current Biology*, **7**, 1–11.

Kopf, S. R., Melani, A., Pedata, F., and Pepeu, G. (1999). Adenosine and memory storage: effect of A(1) and A(2) receptor antagonists. *Psychopharmacology* (Berlin), **146**, 214–219.

Kudrimoti, H. S., Barnes, C. A., and McNaughton, B. L. (1999). Reactivation of hippocampal cell assemblies: effects of behavioral state, experience, and EEG dynamics. *Journal of Neuroscience*, **19**, 4090–4101.

LeDoux, J. E. (2000). Emotional circuits and the brain. *Annual Review of Neuroscience*, **23**, 155–184.

Lelkes, Z., Alfoldi, P., Erdos, A., and Benedek, G. (1998). Rolipram, an antidepressant that increases the availability of cAMP, transiently enhances wakefulness in rats. *Pharmacology, Biochemistry, and Behavior*, **60**, 835–839.

Levin, E. D. and Rose, J. E. (1991). Nicotinic and muscarinic interactions and choice accuracy in the radial-arm maze. *Brain Research Bulletin*, **27**, 125–128.

Li, X. F., Stutzman, G. E., and LeDoux, J. E. (1996). Convergent but temporally separated inputs to lateral amygdala neurons from the auditory thalamus and auditory cortex use different postsynaptic receptors: *in vivo* intracellular and extracellular recordings in fear conditioning pathways. *Learning and Memory*, 3, 229–242.

Lin, A. S., Udhe, T. W., Slate, S. O., and McCann, U. D. (1997). Effects of intravenous caffeine administered to healthy males during sleep. *Depression and Anxiety*, 5,

Louie, K. and Wilson, M. A. (2001). Temporally structured replay of awake hippocampal ensemble activity during rapid eye movement sleep. *Neuron*, 29, 145–156.

Maren, S. (2001). Neurobiology of Pavlovian fear conditioning. *Annual Review of Neuroscience*, 24, 897–931.

Martin, S. J., Grimwood, P. D., and Morris, R. G. (2000). Synaptic plasticity and memory: an evaluation of the hypothesis. *Annual Review of Neuroscience*, 23, 649–711.

McCormick, D. A. (1992). Cellular mechanisms underlying cholinergic and noradrenergic modulation of neuronal firing mode in the cat and guinea pig dorsal lateral geniculate nucleus. *Journal of Neuroscience*, 12, 278–289.

McDonald, R. J. and White, N. M. (1993). A triple dissociation of memory systems: hippocampus, amygdala, and dorsal striatum. *Behavioral Neuroscience*, 107, 3–22.

McGaugh, J. L. (2000). Memory—a century of consolidation. *Science*, 287, 248–251.

Miller, S. and Mayford, M. (1999). Cellular and molecular mechanisms of memory: the LTP connection. *Current Opinion in Genetics and Development*, 9, 333–337.

Milner, B., Squire, L. R., and Kandel, E. R. (1998). Cognitive neuroscience and the study of memory. *Neuron*, 20, 445–468.

Miyakawa, T., Yamada, M., Duttaroy, A., and Wess, J. (2001). Hyperactivity and intact hippocampus-dependent learning in mice lacking the M1 muscarinic acetylcholine receptor. *Journal of Neuroscience*, 21, 5239–5250.

Morris, R. G., Garrud, P., Rawlins, J. N., and O'Keefe, J. (1982). Place navigation impaired in rats with hippocampal lesions. *Nature*, 297, 681–683.

Müller, G. E. and Pilzecker, A. (1900). *Experimentelle Beiträge zur Lehre vom Gedächtnis Zeitschrift für Psychologie*, 1, 1–288.

Nadasdy, Z., Hirase, H., Czurko, A., Csicsvari, J., and Buzsáki, G. (1999). Replay and time compression of recurring spike sequences in the hippocampus. *Journal of Neuroscience*, 19, 9497–9507.

Nail-Boucherie, K., Dourmap, N. R. J., and Costentin, J. (2000). Contextual fear conditioning is associated with an increase of acetylcholine release in the hippocampus of rat. *Cognitive Brain Research*, 9, 193–197.

Nestler, E. J., Hyman, S. E., and Malenka, R. C. (2001). *Molecular neuropharmacology*. McGraw-Hill, New York. p. 539.

Nguyen, P. V., Abel, T., and Kandel, E. R. (1994). Requirement of a critical period of transcription for induction of a late phase of LTP. *Science*, 265, 1104–1107.

O'Keefe, J. and Dostrovsky, J. (1971). The hippocampus as a spatial map. Preliminary evidence from unit activity in the freely-moving rat. *Brain Research*, 34, 171–175.

Packard, M. G. and **McGaugh, J. L.** (1992). Double dissociation of fornix and caudate nucleus lesions on acquisition of two water maze tasks: further evidence for multiple memory systems. *Behavioral Neuroscience*, **106**, 439–446.

Partridge, J. G., Tang, K. C., and **Lovinger, D. M.** (2000). Regional and postnatal heterogeneity of activity-dependent long-term changes in synaptic efficacy in the dorsal striatum. *Journal of Neurophysiology*, **84**, 1422–1429.

Pavlides, C. and **Winson, J.** (1989). Influences of hippocampal place cell firing in the awake state on the activity of these cells during subsequent sleep episodes. *Journal of Neuroscience*, **9**, 2907–2918.

Perez, E., Zamboni, G., and **Parmeggiani, P. L.** (1982). cAMP concentration in the rat's pre-optic region and cerebral cortex during sleep deprivation and recovery induced by ambient temperature. *Experimental Brain Research*, **47**, 114–118.

Phillips, R. G. and **LeDoux, J. E.** (1992). Differential contribution of amygdala and hippocampus to cued and contextual fear conditioning. *Behavioral Neuroscience*, **106**, 274–285.

Pittenger, C., Huang, Y. Y., Paletzki, R. F., Bourtchouladze, R., Scanlin, H., Vronskaya, S., and **Kandel, E. R.** (2002). Reversible inhibition of CREB/ATF transcription factors in region CA1 of the dorsal hippocampus disrupts hippocampus-dependent spatial memory. *Neuron*, **34**, 447–462.

Plihal, W. and **Born, J.** (1999). Effects of early and late nocturnal sleep on priming and spatial memory. *Psychophysiology*, **36**, 571–582.

Poe, G. R., Nitz, D. A., McNaughton, B. L., and **Barnes, C. A.** (2000). Experience-dependent phase-reversal of hippocampal neuron firing during REM sleep. *Brain Research*, **855**, 176–180.

Porkka-Heiskanen, T., Strecker, R. E., Thakkar, M. M., Bjorkum, A. A., and **Greene, R. W.** (1997). Adenosine: a mediator of the sleep-inducing effects of prolonged wakefulness. *Science*, **276**, 1265–1268.

Portas, C. M., Thakkar, M. M., Rainnie, D. G., Greene, R. W., and **McCarley, R. W.** (1997). Role of adenosine in behavioral state modulation: a microdialysis study in the freely moving cat. *Neuroscience*, **79**, 225–235.

Rainnie, D. G., Grunze, H. C., McCarley, R. W., and **Greene, R. W.** (1994). Adenosine inhibition of mesopontine cholinergic neurons: implications for EEG arousal. *Science*, **263**, 689–692.

Rampon, C., Tang, Y. P., Goodhouse, J., Shimizu, E., Kyin, M., and **Tsien, J. Z.** (2000). Enrichment induces structural changes and recovery from nonspatial memory deficits in CA1 NMDAR1-knockout mice. *Nature Neuroscience*, **3**, 238–244.

Rezvani, A. H. and **Levin, E. D.** (2001). Cognitive effects of nicotine. *Biological Psychiatry*, **49**, 258–267.

Ribot, T. (1901). *Les maladies de la mémoire*. F. Alcan, Paris. p. 169.

Riedel, G., Micheau, J., Lam, A. G., Roloff, E., Martin, S. J., Bridge, H., Hoz, L., Poeschel, B., McCulloch, J., and **Morris, R. G.** (1999). Reversible neural inactivation reveals hippocampal participation in several memory processes. *Nature Neuroscience*, **2**, 898–905.

Riekkeinen, M. and **Riekkeinen, P.** (1997). Dorsal hippocampal muscarinic acetylcholine and NMDA receptors disrupt water maze navigation. *Neuroreport*, **8**(3), 645–648.

Roldan, G., Bolanos-Badillo, E., Gonzalez-Sanchez, H., Quirarte, G. L., and Prado-Alcala, R. A. (1997). Selective M1 muscarinic receptors antagonists disrupt memory consolidation of inhibitory avoidance in rats. *Neuroscience Letters*, **230**, 93–96.

Rotenberg, A., Abel, T., Hawkins, R. D., Kandel, E. R., and Muller, R. U. (2000). Parallel instabilities of long-term potentiation, place cells, and learning caused by decreased protein kinase A activity. *Journal of Neuroscience*, **20**, 8096–8102.

Rudy, J. W. (1996). Scopolamine administered before and after training impairs both contextual and auditory-cue fear conditioning. *Neurobiology of Learning and Memory*, **65**, 73–81.

Saint-Cyr, J. A., Taylor, A. E., and Lang, A. E. (1988). Procedural learning and neostriatal dysfunction in man. *Brain*, **111**, 941–959.

Sebastiao, A. M. and Ribeiro, J. A. (1996). Adenosine A2 receptor mediated excitatory actions on the nervous system. *Progress in Neurobiology*, **48**, 167–189.

Segal, M. and Bloom, F. E. (1974). The action of norepinephrine in the rat hippocampus. I. Iontophoretic studies. *Brain Research*, **72**, 79–97.

Seidenberg, M., Griffith, R., Sabsevitz, D., Moran, M., Haltiner, A., Bell, B., Swanson, S., Hammeke, T., and Hermann, B. (2002). Recognition and identification of famous faces in patients with unilateral temporal lobe epilepsy. *Neuropsychologia*, **40**, 446–456.

Shimizu, E., Tang, Y. P., Rampon, C., and Tsien, J. Z. (2000). NMDA receptor-dependent synaptic reinforcement as a crucial process for memory consolidation. *Science*, **290**, 1170–1174.

Siapas, A. G. and Wilson, M. A. (1998). Coordinated interactions between hippocampal ripples and cortical spindles during slow-wave sleep. *Neuron*, **21**, 1123–1128.

Silva, A. J., Kogan, J. H., Frankland, P. W., and Kida, S. (1998). CREB and memory. *Annual Review of Neuroscience*, **21**, 127–148.

Smith, C. (1995). Sleep states and memory processes. *Behavioral Brain Research*, **69**, 137–145.

Smith, C. and Rose, G. M. (1996). Evidence for a paradoxical sleep window for place learning in the Morris water maze. *Physiology and Behavior*, **59**, 93–97.

Smith, C. and Rose, G. M. (1997). Posttraining paradoxical sleep in rats is increased after spatial learning in the Morris water maze. *Behavioral Neuroscience*, **111**, 1197–1204.

Smith, C. T., Conway, J. M., and Rose, G. M. (1998). Brief paradoxical sleep deprivation impairs reference, but not working, memory in the radial arm maze task. *Neurobiology of Learning and Memory*, **69**, 211–217.

Socci, D. J., Sanberg, P. R., and Arendash, G. W. (1995). Nicotine enhances Morris water maze performance of young and aged rats. *Neurobiology of Aging*, **16**, 857–860.

Squire, L. R., Clark, R. E., and Knowlton, B. J. (2001). Retrograde amnesia. *Hippocampus*, **11**, 50–55.

Stefanacci, L., Buffalo, E. A., Schmolck, H., and Squire, L. R. (2000). Profound amnesia after damage to the medial temporal lobe: a neuroanatomical and neuropsychological profile of patient E. P. *Journal of Neuroscience*, **20**, 7024–7036.

Stewart, L. S. and McKay, B. E. (2000). Acquisition deficit and time-dependent retrograde amnesia for contextual fear conditioning in agmatine-treated rats. *Behavioral Pharmacology*, **11**, 93–97.

Stickgold, R., Hobson, J., Fosse, R., and **Fosse, M.** (2001). Sleep, learning, and dreams: off-line memory reprocessing. *Science*, **294**, 1052–1057.

Stickgold, R., James, L., and **Hobson, J. A.** (2000). Visual discrimination learning requires sleep after training. *Nature Neuroscience*, **3**, 1237–1238.

Toumane, A. and **Durkin, T. P.** (1993). Time gradient for post-test vulnerability to scopolamine-induced amnesia following the initial acquisition session of a spatial reference memory task in mice. *Behavioral and Neural Biology*, **60**, 139–151.

Tsien, J. Z., Huerta, P. T., and **Tonegawa, S.** (1996). The essential role of hippocampal CA1 NMDA receptor-dependent synaptic plasticity in spatial memory. *Cell*, **87**, 1327–1338.

Vanderwolf, C. H. (1969). Hippocampal electrical activity and voluntary movement in the rat. *Electroencephalography and Clinical Neurophysiology*, **26**, 407–418.

Wallenstein, G. V. and **Vago, D. R.** (2001). Intrahippocampal scopolamine impairs both acquisition and consolidation of contextual fear conditioning. *Neurobiology of Learning and Memory*, **75**, 245–252.

Woo, N. H., Duffy, S. N., Abel, T., and **Nguyen, P. V.** (2000). Genetic and pharmacological demonstration of differential recruitment of cAMP-dependent protein kinases by synaptic activity. *Journal of Neurophysiology*, **84**, 2739–2745.

Zola-Morgan, S. M. and **Squire, L. R.** (1990). The primate hippocampal formation: evidence for a time-limited role in memory storage. *Science*, **250**, 288–290.

Zola, S. M. and **Squire, L. R.** (2001). Relationship between magnitude of damage to the hippocampus and impaired recognition memory in monkeys. *Hippocampus*, **11**, 92–98.

Zola-Morgan, S., Squire, L. R., and **Amaral, D. G.** (1986). Human amnesia and the medial temporal region: enduring memory impairment following a bilateral lesion limited to field CA1 of the hippocampus. *Journal of Neuroscience*, **6**, 2950–2967.

Zola-Morgan, S., Squire, L. R., Amaral, D. G., and **Suzuki, W. A.** (1989). Lesions of perirhinal and parahippocampal cortex that spare the amygdala and hippocampal formation produce severe memory impairment. *Journal of Neuroscience*, **9**, 4355–4370.

CHAPTER 16

RECENT EVIDENCE OF MEMORY PROCESSING IN SLEEP

CONSTANTINE PAVLIDES AND SIDARTA RIBEIRO

In every dream we may find some reference to the experiences of the preceding day

Freud, 1900.

Introduction

It is generally thought that memories are initially labile and subject to disruption and loss and that a process of consolidation is necessary for them to become stable and permanent. This consolidation most likely involves an active process and must be occurring at various stages that include changes in cellular/network activity which in turn drive molecular/biochemical/structural processes to finally solidify memories for long-term storage. Memory consolidation could occur on-line, although there is evidence to suggest that it could also be taking place off-line. It has been hypothesized that sleep, and more specifically rapid eye movement (REM) sleep, plays a role in brain plasticity and memory consolidation. Although the initial evidence in support of this hypothesis was indirect or anecdotal, recent experimental evidence showing a direct link between sleep and information processing has been forthcoming. This evidence is derived from a wide variety of sources including behavioral, electrophysiological and molecular studies. We will briefly review evidence from the former, but will concentrate the discussion on our recent molecular studies. Finally, a model of how sleep may act to consolidate memories acquired during wakefulness will be presented.

Behavioral studies

One approach to determine the role of REM sleep in learning and memory has been to sleep deprive animals or humans and to determine the effects on memory consolidation. A number of behavioral studies have reported that REM sleep deprivation significantly impairs short-term or declarative memory (Pearlman and Becker 1974; Fishbein and Gutwein 1977; Grosvenor and Lack 1984; Idzikowski 1984; Smith and Kelly 1988; Hennevin *et al.* 1995; Smith *et al.* 1998). It has also been reported that perceptual learning in humans is disrupted by REM-selective sleep interruption (Karni *et al.* 1994).

Conversely, both behavioral training and exposure to enriched environments have been shown to increase the amount and frequency of subsequent REM sleep in rats (Smith *et al.* 1974, 1977, 1980; Smith and Wong 1991; Smith 1996; Smith and Rose 1997), furthermore, similar effects were observed following intensive learning in humans (Smith and Lapp 1991). Interestingly, a recent study also reported that short naps following training prevent performance fatigue over repeated testing on a perceptual task in humans (Mednick *et al.* 2002). In a series of studies, mainly by Smith and his associates, it has been reported that REM sleep is required for memory consolidation during critical time periods after learning, called "REM sleep windows." A critical REM sleep window appears to occur between 4 and 8 h following the learning, although longer time windows (24 h to a number of days) have also been observed (for review see, Smith 1996).

Electrophysiological studies

Behavioral gating

Other supportive evidence for a role of sleep in memory processes is the phenomenon of *behavioral gating*, initially discovered by Winson and Abzug (1977, 1978*a,b*) (for review see, Winson 1986) and subsequently corroborated by other laboratories (Leung 1980; Leung and Vanderwolf 1980). These studies demonstrated that neuronal transmission through the hippocampal trisynaptic circuit is modulated by the behavioral state of the animal—transmission is enhanced during SWS in comparison to an alert state, while in behaviors associated with theta (in rats exploration and REM sleep) transmission was variable, being high in some instances but low in others. This variability most likely resulted from the fact that stimuli used to evoke the responses were delivered at a different phase of the local theta rhythm (i.e. peak, trough or "in between"). When stimulation was applied in phase with the theta rhythm it was shown that the potentials were indeed modulated by theta (Linster *et al.* 1999; Wyble *et al.* 2000). A number of studies have further reported that the firing of hippocampal neurons is correlated with theta rhythm, although the precise relationship between different cell types or during different behavioral states is rather complex (Rudell *et al.* 1980; Buzsáki and Eidelberg 1983; Fox *et al.* 1986; Otto *et al.* 1991). These findings point to an enhancement of information flow through the hippocampus in sleep that may be related to off-line memory consolidation.

Theta rhythm

One of the most prominent characteristics of REM sleep is the appearance of theta rhythm in the EEG. Theta waves are regular, sinusoidal oscillations in the range of 3–7 Hz that occur in the hippocampal EEG (reviewed in, Bland 1986; Green and Arduini 1954). Theta waves are present in all mammals studied to date (Brown 1968; Vanderwolf 1969; Sainsbury 1970; Harper 1971; Winson 1974), including monkeys (Stewart and Fox 1991) and humans (Arnolds *et al.* 1980). Theta waves were a puzzle for many years after their discovery, because the context of their occurrence varies tremendously across species. During the awake state, in rabbits, theta waves are negligible during movement but abundant when the animals freeze, suggesting that theta rhythm is related to alert immobility (Green *et al.* 1960; Harper 1971). On the other hand, rats (Green *et al.* 1960; Winson 1974) and guinea pigs (Green *et al.* 1960) were found to display exactly the opposite—theta occurs when animals are actively exploring their surroundings, and ceases when they freeze. To complicate things further, cats display a hybrid pattern between rats and rabbits, with theta occurring intermittently during both movement and repose (Brown 1968).

The phenomenon of theta rhythm was paradoxical because it both implied and excluded sensorimotor activity as the source of the oscillations. Theta rhythm was proposed to be a correlate of the orienting reflex (Grastyán *et al.* 1959), of approaching behavior (Grastyán *et al.* 1966) and attentive behavior (Adey *et al.* 1967; Elazar and Adey 1967*a,b*). The discovery that theta also occurs during REM sleep (so reliably as to constitute a REM sleep-signature) only increased the contradictions (Vanderwolf 1969). However, after a careful and comprehensive analysis of the waking behaviors involved with theta waves across many species, a common thread was noticed: theta rhythm only occurred during waking when animals were performing ecologically relevant species-specific behaviors (Winson 1972): *"Predatory behavior in the cat, prey behavior in the rabbit, and exploration in the rat are, respectively, most important to their survival"* (Winson 1990). This proposition led to the hypothesis that theta waves are involved in the acquisition and processing of particularly meaningful environmental information. Support for this interpretation came from lesion experiments showing that theta-deprived rats become amnesic (Winson 1978). Furthermore, hippocampal long-term potentiation (LTP), which is widely accepted as a neuronal model of learning and memory (Bliss and Collingridge 1993), was found to be preferentially induced by high-frequency stimulation (HFS) at theta-rhythm periodicity (Larson and Lynch 1986; Larson *et al.* 1986; Rose and Dunwiddie 1986; Staubli and Lynch 1987; Diamond *et al.* 1988; Greenstein *et al.* 1988). We further showed that weak tetanic stimuli which would normally not be sufficient to induce LTP, produced significant potentiation when applied at the positive phase of the theta wave, while conversely they produced long-term depression (LTD) when applied at the negative phase of the theta wave (Pavlides *et al.* 1988). A similar theta-phase effect in LTP induction was observed by other laboratories both in anesthetized (Holscher *et al.* 1997) and in freely behaving animals (Orr *et al.* 2001) as well as *in vitro* (Huerta and Lisman 1993, 1995, 1996).

As stated above, the firing of hippocampal principal neurons is phase locked to the locally recorded theta rhythm during awake behaviors or under urethane anesthesia (Rudell *et al.* 1980; Buzsáki and Eidelberg 1983; Fox *et al.* 1986; Otto *et al.* 1991). In a rather interesting study (Poe *et al.* 2000*a*), it was reported that the firing of place cells is also correlated with theta phase during REM sleep. Hippocampal place cells were recorded either in a novel or familiar environment. While in the place field, the firing of place cells was shown to occur at the positive phase (peak) of the theta rhythm. Interestingly, in REM sleep the firing of the units from the animals exposed to the novel environment occurred at the peak while the units from the animals exposed to the familiar environment fired at the negative phase (trough) of the theta rhythm. It was further shown that the firing at the positive phase for the novel environment cells lasted for several days, although with each successive day there was a shift in the firing toward the negative phase of the theta rhythm. Together with the above studies showing a biphasic modulation of plasticity dependent on the phase of the theta rhythm these results suggest that theta rhythm is important for memory consolidation, and its occurrence during REM sleep indicates that off-line memory processing likely occurs during sleep (Winson 1993).

Neuronal activity in sleep

A number of studies have shown that sleep is a dynamic state in terms of spontaneous neuronal activity. Enhanced activity has been observed in a number of brain regions, including the hippocampus (Ranck 1973; Delacour 1982) and neocortex (Collins *et al.* 1999; Destexhe *et al.* 1999). Perhaps, the most direct evidence for information processing in sleep is the finding that neuronal activity in sleep reflects neuronal activity during awake states. A while ago, we (Pavlides and Winson 1989) reported that hippocampal neurons (i.e. "place cells") which were active in awake behaviors (i.e. when the animal was exposed to a cell's "place field") were re-activated in sleep states that followed, in comparison to simultaneously recorded cells which were kept away from their place fields and which maintained their low firing rates during sleep. When the second of a pair of cells was exposed to its place field (while the first cell was kept away), the second cell of the pair then showed enhanced activity in the sleep that followed. The enhanced activity occurred both in SWS as well as in REM sleep, although it was short-lived, lasting approximately 2–3 h, spanning a number of SWS–REM sleep cycles. Subsequent studies expanded on this finding by first showing that space is mapped by the correlated firing of ensembles of hippocampal neurons (Wilson and McNaughton 1993) and that this correlated activity is maintained in SWS (Wilson and McNaughton 1994). In different studies it was shown that the temporal relation of hippocampal neuronal firing during awake behaviors is also maintained in subsequent SWS (Skaggs and McNaughton 1996; Kudrimoti *et al.* 1999; Nadasdy *et al.* 1999; Hirase *et al.* 2001) and REM sleep (Louie and Wilson 2001). A similar replay of daytime events has been shown in songbirds (Dave and Margoliash 2000). It has further been reported that interactions between limbic and neocortical structures occur in sleep (Qin *et al.* 1997; Siapas and Wilson 1998) which is of significance since it is generally thought that the long-term storage of memories is in the neocortex. These studies provide strong evidence that the neuronal activity in sleep is not merely an overall enhancement in excitability but rather represents information processing in sleep.

In summary, the behavioral studies suggest that the dreaming phase of sleep (REM sleep) plays a key role in the consolidation of daytime memories. A number of electrophysiological studies have reported that REM sleep is a state of enhanced neuronal activity. More recent studies have shown that hippocampal neuronal activity during sleep recapitulates waking activity, providing strong evidence that this could constitute an initial part of the consolidation process. As will be discussed below, the enhanced neuronal activity could then trigger various molecular cascades to solidify synaptic processes and stabilize the neuronal network encoding for specific memories.

Molecular studies

Activity-dependent gene expression during sleep

Several lines of evidence indicate that the laying down of long-term memories requires the modification of neuronal connections, most likely through the activation of gene expression programs that lead to neuronal plasticity (Madison *et al.* 1991; Bliss and Collingridge 1993). In principle, brain reactivation leading to activity-dependent gene expression during sleep could account for the high rates of protein synthesis encountered during SWS sleep (Ramm and Smith 1990), which have been suggested to underlie memory consolidation (Gutwein *et al.* 1980; Idzikowski and Oswald 1983; Kavanau 1996).

A particularly interesting candidate for mediating the long-lasting effects of experience on the brain is the immediate early gene (IEG) *zif-268* (same as Egr-1, NGFI-A, Krox-24, and ZENK) (Milbrandt 1987), whose expression in mature neurons is triggered by sustained membrane depolarization, NMDA channel opening and calcium influx (Cole *et al.* 1989; Wisden *et al.* 1990; Williams *et al.* 2000). Because *zif-268* mRNA levels sharply peak 30 min after a variety of stimuli (Richardson *et al.* 1992; Cullinan *et al.* 1995; Honkaniemi *et al.* 1995; Mello and Clayton 1995; Tanaka *et al.* 1977), its expression can be used for a snapshot assessment of activation throughout the brain (Chaudhuri 1997). The *zif-268* gene encodes a transcription factor (Sukhatme *et al.* 1988; Christy and Nathans 1989; Cole *et al.* 1990*a*; Worley *et al.* 1993) which integrates a cascade of molecular events implicated in neuronal plasticity and learning (Cole *et al.* 1989; Sheng and Greenberg 1990; Sheng *et al.* 1990; Ghosh and Greenberg 1995), including the upregulation of the synapse-specific proteins synapsin I (Thiel *et al.* 1994) and II (Peterson *et al.* 1995) (Fig. 16.1). In line with a possible role in synaptic plasticity, *zif-268* has been specifically linked to the induction of hippocampal LTP (Cole *et al.* 1989; Wisden *et al.* 1990; Abraham *et al.* 1993; Roberts *et al.* 1996), neuronal morphological changes after exposure to an enriched environment (Wallace *et al.* 1995), and other plasticity-related phenomena (Nedivi *et al.* 1993; Kaplan *et al.* 1995, 1996). Furthermore, *zif-268* is upregulated in a variety of novelty or learning behavioral paradigms, such as two-way active avoidance (Nikolaev *et al.* 1992), and brightness discrimination (Grimm and Tischmeyer 1997). Most compellingly, *zif-268* expression is actually required for the long-term maintenance of hippocampal LTP, as well as spatial and nonspatial long-term memories (Jones *et al.* 2001).

Given its role in information processing through distinct physiological phases, sleep has been proposed to be analogous to the sequential process of food digestion (Lucero 1970; Leconte *et al.* 1974; Ambrosini *et al.* 1988; Winson 1993; Giuditta *et al.* 1995;

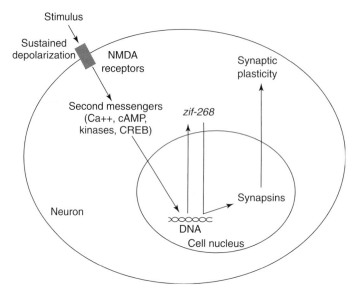

Figure 16.1 Molecular cascade involved in the *zif-268* response. Sustained depolarization opens NMDA channels, leading to calcium entry, phosphorylation of PKA and CREB, and induction of *zif-268*. The immediate-early gene *zif-268* is a plasticity-related transcription factor which has been shown to promote the *in vitro* transcription of synapsins.

Smith 1996). We took this analogy seriously and decided to test whether feeding a rich sensorimotor experience during waking (W) can modulate *zif-268* expression levels in rats during ensuing SWS and REM sleep states (Ribeiro *et al.* 1999).

Animals were handled for 15–20 days so as to decrease the stress response to the experimenter, and were then bilaterally implanted with chronic electrodes in the dentate gyrus (DG) for EEG recording. After a 3-day postoperative recovery period, baseline EEG was recorded for 10–15 consecutive days in order to identify typical W, SW, and REM sleep profiles. Recording was performed inside a soundproof isolation box equipped with one-way mirrors for behavior observation. Figure 16.2 shows the general scheme of the experimental paradigm, which comprised three consecutive phases: an initial exposure to an enriched environment (EE), an intervening period, and a final period of wake/sleep. The EE was novel to all rats and consisted of four cardboard boxes of different sizes, interconnected by PVC tubes that allowed free access of animals to all chambers (total area = 2.5 m^2). Platforms and wooden toys were present in the four chambers. Scented corn flakes of several different flavors were randomly dispersed throughout the labyrinth at semi-hidden places; two water sources were provided.

Behaviors and EEG were continuously monitored throughout the entire experiment; during the EE phase (lights off), behaviors were observed under near-infrared light, to which rats are blind (Neitz and Jacobs 1986). Animals exposed to the EE remained awake throughout the exposure period, engaging in active exploratory behavior of all

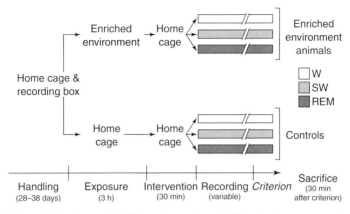

Figure 16.2 Schematic flowchart of the EE experiment. A total of 6 animal groups were studied: 3 EE and 3 unstimulated controls ($n = 6$/group) All rats were allowed to get familiarized with the home cage, experimenter, and recording conditions for several days, during which baseline EEG was recorded. A 12 h/12 h light/darkness schedule was kept, with lights on at 09:00. On the day of the experiment, animals were either exposed for the last 3 h of the darkness period to an enriched environment (EE group), or kept in their home cages as a control (C group). Following an intervening period of 30 min back in the home cages, animals were placed in the recording box for monitoring of wake/sleep states until reaching criterion for W, SWS, or REM sleep; the typical duration of this period was around 90 min. Thirty minutes after criterion, animals were killed and their brains were processed for *zif-268* expression by *in situ* hybridization (from Ribeiro *et al.* 1999).

the EE chambers. Control animals, kept in their home cages instead of the EE, also remained awake for the same 3-h period, displaying grooming and feeding behaviors in addition to a low to moderate degree of locomotion. All animals remained awake during the intervening period. After reaching criterion for W, SWS, or REM sleep, animals were kept awake for an additional 30 min and were then killed. Their brains were processed for *zif-268* expression, which was quantified for 25 brain structures within 6 major brain regions according to the rat atlas (Paxinos and Watson 1986): cerebral cortex, hippocampus, striatum, amygdala, thalamus, and hypothalamus.

Brain *zif-268* expression during REM sleep depends on prior waking experience

Zif-268 expression in control animals generally decreased from the W to the SWS and REM sleep groups (Fig. 16.3, (a)–(a″)); this effect was most prominent in the cerebral cortex (Fig. 16.4). Such a decrease after a single episode of either SWS or REM sleep is consistent with previous studies showing that brain expression of several IEGs (including *zif-268*) is downregulated after several hours of sleep, in comparison to levels found in sleep-deprived animals (Pompeiano *et al.* 1992, 1997; Basheer *et al.* 1997).

A very different picture emerges when one analyzes animals exposed to an EE, and teases apart the specific contributions of SWS and REM sleep: While *zif-268* expression decreased from the W to the SWS group (Fig. 16.3, (b)–(b′)), there was a clear rise from the SWS to the REM sleep group (Fig. 16.3, (b′)–(b″)).

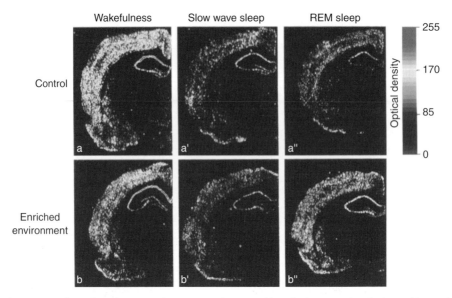

Figure 16.3 Effect of previous sensorimotor experience on *zif-268* brain expression during waking and sleep states. Shown are autoradiograms of representative brain sections for each group studied. In controls, *zif-268* expression decreased from W (a) to SWS (a′) and REM sleep (a″). In enriched environment animals, *zif-268* levels decreased from W (b) to SWS (b′), but increased from the latter to REM sleep (b″). This effect was particularly noticeable in the cerebral cortex and the hippocampus (modified from Ribeiro *et al.* 1999). (See Plate 15.)

As can be seen in Fig. 16.4, this effect was particularly noticeable in the cerebral cortex and hippocampus. For both regions, *zif-268* expression levels in EE animals was significantly higher in the REM sleep group than in the SWS group. In addition, *zif-268* levels during REM sleep were higher for EE than for C animals.

A brief exposure to an EE is known to cause a fast and transient induction of various IEGs, including *zif-268* (Wallace *et al.* 1995). The most parsimonious explanation for our results is that a reinduction of *zif-268* occurs in the brain during REM sleep that follows EE exposure. The following arguments supports this interpretation:

Zif-268 levels in W did not differ significantly between C and EE animals. This is in accord with the well-established transient nature of the *zif-268* response, and argues against the possibility that the high *zif-268* expression seen during REM sleep in EE animals stems from a sustained upregulation (several hours) of *zif-268* after the exposure (Fig. 16.5(a)). Also supportive of this view is the fact that REM sleep is always preceded by SWS sleep (Fishbein and Gutwein 1977; Hennevin *et al.* 1995; Smith 1996), and the SWS group had consistently low *zif-268* levels (Figs 16.3 and 16.4). In EE animals, the time between exposure to the EE and the moment of sacrifice did not differ significantly among the W, SWS, and REM sleep groups (W $= 311 \pm 8$, SW $= 322 \pm 10$, REM sleep $= 325 \pm 7$; means $\pm$ SEM, in min). This rules out the possibility that the high *zif-268* expression in the latter represents a putative late wave of gene expression that would be

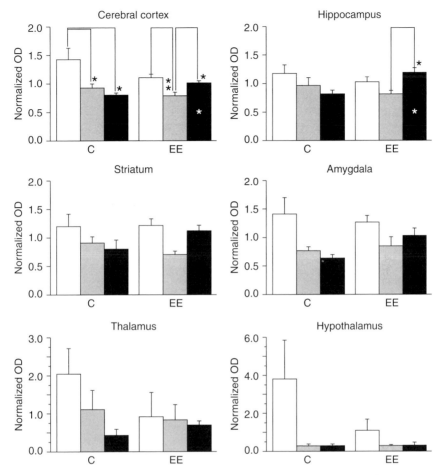

Figure 16.4 Analysis of *zif-268* expression during waking and sleep states in six major brain regions: cerebral cortex, hippocampus, striatum, amygdala, thalamus, and hypothalamus. Statistically significant interactions (ANOVA) between expression profiles occurred for the cerebral cortex ($p = 0.04$) and the hippocampus ($p = 0.03$). Whereas *zif-268* expression in controls decreased from W (white bar) to SWS (shaded bar) and to REM sleep (black bar), *zif-268* levels in animals exposed to the EE decreased from W to SWS but increased from SWS to REM sleep. Similar although not significant trends were observed for the striatum and the amygdala, while the thalamus and the hypothalamus showed no upregulation. Values on the y-axis represent normalized optical density (OD) measurements (means ± SEM) of X-ray film autoradiograms; statistically significant differences (Bonferroni post hoc tests) are indicated by one ($p < 0.05$) or two ($p < 0.01$) asterisks. Asterisks inside columns indicate state differences between C and EE groups (from Ribeiro *et al.* 1999).

independent of the behavioral state, but simply associated with a longer survival of the REM sleep group after exposure to the EE (Fig. 16.5(b)).

The duration of REM sleep did not differ significantly between C and EE animals (148 ± 40 and 137 ± 24, respectively; means ± SEM, in s). This precludes the possibility

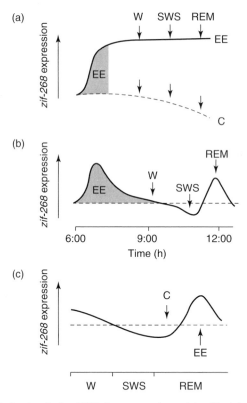

Figure 16.5 *Zif-268* reinduction during REM sleep cannot be explained by (a) a generalized sustained upregulation after enriched environment exposure; (b) a possible late wave of gene expression associated with a presumed longer survival of the REM sleep/EE group and independent of sleep states; (c) or a putative increased REM sleep time in the EE group.

that differences in the amount of REM sleep could account for the observed effects (Fig. 16.5(c)).

For both the cerebral cortex and the hippocampus, *zif-268* expression during REM sleep was significantly higher in EE than in C animals (Figs 16.3 and 16.4). Thus, the high *zif-268* levels during REM sleep in the former are not just a reflection of a relative increase with respect to W and SWS levels, but represent a real increase in *zif-268* expression during REM sleep from unexposed controls to exposed animals.

The experience provided by exposure to an enriched environment such as the one we used is very complex and contains sensory and motor aspects, both of which may have contributed to the gene reinduction observed during REM sleep. Increased motor and somatosensory activities are intrinsic to the exploration of a new environment, and most probably account for a substantial portion of *zif-268* reinduction, particularly that occurring in the frontal cortex (Donoghue *et al.* 1979; Donoghue and Wise 1982). In contrast, the effect observed in the piriform cortex and the hippocampus is likely related to the involvement of these areas in olfaction (Haberly and Price 1978; Schwob *et al.* 1984) and spatial navigation (Olton *et al.* 1978; O'Keefe 1993) respectively. Multimodal responses during the exposure period may also have influenced the reinduction pattern that we found.

The results discussed above constitute a first demonstration that brain gene expression during REM sleep depends on prior waking experience. This finding is seemingly at odds with several studies showing that sleep downregulates the expression of *zif-268* and other activity-dependent genes (Pompeiano *et al.* 1992, 1994, 1997; O'Hara *et al.* 1993; Basheer *et al.* 1997; Cirelli and Tononi 1998). Two factors might explain this apparent discrepancy: First, none of the studies mentioned above attempted to separate the specific contributions of SWS and REM sleep for activity-dependent gene expression. In our studies we have found that SWS is indeed concomitant with marked *zif-268* downregulation, irrespective of preceding W experience. Therefore, the post-sleep downregulation of *zif-268* expression extensively reported by other research groups (O'Hara *et al.* 1993; Pompeiano *et al.* 1994; Cirelli and Tononi 1998, 1999, 2000) could well reflect the natural predominance of SWS over REM sleep in uncontrolled sleep episodes (Timo-Iaria *et al.* 1970; Hobson 1995). Second, none of the studies in question attempted to expose the experimental animals to relevant W experience a few hours prior to the sleep episodes investigated. Thus, the results reported in those papers very likely correspond to the *zif-268* down-regulation we observe in unstimulated SWS and REM sleep control groups (Fig. 16.3, (a)–(a″)).

Is REM sleep a window of increased synaptic plasticity?

Given the association between *zif-268* expression and neuronal plasticity, experience-dependent *zif-268* reinduction during REM sleep may represent a window of increased plasticity whereby previous waking experience can contribute to long-lasting changes in the brain. In order to explore the mechanisms underlying this phenomenon, we decided to extend our experiment by substituting unilateral HFS leading to hippocampal LTP for the EE exposure (Ribeiro 2000; Ribeiro *et al.* 2002).

The use of HFS as a W stimulus offered a number of advantages over the use of EE exposure: standardization of stimulation parameters, specificity of the anatomical path under stimulation, and presence of an internal control (unstimulated) hemisphere. Briefly, rats were subjected to bilateral implantation of recording electrodes in the DG and stimulating electrodes in the medial perforant pathway (mPP). After recovery from surgery, baseline evoked field potentials and EEG were recorded from both hemispheres for a number of days until stable. On the day of the experiment, baseline recordings were again taken from both hemispheres and then one hemisphere (randomized) was tetanized with ten 50 ms trains of 0.25 ms pulses at 400 Hz, one train every 10 s (Winson and Dahl 1986), while the contralateral hemisphere received no stimulation. Brain *zif-268* expression associated with early and late episodes of W, SWS, and REM sleep was assessed in 10 groups of animals: 3 unstimulated control groups (Fig. 16.6; the top 3 bars)

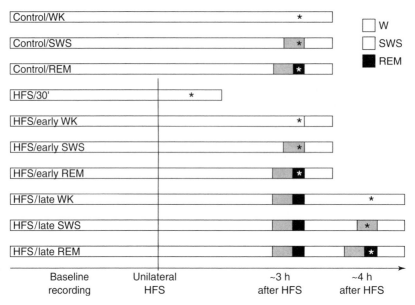

Figure 16.6 Schematic flowchart of the LTP experiment. A total of 10 animal groups were studied: 7 HFS and 3 unstimulated controls ($n = 4$/group). Acquisition of baseline field potentials was followed by HFS of one hemisphere in order to produce unilateral LTP. The first stimulated group consisted of animals kept awake for 30 min after unilateral HFS and then killed; this group served as a positive control for the unilateral DG induction of *zif-268* under our stimulation protocol. The 6 remaining stimulated groups were studied according to the cumulative waking/sleep states reached: early W, early SWS, early REM sleep, late W, late SWS and late REM sleep. Animals were killed 30 min after reaching criteria (indicated by *). All animals were kept awake in the last 30 min of the experiment; animals in the late groups had one full sleep cycle followed by about 1 h of W before being randomly sorted according to wake/sleep states.

and 7 experimental groups, the latter consisting of rats that experienced unilateral LTP induction during W (Fig. 16.6; the bottom 7 bars).

As expected (Cole *et al.* 1989; Wisden *et al.* 1990; Worley *et al.* 1993; Abraham *et al.* 1993), the unilateral HFS protocol we used specifically induced LTP in ipsilateral mPP–DG synapses (Fig. 16.7(a)), as well as marked *zif-268* up-regulation in ipsilateral DG granule neurons 30 min after stimulation (Fig. 16.7(b)). Also in line with previous findings (Ribeiro *et al.* 1999), unstimulated animals showed decreased expression of *zif-268* upon entering SWS sleep in all brain areas studied, and an additional decrease upon entering REM sleep (Figs 16.7(c) and 16.8(a); unstimulated control groups).

Three hours after HFS, hippocampal *zif-268* expression returned to low basal levels (Figs 16.7(c) and 16.8(a), HFS/early W group), but extra-hippocampal regions showed a bilateral increase of *zif-268* expression in all stimulated animals as compared to their corresponding controls (Figs 16.7(c) and 16.8(a)). In spite of the latter effect, the unstimulated hemispheres of all animals that received HFS (Figs 16.7(c) and 16.8(a),

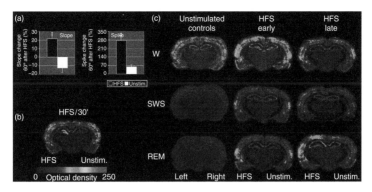

Figure 16.7 (a) HFS produced significant LTP that was long-lasting and unilateral to the stimulated (ipsilateral) hemisphere. Plotted are population spike and slope functions (mean ± SEM) percent change over baseline levels, across all groups) recorded 60 min after HFS (30 min for the HFS30' group) in ipsi- and contralateral hemispheres. Slope and spike values in ipsilateral hemispheres were significantly higher than both baseline and contralateral values (Student's *t*-test, $p < 0.01$), as indicated by asterisks. No significant differences occurred in the amount of potentiation among HFS groups (ANOVA of slope values, $P = 0.36$). (b) Phosphorimager autoradiogram of a representative *zif-268*-hybridized section. The ipsilateral (but not contralateral) DG shows marked *zif-268* up-regulation 30 min after unilateral HFS. Average *zif-268* expression in stimulated (ipsilateral) DG was 4.8 ± 0.4 (mean ± SEM) times higher than the average in unstimulated (contralateral) DG. (c) *Zif-268* brain expression levels during early and late W, SW, and REM sleep depend on prior waking stimulation. HFS groups showed higher bilateral levels of gene expression than controls within each state. Notice the marked *zif-268* upregulation in HFS hemispheres of REM sleep groups. (See Plate 16.)

HFS/early and late, contralateral hemispheres) showed a sleep-related down-regulation of *zif-268* expression similar to the down-regulation found in unstimulated animals.

In contrast, *zif-268* expression in the stimulated (ipsilateral) hemispheres of animals that received HFS was reduced during SWS but markedly increased during REM sleep, often reaching the same levels seen during W (Figs 16.7(c) and 16.8(a), HFS/early and Late, ipsilateral hemispheres; notice in Fig. 16.8(a) that for many brain regions the REM sleep black bars have heights comparable to the W white bars). This unilateral increase during REM sleep in HFS animals can be clearly seen in Fig. 16.8(b): While no appreciable inter-hemispheric *zif-268* expression differences were seen in unstimulated controls (left/right ratios around 1), HFS animals showed significantly higher inter-hemispheric *zif-268* expression ratios during REM sleep in several cortical regions and in the laterodorsal nucleus of the amygdala (LaD) (HFS/unstimulated ratios significantly above 1).

These data indicate that *zif-268* expression is reinduced in the brain during REM sleep that follows HFS of the hippocampus during W, providing additional evidence for brain gene reinduction during REM sleep that follows a relevant waking experience (in this case, hippocampal LTP). Importantly, the survival interval between the application of HFS and sacrifice did not differ significantly across W/SWS/REM sleep groups

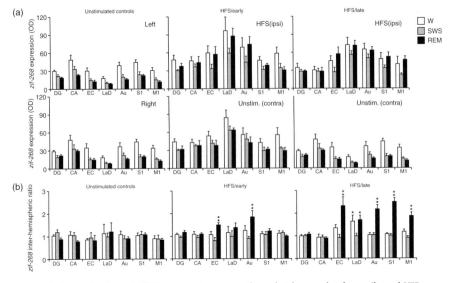

Figure 16.8 Quantification of *zif-268* expression across the wake/sleep cycle after unilateral LTP induction. Seven brain regions of interest were selected according to the rat atlas (Paxinos and Watson, 1997) for quantification of *zif-268* expression: dentate gyrus (DG), Ammon's horn (CA), entorhinal cortex (EC), dorsolateral nucleus of the amygdala (LaD), auditory (Au), primary somatosensory (S1) and primary motor (M1) cortices. (a) Absolute levels of *zif-268* expression. Within each state, all HFS groups had significantly higher levels of *zif-268* expression than controls (ANOVA, $p < 0.01$). Observe that several brain structures in HFS (ipsilateral) hemispheres show high *zif-268* expression during W and REM sleep, and low *zif-268* expression during SWS; in contrast, unstimulated (contralateral) hemispheres of HFS animals show high *zif-268* expression during W but decreased *zif-268* levels during both SWS and REM sleep, similar to the pattern found in unstimulated controls. (b) Inter-hemispheric *zif-268* expression ratios. Histograms are colored according to key on panel a. While controls did not show differences between left and right hemispheres (ANOVA, $p = 0.98$), significant interactions were detected in HFS groups (ANOVA $p < 0.0001$), owing to higher *zif-268* inter-hemispheric ratios (HFS/unstimulated) during REM sleep than during preceding episodes of SWS in the EC, LaD, Au, S1, and M1 (Bonferroni post-hoc tests, $^*p < 0.05$, and $^{**}p < 0.01$). Notice that the LaD showed significantly higher *zif-268* expression in the late W group than in the late SWS group.

($p = 0.69$ and 0.44 for Early and Late groups, respectively); therefore, the observed effect cannot be explained by differences in the survival intervals after stimulation. Additional controls ($n = 4$; data not shown) that received HFS in one hemisphere and low-frequency stimulation (LFS, ten 10 Hz trains lasting 1 s; once every 10 s) in the other hemisphere showed no significant difference in gene expression profile from that of HFS/unstimulated animals, indicating that specific patterns of W electrical stimulation such as HFS are required for the reinduction of *zif-268* during ensuing REM sleep. Notably, HFS of the mPP is reported to induce both *zif-268* primary induction and LTP in the DG, whereas LFS fails to produce either effect (Cole *et al.* 1989).

The reactivation of *zif-268* expression during early REM sleep was observed in the entorhinal (EC) and the auditory (Au) cortices, whereas during late REM sleep the effect reached further distal areas such as the primary sensory (S1) and motor (M1) cortices, and the dorsolateral nucleus of the amygdala (LaD), several synapses away from the site of HFS application. This raised the question of whether extra-hippocampal *zif-268* reinduction during REM sleep is dependent on concurrent hippocampal activity. To investigate this issue, we assessed whether the unihemispheric inactivation of the hippocampus during early REM sleep disrupts post-HFS *zif-268* reinduction in extra-hippocampal regions. Animals ($n = 4$) were implanted with chronic bilateral stimulating electrodes in the mPP, recording electrodes in the DG, and bilateral guide cannulas 1.5 mm above the DG. On the day of the experiment, animals were subjected to bilateral HFS in order to induce comparable LTP in both hemispheres (average spike change 582.3% $\pm$ 70.9 and 422.2% $\pm$ 167.1 for left and right hemispheres, respectively; mean $\pm$ SEM). Rats were kept awake for a minimum of 2 h, and then allowed to sleep (Fig. 16.9(a)). Shortly after the onset of REM sleep (2.4 $\pm$ 0.7 min, mean duration $\pm$ SEM), the anesthetic tetracaine (Poe *et al.* 2000*b*) was infused into the left DG. Thirty minutes after REM sleep offset, animals were sacrificed and their brains processed for *zif-268* expression. Unstimulated controls ($n = 4$) that were infused unilaterally with tetracaine during W were also analyzed (Fig. 16.9(a)).

Tetracaine administration strongly reduced EEG power (Fig. 16.9(b)) and evoked potentials (Fig. 16.9(c)), confirming the effectiveness of the treatment to inactivate the hippocampus during REM sleep. Tetracaine application also resulted in the blockade of *zif-268* reinduction during REM sleep in the cortex and amygdala (EC, Au, and LaD) of the injected hemisphere (Fig. 16.9(d) and 16.9(e)). This blockade was not seen in saline-injected hemispheres, which displayed high levels of *zif-268* in the same regions (Fig. 16.9(d) and 16.9(e)). The lack of a significant reduction in *zif-268* expression in these areas when comparable tetracaine injections were applied during W (Fig. 16.9(f) and 16.9(g)) argues for the blockade of *zif-268* reinduction seen in tetracaine-injected animals during REM sleep not being simply due to tetracaine diffusion from the injection site. These results indicate that hippocampal activity during early REM sleep that follows HFS is essential for REM sleep-associated *zif-268* reinduction in the cerebral cortex and the amygdala.

Hippocampal interactions with the cortex and amygdala during REM sleep

To the extent that the analysis of *zif-268* expression yields an average estimate of synaptic activity occurring ~30 min before sacrifice (Cole *et al.* 1989, 1990*b*; Wisden *et al.* 1990; Richardson *et al.* 1992; Abraham *et al.* 1993; Worley *et al.* 1993; Cullinan *et al.* 1995; Mello and Clayton 1995; Ribeiro *et al.* 1999), our observations provide evidence for the sequential activation of the cortex and amygdala during REM sleep that follows induction of hippocampal LTP. We also show that cortical and amygdalar activation during REM sleep is strongly dependent on concurrent hippocampal activity, which points to the existence of a hippocampofugal process of cortical activation during REM sleep. It has been found that while several kinds of memory initially depend on the hippocampus, they become gradually independent of that brain structure and correspondingly more reliant

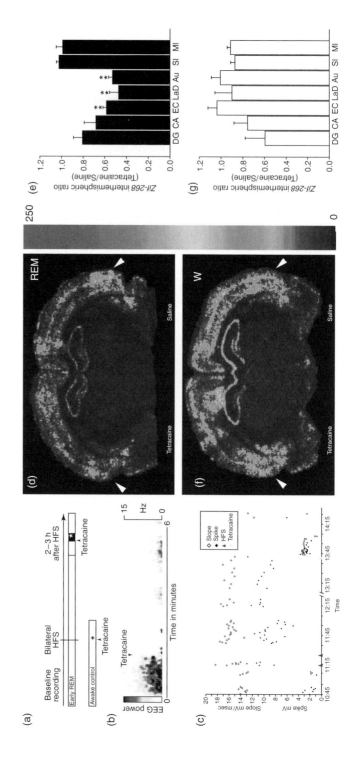

Figure 16.9 Effect on *zif-268* expression of hippocampus inactivation during REM sleep. (a) Experimental design of the hippocampal inactivation experiment. After baseline recordings of EEG and evoked potentials, experimental animals ($n = 4$) received bilateral HFS and were kept awake for 2 h before being allowed to sleep. At the beginning of REM sleep and without waking the animals, tetracaine was unilaterally infused in the left hemispheres (saline in right hemispheres), followed by further recording of evoked potentials. Animals were sacrificed 30 min after the end of REM sleep. Control animals ($n = 4$) were not subjected to HFS; they were kept awake and were killed 30 min after unilateral tetracaine infusion. (b) Tetracaine effects on EEG. Plotted is a spectrogram (frequency and power over time) of a representative EEG segment, showing that tetracaine infusion strongly reduced EEG power in the DG immediately after beginning of injection. Power is coded according to the color bar to the left, which runs linearly between −10 and +13 SD of the logarithm of the power between 6 and 9 Hz. Frequencies are depicted in a linear scale according to the references on the right. (c) Tetracaine effects on evoked potentials. A representative experiment is shown. Tetracaine produced an immediate and robust reduction of evoked potentials in the tetracaine-infused (left) DG (spike values decreased 73.1% ± 11.6; mean ± SEM), while minor effects were observed in the vehicle-infused (right) DG (spike values decreased 3.6% ± 2.6; mean ± SEM). Tetracaine effects lasted for approximately 30 min, keeping the hippocampus silenced during most of the REM sleep and ensuing W. The potentials almost recovered to their previous potentiated levels right before sacrifice, at 14:15 h. Each datapoint is an average of 4 evoked potentials. (d) *Zif-268* brain expression levels during early REM sleep, following bilateral HFS and unilateral tetracaine infusion. Shown is a Phosphorimager autoradiogram of a representative brain section hybridized for *zif-268*. There is a marked reduction of *zif-268* expression in the left EC, Au, and LaD, as compared to the right hemisphere. Arrows point to Au. (e) *Zif-268* expression inter-hemispheric ratios (tetracaine/saline) in bilateral HFS, early REM sleep animals. Significantly lower ratios were found in the EC, Au, and LaD (ANOVA, $p < 0.0001$, followed by Bonferroni post hoc tests, $*p < 0.05$, and $**p < 0.01$). These results reflect *zif-268* downregulation in tetracaine-infused hemispheres, and indicate that extra-hippocampal *zif-268* reinduction during REM sleep requires an active hippocampus. (f) *Zif-268* brain expression levels during W, following unilateral tetracaine infusion. *Zif-268* expression levels are comparable between hemispheres. Arrows point to Au. (g) *Zif-268* expression interhemispheric ratios (tetracaine/saline) in W control animals. No significant differences in *zif-268* levels were found between tetracaine and saline-infused hemispheres in the control group (ANOVA, $p = 0.15$). Extra-hippocampal *zif-268* expression during W appears to be largely independent of hippocampal activity, presumably owing to the intense thalamocortical processing that characterizes W. (See Plate 17.)

on the cerebral cortex for long-term storage (Scoville and Milner 1957; Mishkin 1978; Kesner and Novak 1982; Buzsáki *et al.* 1990; Zola-Morgan and Squire 1990; Squire 1992; Kim *et al.* 1995; Izquierdo and Medina 1997; Bontempi *et al.* 1999; Lavenex and Amaral 2000; Wincour *et al.* 2001). Therefore, our results establish a link between hippocampo–cortical interactions postulated for memory consolidation and the mnemonic role of REM sleep.

We suggest that REM sleep constitutes a privileged window for hippocampus-driven cortical activation, free from waking interference and, in principle, capable of playing an instructive role in the communication of memory traces from the hippocampus to the cortex. In this regard, the fact that *zif-268* reinduction is anatomically more extensive in late than in early REM sleep is especially interesting, considering that late but not early post-training REM sleep episodes are crucial for learning (Smith and Rose 1996; Stickgold *et al.* 2000). Special mention should also be made to the fact that the LaD shows significantly high levels of *zif-268* expression during late W and REM sleep, adding to the evidence that the amygdala plays a sustained role in information processing after the initial phase of LTP or behavioral learning (Ben-Ari and Le Gal la Salle 1972; Maren *et al.* 1991; Izquierdo and Medine 1997; Rogan *et al.* 1997; McGaugh 2000).

In summary, the results presented above are consistent with the notion that experience-dependent brain reactivation during REM sleep contributes to the formation of long-lasting memories through the up-regulation of activity-dependent genes associated with synaptic plasticity. Thus, it is possible that *zif-268* itself plays a role in memory consolidation during REM sleep by promoting genomic events associated with long-term synaptic plasticity. According to this hypothesis, brain reactivation during REM sleep (Pavlides and Winson 1989; Maquet *et al.* 2000; Poe *et al.* 2000*a*; Louie and Wilson 2001) contributes to the formation of long-lasting memories by propagating calcium-dependent post-synaptic changes from the hippocampus to cortical and amygdalar networks, as recently suggested (Frankland *et al.* 2001).

A model of memory consolidation during sleep

Based on our data and on the existing literature, we would like to propose a model of how sleep contributes to memory consolidation in warm-blooded amniotes.[1] The first part of the model (Fig. 16.10(a)) concerns the mechanisms underlying experience-dependent gene expression across the wake-sleep cycle.

When an awake animal is presented with a stimulus to which it is habituated (Fig. 16.10a, left panel), no appreciable increases are seen in the magnitudes of cellular calcium influx (Nicholson *et al.* 1978; Llinas and Lopez-Barneo 1988; Martin and Koshland 1991; Li *et al.* 1996) and monoaminergic/cholinergic neuromodulation (Rasmusson and Szerb 1976; Dunant *et al.* 1980; Rasmussen *et al.* 1986*a,b*; McFadden

---

1   REM sleep is thought to be absent in reptiles, with the possible exception of crocodilians Hobson (1989).

(a)

Habitual/poor
stimulus

Novel/rich
stimulus

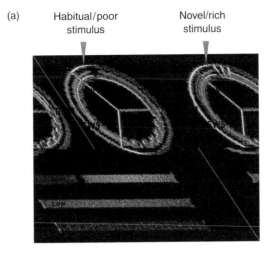

(b)

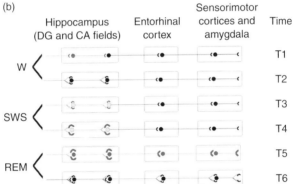

	Hippocampus (DG and CA fields)	Entorhinal cortex	Sensorimotor cortices and amygdala	Time

Figure 16.10 A model of memory consolidation across the wake–sleep cycle. (a) Cellular mechanisms underlying experience-dependent gene expression during W, SWS, and REM sleep. Three biological variables are represented: cellular calcium influx, monoaminergic/cholinergic neuromodulation, and activity-dependent gene expression. The left and right panels represent brain processes in animals exposed to habitual/poor or novel/rich stimulus, respectively. (b) Spatiotemporal dynamics of experience-dependent synaptic changes across the wake–sleep cycle. For the sake of simplicity, the amniote telencephalon is represented as a unidirectional neuronal circuit encompassing the hippocampus, the entorhinal cortex, the sensorimotor cortices, and the amygdala. A minimum of synapses is represented, and the hippocampus is depicted as the startpoint for information input. Calcium-dependent gene expression is shown in red, calcium-influx without genomic activation is represented in yellow, synaptic sprouting is indicated by the addition of synapses, and increases in synaptic efficacy are depicted as an enlargement in the sizes of synapses. (See Plate 18.)

and Koshland 1990), presumably reflecting a relatively small change in ongoing brain activity. Since increases in calcium influx (Cole *et al.* 1989; Wisden *et al.* 1990; Williams *et al.* 2000) and monoaminergic/cholinergic neuromodulation (Greenberg *et al.* 1986; Shiromani *et al.* 1992; Cirelli *et al.* 1996; Power and Sah 2002) seem to be required for the up-regulation of several activity-dependent genes, it would be expected that the expression levels of activity-dependent genes in animals exposed to habitual stimuli during W would not increase above baseline levels (Greenberg *et al.* 1992; Ennulat *et al.* 1994; Mello *et al.* 1995; Xia *et al.* 1996). Given the role of calcium signaling pathways and gene regulation for synaptic plasticity (Madison *et al.* 1991; Bliss and Collingridge 1993), one would conclude that synaptic efficacies remain unaltered by exposure to habitual stimuli. Without W changes in synaptic efficacy, no experience-dependent neuronal reactivation is expected to occur in the sleeping brain (Pavlides and Winson 1989; Wilson and McNaughton 1993, 1994; Skaggs and McNaughton 1996; Kudrimoti *et al.* 1999; Nadasdy *et al.* 1999; Dave and Margoliash 2000; Maquet *et al.* 2000; Hirase *et al.* 2001; Louie and Wilson 2001) and, therefore, it is not surprising that the expression levels of activity-dependent genes should fall dramatically during ensuing SWS and REM sleep (Pompeiano *et al.* 1992, 1994, 1997; O'Hara *et al.* 1993; Basheer *et al.* 1997; Cirelli and Tononi 1998, 1999, 2000; Ribeiro *et al.* 1999). In summary: When animals are habituated to the stimulus, no new memories are acquired, much less consolidated.

In contrast, the presentation of a novel/rich stimulus to an awake animal (Fig. 16.10(a), right panel) produces a marked increase in cellular calcium influx (Klein and Kandel 1980; Hernandez-Cruz *et al.* 1990; Eliot *et al.* 1993; Li *et al.* 1996; Izquierdo *et al.* 1999; Vianna *et al.* 2000; Meuth *et al.* 2002), monoaminergic/cholinergic neuromodulation (Rasmusson and Szerb 1976; Foote *et al.* 1980; Aston-Jones and Bloom 1981*a*; Moroni *et al.* 1981; Rasmussen *et al.* 1986*a,b*; Sara *et al.* 1994), and activity-dependent gene expression (Dragunow and Robertson 1987; Sukhatme *et al.* 1988; Anokhin *et al.* 1991; Mello *et al.* 1992; Ghosh *et al.* 1994; Wallace *et al.* 1995; Bertini *et al.* 2002). Presumably, this chain of plasticity-related events carves novel memory traces in the brain by potentiating specific synapses (Madison *et al.* 1991; Bliss and Collingridge 1993), triggering protein synthesis (Lossner *et al.* 1990; Fazeli *et al.* 1993; Barea-Rodriguez *et al.* 2000; Mochida *et al.* 2001) and eventually determining morphological synaptic changes such as synaptic sprouting (Wallace *et al.* 1995; Adams *et al.* 1997; Klintsova and Greenough 1999; Hassan *et al.* 2000). Upon entering SWS, the large-amplitude oscillations that characterize this state will generate long alternating transients of high and low calcium (Massimini and Amzica 2001), likely leading to the periodic activation of calcium-dependent second-messenger cascades, such as the phosphorylation of CaMKII, PKA, and CREB. (Frankland *et al.* 2001; Deisseroth and Tsien 2002; Lisman *et al.* 2002). Still, SWS does not seem to be concomitant with plasticity-related gene expression capable of consolidating the newly acquired synaptic changes (Pompeiano *et al.* 1992, 1994, 1997; O'Hara *et al.* 1993; Basheer *et al.* 1997; Cirelli and Tononi 1998, 1999, 2000; Ribeiro *et al.* 1999), which reappears in association with REM sleep (Ribeiro 2000; Ribeiro *et al.* 1999, 2001). Given the natural alternation of SWS and REM sleep, and the intrinsic temporal delay between mRNA synthesis and protein translation, it is easy to conceive how increased gene expression during REM sleep leads to an augmentation of protein synthesis during SWS (Ramm and Smith 1990).

The model compels the discussion of some current gaps in our knowledge. For instance, the mechanisms underlying the lack of activity-dependent gene expression during SWS are unknown. Perhaps the neuronal firing rates during SWS are below a putative gene expression threshold. Alternatively, calcium transients during SWS may be too short to generate measurable transcriptional responses (Chawla and Bading 2001). Finally, there is the interesting hypothesis—which we chose to present in Fig. 16.10(a)—that activity-dependent gene expression during SWS may be halted because of a putative asynchrony between calcium inflow and noradrenergic input during SWS (Sejnowski and Destexhe 2000).

Also controversial are the mechanisms underlying activity-dependent gene up-regulation during REM sleep. It has been shown that activity-dependent gene expression in the brains of rats is highly dependent on the integrity of noradrenergic modulation from the locus coeruleus (Cirelli *et al.* 1996), leading to the proposition that sleep-related decrease in IEG expression in unstimulated animals (Pompeiano *et al.* 1992, 1997; Basheer *et al.* 1997), reflects a lack of noradrenergic modulation caused by the silencing of the locus coeruleus during sleep (Aston-Jones and Bloom 1981*a,b*). Such a rationale accounts well for the SWS/REM sleep downregulation of activity-dependent genes observed in unstimulated animals, but not for the gene upregulation seen during REM sleep in exposed animals (Ribeiro 2000; Ribeiro *et al.* 1999, 2001). At least three hypotheses can be formulated to reconcile the lack of locus coeruleus activity during REM sleep with concurrent activity-dependent gene upregulation. The most parsimonious has to do with cholinergic transmission, which is very robust during REM sleep (Hobson 1992; Reid *et al.* 1994; Williams *et al.* 1994). In principle, abundant cholinergic release could compensate for the lack of noradrenergic transmission, setting in motion the same molecular cascades that lead to the noradrenaline-induced upregulation of *zif-268* and other IEGs (Greenberg *et al.* 1992; Shiromani *et al.* 1992; Power and Sah 2002). Another possibility is that the locus coeruleus actually releases noradrenaline during REM sleep that follows relevant W experience, either via subthreshold activity or through experience-dependent neuronal firing. Though less likely than the previous one, this specific hypothesis has yet to be tested. Finally, it is possible that the activity-dependent gene reinduction we observed during REM sleep is triggered during the transition between REM sleep and W, a brief moment in which REM sleep-specific neuronal activity and noradrenaline should coexist in space and time. Further experimentation is needed to explore these possibilities.

The second part of our model attempts to apply the concepts discussed above to a schematic amniote telencephalon (Fig. 16.10(b)) (Lopes da Silva *et al.* 1990; Paxinos 1995; Butler and Hodos 1996). Given that most memories are highly dependent on the hippocampus in the initial post-acquisition waking phase (Scoville and Milner 1957; Mishkin 1978; Kesner and Novak 1982; Buzsáki *et al.* 1990; Zola-Morgan and Squire 1990; Squire 1992; Kim *et al.* 1995; Izquierdo and Medina 1997; Bontempi *et al.* 1999; Lavenex and Amaral 2000; Winocur *et al.* 2001), we assume that memory traces are initially either stored in the hippocampus or dispersed across the cerebral cortex in fragments that require the hippocampus to be associatively assembled. Therefore, in the initial phase of memory acquisition (Fig. 16.10(b), W), traces derived from the waking experience should be encoded by the potentiation of hippocampal synapses, leading to calcium-dependent gene expression (Fig. 16.10(b), T1, represented in red), and to morphological plasticity such as synaptic sprouting (Fig. 16.10(b), T2).

As SWS begins (Fig. 16.10(b), SWS), a progressive synchronization of endogenous neuronal activity takes place, likely reflecting the entrainment, as time goes by, of larger and larger neuronal ensembles to the low-frequency oscillations typical of SWS (mostly <4 Hz) (Hobson 1989). We postulate that endogenous activity will flow preferentially through previously potentiated synapses, generating firing patterns that replay those most observed during wakefulness (Pavlides and Winson 1989; Wilson and McNaughton 1994; Skaggs and McNaughton 1996; Louie and Wilson 2001). This should elicit increased calcium influx in the reactivated neurons, but no activity-dependent gene expression, as discussed above (Fig. 16.10(b), T3, represented in yellow). Typically, replayed SWS firing sequences in the hippocampus are fairly short-lived (hundreds of milliseconds), suggesting that neuronal processing during SWS occurs at the level of the local circuitry (Louie and Wilson 2001). In principle, this process should result in a calcium-dependent local amplification of synaptic changes acquired during W (Fig. 16.10(b), T4, represented by enlarged synapses). However, since SWS is not concomitant with activity-dependent gene expression, changes in synaptic efficacies introduced during this phase should not yet be consolidated, relying on the temporary activation of calcium signaling pathways.

In contrast with SWS, the cortical EEG activity during REM sleep (Fig. 16.10(b), REM sleep) shifts to much higher frequency bands (up to 80 Hz), and observed correlations between hippocampal neurons expand two orders of magnitude so as to span seconds and even minutes (Louie and Wilson 2001). These very long temporal correlations of neuronal firing during REM sleep can be interpreted as representing activity reverberation between the hippocampus and distal areas in the limbic system and the cerebral cortex (Louie and Wilson 2001), perhaps through the lift of sensory gates (Dave et al. 1998). The notion of REM sleep as a global brain process is supported by our own data, which reveals waves of activity-dependent gene expression that propagate from the hippocampus to cortical and amygdalar sites as REM sleep recurs (Figs 16.7–16.9).

Based on the existing evidence, we propose two separate but related functions for REM sleep: First, it propagates synaptic changes within the hippocampus to downstream cortical and amygdalar neurons, via the activation of calcium-dependent signaling cascades. We suggest that this process binds together, in the appropriate temporal sequence, short memory traces stored in the hippocampus and cerebral cortex as increased firing correlations among neuronal ensembles. Second, REM sleep triggers plasticity-related gene expression along the activated circuit, leading to the addition (and removal) of synapses, and therefore to the effective consolidation in extra-hippocampal regions of the new memory traces acquired during W (Fig. 16.10(b), REM sleep).

According to this view, the ultimate role of REM sleep in memory processing would be to transcriptionally "freeze" the pre-genomic changes in synaptic efficacies evolved locally during SWS and then globally during REM sleep, so as to convert biochemical changes into morphological ones. Such a mechanism for the consolidation of synaptic changes during REM sleep predicts a homeostatic renormalization of synaptic efficacies through the brain after a certain number of sleep–wake cycles (in computational neuroscience jargon, "network renormalization"), at the expense of the addition and removal of synapses. Also implicit in the model is the idea that the repetition of the SWS/REM sleep cycle and the proportional increase of the latter as the subjective night progresses should allow for the evolution of longer and longer correlated firing chains across the neuronal matrix, that is, for the evolution of increasingly more complex memory traces as the sleep–wake cycle recurs.

Our model raises some testable predictions: (i) blockade of plasticity-related gene expression during REM sleep should disrupt memory formation, but not during SWS; (ii) calcium depletion should be detrimental to memory formation during both phases of sleep; (iii) late REM sleep should display temporally longer correlations of neuronal firing than early REM sleep; (iv) the rate of change in synaptic efficacies during REM sleep should be higher that during SWS, due to the higher frequencies of REM sleep neuronal processing.

Acknowledgments

This work has been supported by NHLBI grant 1 R01 HL69699-01 to C. P, and a Pew Latin American Fellowship to S. R.

References

Abraham, W. C., Mason, S. E., Demmer, J., Williams, J. M., Richardson, C. L., Tate, W. P., Lawlor, P. A., and Dragunow, M. (1993). Correlations between immediate early gene induction and the persistence of long-term potentiation. *Neuroscience*, **56**, 717–727.

Adams, B., Lee, M., Fahnestock, M., and Racine, R. J. (1997). Long-term potentiation trains induce mossy fiber sprouting. *Brain Research*, **775**, 193–197.

Adey, W. R., Elul, R., Walter, R. D., and Crandall, P. H. (1967). The cooperative behavior of neuronal populations during sleep and mental tasks. *Electroencephalography and Clinical Neurophysiology*, **23**, 88.

Ambrosini, M. V., Sadile, A. G., Gironi Carnevale, U. A., Mattiaccio, M., and Giuditta, A. (1988). The sequential hypothesis on sleep function. I. Evidence that the structure of sleep depends on the nature of the previous waking experience. *Physiology and Behavior*, **43**, 325–337.

Anokhin, K. V., Mileusnic, R., Shamakina, I. Y., and Rose, S. P. (1991). Effects of early experience on c-fos gene expression in the chick forebrain. *Brain Research*, **544**, 101–107.

Arnolds, D. E., Lopes da Silva, F. H., Aitink, J. W., Kamp, A., and Boeijinga, P. (1980). The spectral properties of hippocampal EEG related to behaviour in man. *Electroencephalography and Clinical Neurophysiology*, **50**, 324–328.

Aston-Jones, G. and Bloom, F. E. (1981*a*). Activity of norepinephrine-containing locus coeruleus neurons in behaving rats anticipates fluctuations in the sleep–waking cycle. *Journal of Neuroscience*, **1**, 876–886.

Aston-Jones, G. and Bloom, F. E. (1981*b*). Nonrepinephrine-containing locus coeruleus neurons in behaving rats exhibit pronounced responses to non-noxious environmental stimuli. *Journal of Neuroscience*, **1**, 887–900.

Barea-Rodriguez, E. J., Rivera, D. T., Jaffe, D. B., and Martinez, J. L., Jr. (2000). Protein synthesis inhibition blocks the induction of mossy fiber long-term potentiation *in vivo*. *Journal of Neuroscience*, **20**, 8528–8532.

Basheer, R., Sherin, J. E., Saper, C. B., Morgan, J. I., McCarley, R. W., and Shiromani, P. J. (1997). Effects of sleep on wake-induced c-fos expression. *Journal of Neuroscience*, **17**, 9746–9750.

Ben-Ari, Y. and Le Gal la Salle, G. (1972). Plasticity at unitary level. II. Modifications during sensory–sensory association procedures. *Electroencephalography and Clinical Neurophysiology*, **32**, 667–679.

Bertini, G., Peng, Z. C., Fabene, P. F., Grassi-Zucconi, G., and Bentivoglio, M. (2002). Fos induction in cortical interneurons during spontaneous wakefulness of rats in a familiar or enriched environment. *Brain Research Bulletin*, **57**, 631–638.

Bland, B. H. (1986). The physiology and pharmacology of hippocampal formation theta rhythm. *Progress in Neurobiology*, **26**, 1–54.

Bliss, T. V. P. and Collingridge, G. L. (1993). A synaptic model of memory: long-term potentiation in the hippocampus. *Nature*, **361**, 31–39.

Bontempi, B., Laurent-Demir, C., Destrade, C., and Jaffard, R. (1999). Time-dependent reorganization of brain circuitry underlying long-term memory storage. *Nature*, **400**, 671–675.

Brown, B. B. (1968). Frequency and phase of hippocampal theta activity in the spontaneously behaving cat. *Electroencephalography and Clinical Neurophysiology*, **24**, 53–62.

Butler, A. and Hodos, W. (1996). *Comparative vertebrate anatomy: evolution and adaptation*. Wiley-Liss Press, New York.

Buzsáki, G., Chen, L. S., and Gage, F. H. (1990). Spatial organization of physiological activity in the hippocampal region: relevance to memory formation. *Progress in Brain Research*, **83**, 257–268.

Buzsáki, G. and Eidelberg, E. (1983). Phase relations of hippocampal projection cells and interneurons to theta activity in the anesthetized rat. *Brain Research*, **266**, 334.

Chaudhuri, A. (1997). Neural activity mapping with inducible transcription factors. *Neuroreport*, **8**, iii–vii.

Chawla, S. and Bading, H. (2001). CREB/CBP and SRE-interacting transcriptional regulators are fast on-off switches: duration of calcium transients specifies the magnitude of transcriptional responses. *Journal of Neurochemistry*, **79**, 849–858.

Christy, B. and Nathans, D. (1989). DNA binding site of the growth factor-inducible protein Zif268. *Proceedings of the National Academy of Sciences, USA*, **86**, 8737–8741.

Cirelli, C., Pompeiano, M., and Tononi, G. (1996). Neuronal gene expression in the waking state: a role for the locus coeruleus. *Science*, **274**, 1211–1215.

Cirelli, C. and Tononi, G. (1998). Differences in gene expression between sleep and waking as revealed by mRNA differential display. *Molecular Brain Research*, **56**, 293–305.

Cirelli, C. and Tononi, G. (1999). Differences in brain gene expression between sleep and waking as revealed by mRNA differential display and cDNA microarray technology. *Journal of Sleep Research*, **8** (Suppl. 1), 44–52.

Cirelli, C. and Tononi, G. (2000). Gene expression in the brain across the sleep–waking cycle. *Brain Research*, **885**, 303–321.

Cole, A. J., Abu-Shakra, S., Saffen, D. W., Baraban, J. M., and Worley, P. F. (1990*a*). Rapid rise in transcription factor mRNAs in rat brain after electroshock-induced seizures. *Journal of Neurochemistry*, **55**, 1920–1927.

Cole, A. J., Saffen, D. W., Baraban, J. M., and Worley, P. F. (1990*b*). Synaptic regulation of transcription factor mRNA in the rat hippocampus. *Advances in Neurology*, **51**, 103–108.

Cole, A. J., Saffen, D. W., Baraban, J. M., and Worley, P. F. (1989). Rapid increase of an immediate early gene messenger RNA in hippocampal neurons by synaptic NMDA receptor activation. *Nature*, **340**, 474–476.

Collins, D. R., Lang, E. J., and Pare, D. (1999). Spontaneous activity of the perirhinal cortex in behaving cats. *Neuroscience*, **89**, 1025–1039.

Cullinan, W. E., Herman, J. P., Battaglia, D. F., Akil, H., and Watson, S. J. (1995). Pattern and time course of immediate early gene expression in rat brain following acute stress. *Neuroscience*, **64**, 477–505.

Dave, A. S. and Margoliash, D. (2000). Song replay during sleep and computational rules for sensorimotor vocal learning. *Science*, **290**, 812–816.

Dave, A. S., Yu, A. C., and Margoliash, D. (1998). Behavioral state modulation of auditory activity in a vocal motor system. *Science*, **282**, 2250–2254.

Deisseroth, K. and Tsien, R. W. (2002). Dynamic multiphosphorylation passwords for activity-dependent gene expression. *Neuron*, **34**, 179–182.

Delacour, J. (1982). Associative and non-associative changes in unit activity of the rat hippocampus. *Brain Research Bulletin*, **8**, 367–373.

Destexhe, A., Contreras, D., and Steriade, M. (1999). Spatiotemporal analysis of local field potentials and unit discharges in cat cerebral cortex during natural wake and sleep states. *Journal of Neuroscience*, **19**, 4595–4608.

Diamond, D. M., Dunwiddie, T. V., and Rose, G. M. (1988). Characteristics of hippocampal primed burst potentiation *in vitro* and in the awake rat. *Journal of Neuroscience*, **8**, 4079–4088.

Donoghue, J. P., Kerman, K. L., and Ebner, F. F. (1979). Evidence for two organizational plans within the somatic sensory-motor cortex of the rat. *Journal of Comparative Neurology*, **183**, 647–663.

Donoghue, J. P. and Wise, S. P. (1982). The motor cortex of the rat: cytoarchitecture and microstimulation mapping. *Journal of Comparative Neurology*, **212**, 76–88.

Dragunow, M. and Robertson, H. A. (1987). Kindling stimulation induces c-fos protein(s) in granule cells of the rat dentate gyrus. *Nature*, **329**, 441–442.

Dunant, Y., Eder, L., and Servetiadis-Hirt, L. (1980). Acetylcholine release evoked by single or a few nerve impulses in the electric organ of Torpedo. *Journal of Physiology*, **298**, 185–203.

Elazar, Z. and Adey, W. R. (1967*a*). Electroencephalographic correlates of learning in subcortical and cortical structures. *Electroencephalography and Clinical Neurophysiology*, **23**, 306–319.

Elazar, Z. and Adey, W. R. (1967*b*). Spectral analysis of low frequency components in the electrical activity of the hippocampus during learning. *Electroencephalography and Clinical Neurophysiology*, **23**, 225–240.

Eliot, L. S., Kandel, E. R., Siegelbaum, S. A., and Blumenfeld, H. (1993). Imaging terminals of Aplysia sensory neurons demonstrates role of enhanced Ca^{2+} influx in presynaptic facilitation. *Nature*, **361**, 634–637.

Ennulat, D. J., Babb, S., and Cohen, B. M. (1994). Persistent reduction of immediate early gene mRNA in rat forebrain following single or multiple doses of cocaine. *Molecular Brain Research*, **26**, 106–112.

Fazeli, M. S., Corbet, J., Dunn, M. J., Dolphin, A. C., and Bliss, T. V. P. (1993). Changes in protein synthesis accompanying long-term potentiation in the dentate gyrus *in vivo*. *Journal of Neuroscience*, **13**, 1346–1353.

Fishbein, W. and Gutwein, B. M. (1977). Paradoxical sleep and memory storage processes. *Behavioral Biology*, **19**, 425–464.

Foote, S. L., Aston-Jones, G., and Bloom, F. E. (1980). Impulse activity of locus coeruleus neurons in awake rats and monkeys is a function of sensory stimulation and arousal. *Proceedings of the National Academy Sciences, USA*, **77**, 3033–3037.

Fox, S. F., Wolfson, S., and Ranck, J. B., Jr. (1986). Hippocampal theta rhythm and the firing of neurons in walking and urethane anesthetized rats. *Experimental Brain Research*, **62**, 495–508.

Frankland, P. W., O'Brien, C., Ohno, M., Kirkwood, A., and Silva, A. J. (2001). Alpha-CaMKII-dependent plasticity in the cortex is required for permanent memory. *Nature*, **411**, 309–313.

Ghosh, A., Ginty, D. D., Bading, H., and Greenberg, M. E. (1994). Calcium regulation of gene expression in neuronal cells. *Journal of Neurobiology*, **25**, 294–303.

Ghosh, A. and Greenberg, M. E. (1995). Calcium signaling in neurons: molecular mechanisms and cellular consequences. *Science*, **268**, 239–247.

Giuditta, A., Ambrosini, M. V., Montagnese, P., Mandile, P., Cotugno, M., Zucconi, G. G., and Vescia, S. (1995). The sequential hypothesis of the function of sleep. *Behavioral Brain Research*, **69**, 157–166.

Grastyán, E., Karmos, G., Vereczkey, L., and Kellenyi, L. (1966). The hippocampal electrical correlates of the homeostatic regulation of motivation. *Electroencephalography and Clinical Neurophysiology*, **21**, 34–53.

Grastyán, E., Lissak, K., Madarász, I., and **Donhoffer, H.** (1959). Hippocampal Electrical activity during the development of conditioned reflexes. *Electroencephalography and Clinical Neurophysiology*, **11**, 409–430.

Green, J. D. and **Arduini, A. A.** (1954). Hippocampal electrical activity in arousal. *Journal of Neurophysiology*, **17**, 533–557.

Green, J. D., Maxwell, D. S., Schindler, W. J., and **Stumpf, C.** (1960). Rabbit EEG "theta" rhythm: its anatomical source and relation to activity in singulate nucleus. *Journal of Neurophysiology*, **23**, 403.

Greenberg, M. E., Thompson, M. A., and **Sheng, M.** (1992). Calcium regulation of immediate early gene transcription. *Journal of Physiology, Paris*, **86**, 99–108.

Greenberg, M. E., Ziff, E. B., and **Greene, L. A.** (1986). Stimulation of neuronal acetylcholine receptors induces rapid gene transcription. *Science*, **234**, 80–83.

Greenstein, Y. J., Pavlides, C., and **Winson, J.** (1988). Long-term potentiation in the dentate gyrus is preferentially induced at theta rhythm periodicity. *Brain Research*, **438**, 331–334.

Grimm, R. and **Tischmeyer, W.** (1997). Complex patterns of immediate early gene induction in rat brain following brightness discrimination training and pseudotraining. *Behavioral Brain Research*, **84**, 109–116.

Grosvenor, A. and **Lack, L. C.** (1984). The effect of sleep before or after learning on memory. *Sleep*, **7**, 155–167.

Gutwein, B. M., Shiromani, P. J., and **Fishbein, W.** (1980). Paradoxical sleep and memory: long-term disruptive effects of Anisomycin. *Pharmacology, Biochemistry and Behavior*, **12**, 377–384.

Haberly, L. B. and **Price, J. L.** (1978). Association and commissural fiber systems of the olfactory cortex of the rat. *Journal of Comparative Neurology*, **178**, 711–740.

Harper, R. M. (1971). Frequency changes in hippocampal electrical activity during movement and tonic immobility. *Physiology and Behavior*, **7**, 55–58.

Hassan, H., Pohle, W., Ruthrich, H., Brodemann, R., and **Krug, M.** (2000). Repeated long-term potentiation induces mossy fibre sprouting and changes the sensibility of hippocampal granule cells to subconvulsive doses of pentylenetetrazol. *European Journal of Neuroscience*, **12**, 1509–1515.

Hennevin, E., Hars, B., Maho, C., and **Bloch, V.** (1995). Processing of learned information in paradoxical sleep: relevance for memory. *Behavioral Brain Research*, **69**, 125–135.

Hernandez-Cruz, A., Sala, F., and **Adams, P. R.** (1990). Subcellular calcium transients visualized by confocal microscopy in a voltage-clamped vertebrate neuron. *Science*, **247**, 858–862.

Hirase, H., Leinekugel, X., Czurko, A., Csicsvari, J., and **Buzsáki, G.** (2001). Firing rates of hippocampal neurons are preserved during subsequent sleep episodes and modified by novel awake experience. *Proceedings of the National Academy Sciences, USA*, **98**, 9386–9390.

Hobson, A. J. (1989). *Sleep*. Scientific American Library, New York (distributed by W.H. Freeman).

Hobson, J. A. (1992). Sleep and dreaming: induction and mediation of REM sleep by cholinergic mechanisms. *Current Opinion in Neurobiology*, **2**, 759–763.

Hobson, J. A. (1995). *Sleep*. Scientific American Library, New York (distributed by W.H. Freeman).

Holscher, C., Anwyl, R., and Rowan, M. J. (1997). Stimulation on the positive phase of hippo-campal theta rhythm induces long-term potentiation that can be depotentiated by stimulation on the negative phase in area CA1 *in vivo*. *Journal of Neuroscience*, **17**, 6470–6477.

Honkaniemi, J., Sagar, S. M., Pyykonen, I., Hicks, K. J., and Sharp, F. R. (1995). Focal brain injury induces multiple immediate early genes encoding zinc finger transcription factors. *Molecular Brain Research*, **28**, 157–163.

Huerta, P. T. and Lisman, J. E. (1993). Heightened synaptic plasticity of hippocampal CA1 neurons during a cholinergically induced rhythmic state. *Nature*, **364**, 723–725.

Huerta, P. T. and Lisman, J. E. (1995). Bidirectional synaptic plasticity induced by a single burst during cholinergic theta oscillation in CAl *in vitro*. *Neuron*, **15**, 1053–1063.

Huerta, P. T. and Lisman, J. E. (1996). Synaptic plasticity during the cholinergic theta-frequency oscillation *in vitro*. *Hippocampus*, **6**, 58–61.

Idzikowski, C. (1984). Sleep and memory. *British Journal of Psychology*, **75** (Pt. 4), 439–449.

Idzikowski, C. and Oswald, I. (1983). Interference with human memory by an antibiotic. *Psychopharmacology*, (Berlin) **79**, 108–110.

Izquierdo, I. and Medina, J. H. (1997). Memory formation: the sequence of biochemical events in the hippocampus and its connection to activity in other brain structures. *Neurobiology of Learning and Memory*, **68**, 285–316.

Izquierdo, I., Schroder, N., Netto, C. A., and Medina, J. H. (1999). Novelty causes time-dependent retrograde amnesia for one-trial avoidance in rats through NMDA receptor- and CaMKII-dependent mechanisms in the hippocampus. *European Journal of Neuroscience*, **11**, 3323–3328.

Jones, M. W., Errington, M. L., French, P. J., Fine, A., Bliss, T. V., Garel, S., Charnay, P., Bozon, B., Laroche, S., and Davis, S. (2001). A requirement for the immediate early gene Zif268 in the expression of late LTP and long-term memories. *Nature Neuroscience*, **4**, 289–296.

Kaplan, I. V., Guo, Y., and Mower, G. D. (1995). Developmental expression of the immediate early gene EGR-1 mirrors the critical period in cat visual cortex. *Developmental Brain Research*, **90**, 174–179.

Kaplan, I. V., Guo, Y., and Mower, G. D. (1996). Immediate early gene expression in cat visual cortex during and after the critical period: differences between EGR-1 and Fos proteins. *Molecular Brain Research*, **36**, 12–22.

Karni, A., Tanne, D., Rubenstein, B. S., Askenasy, J. J. M., and Sagi, D. (1994). Dependence on REM sleep of overnight improvement of a perceptual skill. *Science*, **265**, 679–682.

Kavanau, J. L. (1996). Memory, sleep, and dynamic stabilization of neural circuitry: evolutionary perspectives. *Neuroscience and Biobehavioral Reviews*, **20**, 289–311.

Kesner, R. P. and Novak, J. M. (1982). Serial position curves in rats: role of the dorsal hippocampus. *Science*, **218**, 173–174.

Kim, J. J., Clark, R. E., and Thompson, R. F. (1995). Hippocampectomy impairs the memory of recently, but not remotely, acquired trace eyeblink conditioned responses. *Behavioral Neuroscience*, **109**, 195–203.

Klein, M. and Kandel, E. R. (1980). Mechanism of calcium current modulation underlying presynaptic facilitation and behavioral sensitization in Aplysia. *Proceedings of the National Academy of Sciences, USA*, **77**, 6912–6916.

Klintsova, A. Y. and Greenough, W. T. (1999). Synaptic plasticity in cortical systems. *Current Opinion in Neurobiology*, **9**, 203–208.

Kudrimoti, H. S., Barnes, C. A., and McNaughton, B. L. (1999). Reactivation of hippocampal cell assemblies: effects of behavioral state, experience, and EEG dynamics. *Journal of Neuroscience*, **19**, 4090–4101.

Larson, J. and Lynch, G. (1986). Induction of synaptic potentiation in hippocampus by patterned stimulation involves two events. *Science*, **232**, 985–988.

Larson, J., Wong, D., and Lynch, G. (1986). Patterned stimulation at the theta frequency is optimal for the induction of hippocampal long-term potentiation. *Brain Research*, **368**, 347–350.

Lavenex, P. and Amaral, D. G. (2000). Hippocampal-neocortical interaction: a hierarchy of associativity. *Hippocampus*, **10**, 420–430.

Leconte, P., Hennevin, E., and Bloch, V. (1974). Duration of paradoxical sleep necessary for the acquisition of conditioned avoidance in the rat. *Physiology and Behavior*, **13**, 675–681.

Leung, L. S. (1980). Behavior-dependent evoked potentials in the hippocampal CA1 region of the rat. I. Correlation with behavior and EEG. *Brain Research*, **198**, 95–117.

Leung, L. S. and Vanderwolf, C. H. (1980). Behavior-dependent evoked potentials in the hippocampal CA1 region of the rat. II. Effect of eserine, atropine, ether and pentobarbital. *Brain Research*, **198**, 119–133.

Li, M., Jia, M., Fields, R. D., and Nelson, P. G. (1996). Modulation of calcium currents by electrical activity. *Journal of Neurophysiology*, **76**, 2595–2607.

Linster, C., Wyble, B. P., and Hasselmo, M. E. (1999). Electrical stimulation of the horizontal limb of the diagonal band of broca modulates population EPSPs in piriform cortex. *Journal of Neurophysiology*, **81**, 2737–2742.

Lisman, J., Schulman, H., and Cline, H. (2002). The molecular basis of CaMKII function in synaptic and behavioural memory. *Nature Neuroscience*, **3**, 175–190.

Llinas, R. and Lopez-Barneo, J. (1988). Electrophysiology of mammalian tectal neurons *in vitro*. II. Long-term adaptation. *Journal of Neurophysiology*, **60**, 869–878.

Lopes da Silva, F. H., Witter, M. P., Boeijinga, P. H., and Lohman, A. H. (1990). Anatomic organization and physiology of the limbic cortex. *Physiology Reviews*, **70**, 453–511.

Lossner, B., Schweigert, C., Krug, M., and Matthies, H. K. (1990). Posttetanic long-term potentiation in the dentate gyrus of freely moving rats is accompanied by an increase in protein synthesis. *Biomedica Biochimica Acta*, **49**, 385–392.

Louie, K. and Wilson, M. A. (2001). Temporally structured replay of awake hippocampal ensemble activity during rapid eye movement sleep. *Neuron*, **29**, 145–156.

Lucero, M. A. (1970). Lengthening of REM sleep duration consecutive to learning in the rat. *Brain Research*, **20**, 319–322.

Madison, D. V., Malenka, R. C., and Nicoll, R. A. (1991). Mechanisms underlying long-term potentiation of synaptic transmission. *Annual Review of Neuroscience*, **14**, 379–397.

Maquet, P., Laureys, S., Peigneux, P., Fuchs, S., Petiau, C., Phillips, C., Aerts, J., Del Fiore, G., Degueldre, C., Meulemans, T. *et al.* (2000). Experience-dependent changes in cerebral activation during human REM sleep. *Nature Neuroscience*, **3**, 831–836.

Maren, S., Poremba, A., and Gabriel, M. (1991). Basolateral amygdaloid multi-unit neuronal correlates of discriminative avoidance learning in rabbits. *Brain Research*, **549**, 311–316.

Martin, P. T. and Koshland, D. E., Jr. (1991). The biochemistry of the neuron. Neurosecretory habituation to repetitive depolarizations in PC12 cells. *Journal of Biological Chemistry*, **266**, 7388–7392.

Massimini, M. and Amzica, F. (2001). Extracellular calcium fluctuations and intracellular potentials in the cortex during the slow sleep oscillation. *Journal of Neurophysiology*, **85**, 1346–1350.

McFadden, P. N. and Koshland, D. E., Jr. (1990). Habituation in the single cell: diminished secretion of norepinephrine with repetitive depolarization of PC12 cells. *Proceedings of the National Academy Sciences, USA*, **87**, 2031–2035.

McGaugh, J. L. (2000). Memory—a century of consolidation. *Science*, **287**, 248–251.

Mednick, S. C., Nakayama, K., Cantero, J. L., Atienza, M., Levin, A. A., Pathak, N., and Stickgold, R. (2002). The restorative effect of naps on perceptual deterioration. *Nature Neuroscience*, **5**, 677–681.

Mello, C., Nottebohm, F., and Clayton, D. (1995). Repeated exposure to one song leads to a rapid and persistent decline in an immediate early gene's response to that song in zebra finch telencephalon. *Journal of Neuroscience*, **15**, 6919–6925.

Mello, C. V. and Clayton, D. F. (1995). Differential induction of the ZENK gene in the avian forebrain and song control circuit after metrazole-induced depolarization. *Journal of Neurobiology*, **26**, 145–161.

Mello, C. V., Vicario, D. S., and Clayton, D. F. (1992). Song presentation induces gene expression in the songbird forebrain. *Proceedings of the National Academy of Sciences, USA*, **89**, 6818–6822.

Meuth, S., Pape, H. C., and Budde, T. (2002). Modulation of Ca2+ currents in rat thalamocortical relay neurons by activity and phosphorylation. *European Journal of Neuroscience*, **15**, 1603–1614.

Milbrandt, J. (1987). A nerve growth factor-induced gene encodes a possible transcriptional regulatory factor. *Science*, **238**, 797–799.

Mishkin, M. (1978). Memory in monkeys severely impaired by combined but not by separate removal of amygdala and hippocampus. *Nature*, **273**, 297–298.

Mochida, H., Sato, K., Sasaki, S., Yazawa, I., Kamino, K., and Momose-Sato, Y. (2001). Effects of anisomycin on LTP in the hippocampal CA1: long-term analysis using optical recording. *Neuroreport*, **12**, 987–991.

Moroni, F., Bianchi, C., Tanganelli, S., Moneti, G., and Beani, L. (1981). The release of gamma-aminobutyric acid, glutamate, and acetylcholine from striatal slices: a mass fragmentographic study. *Journal of Neurochemistry*, **36**, 1691–1699.

Nadasdy, Z., Hirase, H., Czurko, A., Csicsvari, J., and Buzsáki, G. (1999). Replay and time compression of recurring spike sequences in the hippocampus. *Journal of Neuroscience*, **19**, 9497–9507.

Nedivi, E., Hevroni, D., Naot, D., Israeli, D., and Citri, Y. (1993). Numerous candidate plasticity-related genes revealed by differential cDNA cloning. *Nature*, **363**, 718–722.

Neitz, J. and Jacobs, G. H. (1986). Reexamination of spectral mechanisms in the rat (Rattus norvegicus). *Journal of Comparative Psychology*, **100**, 21–29.

Nicholson, C., ten Bruggencate, G., Stockle, H., and Steinberg, R. (1978). Calcium and potassium changes in extracellular microenvironment of cat cerebellar cortex. *Journal of Neurophysiology*, **41**, 1026–1039.

Nikolaev, E., Kaminska, B., Tischmeyer, W., Matthies, H., and Kaczmarek, L. (1992). Induction of expression of genes encoding transcription factors in the rat brain elicited by behavioral training. *Brain Research Bulletin*, **28**, 479–484.

O'Hara, B. F., Young, K. A., Watson, F. L., Heller, H. C., and Kilduff, T. S. (1993). Immediate early gene expression in brain during sleep deprivation: preliminary observations. *Sleep*, **16**, 1–7.

O'Keefe, J. (1993). Hippocampus, theta, and spatial memory. *Current Opinion in Neurobiology*, **3**, 917–924.

Olton, D. *et al.* (1978). Hippocampal connections and spatial discrimination. *Brain Research*, **139**, 295–308.

Orr, G., Rao, G., Houston, F. P., McNaughton, B. L., and Barnes, C. A. (2001). Hippocampal synaptic plasticity is modulated by theta rhythm in the fascia dentata of adult and aged freely behaving rats. *Hippocampus*, **11**, 647–654.

Otto, T., Eichenbaum, H., Wiener, S. I., and Wible, C. G. (1991). Learning-related patterns of CA1 spike trains parallel stimulation parameters optimal for inducing hippocampal long-term potentiation. *Hippocampus*, **1**, 181–192.

Pavlides, C., Greenstein, Y. J., Grudman, M., and Winson, J. (1988). Long-term potentiation in the dentate gyrus is induced preferentially on the positive phase of theta-rhythm. *Brain Research*, **439**, 383–387.

Pavlides, C. and Winson, J. (1989). Influences of hippocampal place cell firing in the awake state on the activity of these cells during subsequent sleep episodes. *Journal of Neuroscience*, **9**, 2907–2918.

Paxinos, G. (1995). *The rat nervous system*, 2nd edn. Academic Press, San Diego.

Paxinos, G. and Watson, C. (1986). *The rat brain in stereotaxic coordinates*, Academic Press, New York.

Paxinos, G. and Watson, C. (1997). *The rat brain in stereotaxic coordinates*, Compact 3rd edn. Academic Press, San Diego.

Pearlman, C. and Becker, M. (1974). REM sleep deprivation impairs bar-press acquisition in rats. *Physiology and Behavior*, **13**, 813–817.

Peterson, C. L., Thompson, M. A., Martin, D., and Nadler, J. V. (1995). Modulation of glutamate and aspartate release from slices of hippocampal area CA1 by inhibitors of arachidonic acid metabolism. *Journal of Neurochemistry*, **64**, 1152–1160.

Poe, G. R., Nitz, D. A., McNaughton, B. L., and Barnes, C. A. (2000a). Experience-dependent phase-reversal of hippocampal neuron firing during REM sleep. *Brain Research*, **855**, 176–180.

Poe, G. R., Teed, R. G., Insel, N., White, R., McNaughton, B. L., and Barnes, C. A. (2000b). Partial hippocampal inactivation: effects on spatial memory performance in aged and young rats. *Behavioral Neuroscience*, **114**, 940–949.

Pompeiano, M., Cirelli, C., Ronca-Testoni, S., and Tononi, G. (1997). NGFI-A expression in the rat brain after sleep deprivation. *Molecular Brain Research*, **46**, 143–153.

Pompeiano, M., Cirelli, C., and Tononi, G. (1992). Effects of sleep deprivation on fos-like immunoreactivity in the rat brain. *Archivio Italiano di Anatomia e di Embriologia*. **130**, 325–335.

Pompeiano, M., Cirelli, C., and Tononi, G. (1994). Immediate-early genes in spontaneous wakefulness and sleep: expression of c-fos and NGIF-A mRNA protein. *Journal of Sleep Research*, **3**, 80–96.

Power, J. M. and Sah, P. (2002). Nuclear calcium signaling evoked by cholinergic stimulation in hippocampal CA1 pyramidal neurons. *Journal of Neuroscience*, **22**, 3454–3462.

Qin, Y. L., McNaughton, B. L., Skaggs, W. E., and Barnes, C. A. (1997). Memory reprocessing in corticocortical and hippocampocortical neuronal ensembles. *Philosophical Transactions of the Royal Society, London, Series B: Biological Sciences*, **352**, 1525–1533.

Ramm, P. and Smith, C. T. (1990). Rates of cerebral protein synthesis are linked to slow wave sleep in the rat. *Physiology and Behavior*, **48**, 749–753.

Ranck, J. B., Jr. (1973). Studies on single neurons in dorsal hippocampal formation and septum in unrestrained rats. I. Behavioral correlates and firing repertoires. *Experimental Neurology*, **43**, 461–531.

Rasmussen, K., Morilak, D. A., and Jacobs, B. L. (1986a). Single unit activity of locus coeruleus neurons in the freely moving cat. I. During naturalistic behaviors and in response to simple and complex stimuli. *Brain Research*, **371**, 324–334.

Rasmussen, K., Strecker, R. E., and Jacobs, B. L. (1986b). Single unit response of noradrenergic, serotonergic and dopaminergic neurons in freely moving cats to simple sensory stimuli. *Brain Research*, **369**, 336–340.

Rasmusson, D. and Szerb, J. C. (1976). Acetylcholine release from visual and sensorimotor cortices of conditioned rabbits: the effects of sensory cuing and patterns of responding. *Brain Research*, **104**, 243–259.

Reid, M. S., Siegel, J. M., Dement, W. C., and Mignot, E. (1994). Cholinergic mechanisms in canine narcolepsy–II. Acetylcholine release in the pontine reticular formation is enhanced during cataplexy. *Neuroscience*, **59**, 523–530.

Ribeiro, S. (2000). Song, sleep, and the slow evolution of thoughts: gene expreison studies on brain representation, Ph.D. Dissertation, The Rockefeller University, New York.

Ribeiro, S., Goyal, V., Mello, C. V., and Pavlides, C. (1999). Brain gene expression during REM sleep depends on prior waking experience. *Learning and Memory*, **6**, 500–508.

Ribeiro, S., Mello, C. V., Velho, T., Gardner, T., Jarvis, E., and Pavlides, C. (2001). Experience-dependent zif-268 upregulation during REM sleep that follows hippocampal LTP. *Society of Neuroscience Abstracts*, **27**, 847.

Ribeiro, S., Mello, C. V., Velho, T., Gardner, T., Jarvis, E., and Pavlides, C. (2002). Induction of hippocampal long-term potentiation during waking leads to increased extra-hippocampal zif-268 expression during ensuing REM sleep. *Journal of Neuroscience*, **22**, 10914–10923.

Richardson, C. L., Tate, W. P., Mason, S. E., Lawlor, P. A., Dragunow, M., and Abraham, W. C. (1992). Correlation between the induction of an immediate early gene, zif/268, and long-term potentiation in the dentate gyrus. *Brain Research*, **580**, 147–154.

Roberts, L. A., Higgins, M. J., O'Shaughnessy, C. T., Stone, T. W., and Morris, B. J. (1996). Changes in hippocampal gene expression associated with the induction of long-term potentiation. *Molecular Brain Research*, **42**, 123–127.

Rogan, M. T., Staubli, U. V., and LeDoux, J. E. (1997). Fear conditioning induces associative long-term potentiation in the amygdala. *Nature*, **390**, 604–607.

Rose, G. M. and Dunwiddie, T. V. (1986). Induction of LTP using physiologically patterned stimulation. *Neuroscience Letters*, **69**, 244–248.

Rudell, A. P., Fox, S. E., and Ranck, J. B., Jr. (1980). Hippocampal excitability phase-locked to the theta rhythm in walking rats. *Experimental Neurology*, **68**, 87–96.

Sainsbury, R. S. (1970). Hippocampal activity during natural behavior in the guinea pig. *Physiology and Behavior*, **5**, 317–324.

Sara, S. J., Vankov, A., and Herve, A. (1994). Locus coeruleus-evoked responses in behaving rats: a clue to the role of noradrenaline in memory. *Brain Research Bulletin*, **35**, 457–465.

Schwob, J. E., Haberly, L. B., and Price, J. L. (1984). The development of physiological responses of the piriform cortex in rats to stimulation of the lateral olfactory tract. *Journal of Comparative Neurology*, **223**, 223–237.

Scoville, W. B. and Milner, B. (1957). Loss of recent memory after bilateral hippocampal lesions. *Journal of Neurology, Neurosurgery, and Psychiatry*, **20**, 11–21.

Sejnowski, T. J. and Destexhe, A. (2000). Why do we sleep? *Brain Research*, **886**, 208–223.

Sheng, M. and Greenberg, M. E. (1990). The regulation and function of c-fos and other immediate early genes in the nervous system. *Neuron*, **4**, 477–485.

Sheng, M., McFadden, G., and Greenberg, M. E. (1990). Membrane depolarization and calcium induce c-fos transcription via phosphorylation of transcription factor CREB. *Neuron*, **4**, 571–582.

Shiromani, P. J., Kilduff, T. S., Bloom, F. E., and McCarley, R. W. (1992). Cholinergically induced REM sleep triggers fos-like immunoreactivity in dorsolateral pontine regions associated with REM sleep. *Brain Research*, **580**, 351–357.

Siapas, A. G. and Wilson, M. A. (1998). Coordinated interactions between hippocampal ripples and cortical spindles during slow-wave sleep. *Neuron*, **21**, 1123–1128.

Skaggs, W. E. and McNaughton, B. L. (1996). Replay of neuronal firing sequences in rat hippocampus during sleep following spatial experience. *Science*, **271**, 1870–1873.

Smith, C. (1996). Sleep states, memory processes and synaptic plasticity. *Behavioral Brain Research*, **78**, 49–56.

Smith, C. and Kelly, G. (1988). Paradoxical sleep deprivation applied two days after end of training retards learning. *Physiology and Behavior*, **43**, 213–216.

Smith, C., Kitahama, K., Valatx, J. L., and Jouvet, M. (1974). Increased paradoxical sleep in mice during acquisition of a shock avoidance task. *Brain Research*, **77**, 221–230.

Smith, C. and Lapp, L. (1991). Increases in number of REM S and REM sleep density in humans following an intensive learning period. *Sleep*, **14**, 325–330.

Smith, C., Lowe, D., and Smith, M. J. (1977). Increases in paradoxical and slow sleep during the acquisition of an appetitive task in rats. *Physiology and Psychology*, **5**, 364–372.

Smith, C. and Rose, G. M. (1996). Evidence for a paradoxical sleep window for place learning in the Morris water maze. *Physiology and Behavior*, **59**, 93–97.

Smith, C. and Rose, G. M. (1997). Posttraining paradoxical sleep in rats is increased after spatial learning in the Morris water maze. *Behavioral Neuroscience*, **111**, 1197–1204.

Smith, C. and Wong, P. T. P. (1991). Paradoxical sleep increases predict successful learning in a complex operant task. *Behavioral Neuroscience*, **105**, 282–288.

Smith, C., Young, J., and Young, W. (1980). Prolonged increases in paradoxical sleep during and after avoidance-task acquisition. *Sleep*, **3**, 67–81.

Smith, C. T., Conway, J. M., and Rose, G. M. (1998). Brief paradoxical sleep deprivation impairs reference, but not working, memory in the radial arm maze task [In Process Citation]. *Neurobiology of Learning and Memory*, **69**, 211–217.

Squire, L. R. (1992). Memory and the hippocampus: a synthesis from findings with rats, monkeys, and humans. *Psychological Reviews*, **99**, 195–231.

Staubli, U. and Lynch, G. (1987). Stable hippocampal long-term potentiation elicited by "theta" pattern stimulation. *Brain Research*, **435**, 227–234.

Stewart, M. and Fox, S. E. (1991). Hippocampal theta activity in monkeys. *Brain Research*, **538**, 59–63.

Stickgold, R., Whidbee, D., Schirmer, B., Patel, V., and Hobson, J. A. (2000). Visual discrimination task improvement: A multi-step process occurring during sleep. *Journal of Cognitive Neuroscience*, **12**, 246–254.

Sukhatme, V. P., Cao, X. M., Chang, L. C., Tsai-Morris, C. H., Stamenkovich, D., Ferreira, P. C., Cohen, D. R., Edwards, S. A., Shows, T. B., Curran, T. *et al.* (1988). A zinc finger-encoding gene coregulated with c-fos during growth and differentiation, and after cellular depolarization. *Cell*, **53**, 37–43.

Tanaka, M., de Kloet, E. R., de Wied, D., and Versteeg, D. H. (1977). Arginine8-vasopressin affects catecholamine metabolism in specific brain nuclei. *Life Sciences*, **20**, 1799–1808.

Thiel, G., Schoch, S., and Petersohn, D. (1994). Regulation of synapsin I gene expression by the zinc finger transcription factor zif268/egr-1. *Journal of Biological Chemistry*, **269**, 15294–15301.

Timo-Iaria, C., Negrao, N., Schmidek, W. R., Hoshino, K., Lobato de Menezes, C. E., and Leme da Rocha, T. (1970). Phases and states of sleep in the rat. *Physiology Behavior*, **5**, 1057–1062.

Vanderwolf, C. H. (1969). Hippocampal theta activity and voluntary movement in the rat. *Electroencephalography and Clinical Neurophysiology*, **26**, 407–418.

Vianna, M. R., Alonso, M., Viola, H., Quevedo, J., de Paris, F., Furman, M., de Stein, M. L., Medina, J. H., and Izquierdo, I. (2000). Role of hippocampal signaling pathways in long-term memory formation of a nonassociative learning task in the rat. *Learning and Memory*, **7**, 333–340.

Wallace, C. S., Withers, G. S., Weiler, I. J., George, J. M., Clayton, D. F., and Greenough, W. T. (1995). Correspondence between sites of NGFI-A induction and sites of morphological plasticity following exposure to environmental complexity. *Molecular Brain Research*, **32**, 211–220.

Williams, J. A., Comisarow, J., Day, J., Fibiger, H. C., and Reiner, P. B. (1994). State-dependent release of acetylcholine in rat thalamus measured by *in vivo* microdialysis. *Journal of Neuroscience*, **14**, 5236–5242.

Williams, J. M., Beckmann, A. M., Mason-Parker, S. E., Abraham, W. C., Wilce, P. A., and Tate, W. P. (2000). Sequential increase in Egr-1 and AP-1 DNA binding activity in the dentate gyrus following the induction of long-term potentiation. *Molecular Brain Research*, **77**, 258–266.

Wilson, M. A. and McNaughton, B. L. (1993). Dynamics of the hippocampal ensemble code for space. *Science*, **261**, 1055–1058.

Wilson, M. A. and McNaughton, B. L. (1994). Reactivation of hippocampal ensemble memories during sleep. *Science*, **265**, 676–679.

Winocur, G., McDonald, R. M., and Moscovitch, M. (2001). Anterograde and retrograde amnesia in rats with large hippocampal lesions. *Hippocampus*, **11**, 18–26.

Winson, J. (1972). Interspecies differences in the occurrence of theta. *Behavioral Biology*, **7**, 479–487.

Winson, J. (1974). Patterns of hippocampal theta rhythm in the freely moving rat. *Electroencephalography and Clinical Neurophysiology*, **36**, 291–301.

Winson, J. (1978). Loss of hippocampal theta rhythm results in spatial memory deficit in the rat. *Science*, **201**, 160–163.

Winson, J. (1986). Behavioraly dependent neuronal gating in the hippocampus. In *The hippocampus* (eds R. L. Isaacson and K. H. Pribram), pp. 77–91. Plenum Press, New York.

Winson, J. (1990). The meaning of dreams. *Scientific American*, **263**, 86–96.

Winson, J. (1993). The biology and function of rapid eye movement sleep. *Current Opinion in Neurobiology*, **3**, 243–248.

Winson, J. and Abzug, C. (1977). Gating of neuronal transmission in the hippocampus: efficacy of transmission varies with behavioral state. *Science*, **196**, 1223–1225.

Winson, J. and Abzug, C. (1978*a*). Dependence upon behavior of neuronal transmission from perforant pathway trough entorhinal cortex. *Brain Research*, **147**, 422–427.

Winson, J. and Abzug, C. (1978*b*). Neuronal transmission through hippocampal pathways dependent on behavior. *Journal of Neurophysiology*, **41**, 716–732.

Winson, J. and Dahl, D. (1986). Long-term potentiation in dentate gyrus: induction by asynchronous voleys in separate afferents. *Science*, **234**, 985–988.

Wisden, W., Errington, M. L., Williams, S., Dunnett, S. B., Waters, C., Hitchcock, D., Evan, G., Bliss, T. V. P., and Hunt, S. P. (1990). Differential expression of immediate early genes in the hippocampus and spinal cord. *Neuron*, **4**, 603–614.

Worley, P. F., Bhat, R. V., Baraban, J. M., Erickson, C. A., McNaughton, B. L., and Barnes, C. A. (1993). Thresholds for synaptic activation of transcription factors in hippocampus—correlation with long-term enhancement. *Journal of Neuroscience*, **13**, 4776–4786.

Wyble, B. P., Linster, C. and Hasselmo, M. E. (2000). Size of CA1-evoked synaptic potentials is related to theta rhythm phase in rat hippocampus. *Journal of Neurophysiology*, **83**, 2138–2144.

Xia, Z., Dudek, H., Miranti, C. K., and Greenberg, M. E. (1996). Calcium influx via the NMDA receptor induces immediate early gene transcription by a MAP kinase/ERK-dependent mechanism. *Journal of Neuroscience*, **16**, 5425–5436.

Zola-Morgan, S. M. and Squire, L. R. (1990). The primate hippocampal formation—evidence for a time-limited role in memory storage. *Science*, **250**, 288–290.

CHAPTER 17

SLEEP MODULATION OF THE EXPRESSION OF PLASTICITY MARKERS

JAMES M. KRUEGER, FERENC OBÁL JR.,

JOSEPH W. HARDING, JOHN W. WRIGHT, AND

LYNN CHURCHILL

Introduction

Sleep must have a very robust adaptive value. Sleep is the regulated loss of consciousness. While asleep, one does not eat, drink, engage in social activity, or reproduce and one is vulnerable to predation. Further, if an animal or human survives a lesion, for example, stroke, it sleeps regardless of what was lesioned thereby suggesting that sleep occurs in any surviving group of neurons. Sleep thus seems to be a fundamental property of neuronal networks. Another property of neuronal networks is that the specific connections between neurons, that is, their synapses, are reinforced if activated and are weakened if unused (reviewed Purves 1994). The brain microcircuitry is thus in a constant flux. The notion that sleep may aid synaptic plasticity has been suggested in several theories (e.g. Moruzzi 1972; Smith 1985, 1996; Krueger and Obal 1993, 2002; Giuditta 1995; Kavanau 1996; McNaughton 1998). These represent the first testable theories of sleep function; some of the evidence germane to these theories is reviewed herein.

How does the brain modify its structure through experience, what mediates the neural plasticity underlying learning and memory, and what role might sleep play in facilitating these mechanisms? The specific processes involved include, at a minimum, cellular signaling from the external environment to the internal environment, to the cell nucleus. Presumably, such cellular signaling initiates the expression of those genes necessary for synthesis of specific molecules important to reconfiguration of connections among neurons, and thus underlies the phenomenon of neural plasticity. In order to begin to understand the potential role of sleep in neural plasticity we must identify candidate molecules important to transmembrane signaling, the mediation of neural connections, cell morphology, cytoskeletal protein changes, and cellular growth, and then we have to demonstrate how the activity of these molecules varies with sleep and wakefulness. Several such substances have been identified and many of these are either involved in sleep regulation or are affected by sleep.

Brain organization and sleep

Global outputs of the brain such as the electroencephalogram (EEG) and behavior are usually used to define sleep at the organism level. Further, there is substantial evidence for the involvement of specific networks in the initiation and maintenance of sleep. For instance, there are the well-known thalamic and anterior hypothalamic–basal forebrain circuits involved in non-rapid eye movement (NREM) sleep regulation and the pontine REM sleep mechanisms. Furthermore, there are several arousal systems, which are influenced by the sleep regulatory networks, including raphe serotoninergic, locus coeruleus noradrenergic, posterior hypothalamic histaminergic, and basal forebrain cholinergic networks. The collective body of evidence implicating such structures in sleep–wake regulation is massive and convincing and thereby forms the fundamental paradigm of sleep research; that sleep is actively regulated by these networks and is dependent upon prior duration of wakefulness.

Previously we proposed a fundamental modification of this paradigm, yet one consistent with the literature and the roles that these networks play in sleep regulation (Krueger and Obál 1993, 2002). We posited that sleep is an inherent property of small groups of highly interconnected neurons (neuronal groups). Further, we proposed that sleep is targeted to neuronal groups based on the degree of their prior activity (see Section IV for the mechanisms responsible) rather than on the duration of prior wakefulness. Finally, we envisioned that the role of the sleep regulatory and arousal networks was one of annealing the sleep of individual neuronal groups into a coordinated niche-adapted sleep for the organism. Our view of brain organization as it applies to sleep thus suggests that sleep intensity is targeted disproportionately to areas of brain intensely used during prior waking, that sleep is a distributed process in the brain and that it is not a uniform process of the brain.

There is much evidence for our view of sleep–brain organization (reviewed Krueger *et al.* 1995, 1999a; Krueger and Obál 2002). Very briefly, some of the strongest evidence include the following. Birds and whales are capable of unihemispheric sleep (Oleksenko *et al.* 1992) thereby demonstrating that parts of the brain can be asleep while other parts remain awake. Clinical observations also suggest that sleep and wakefulness can occur simultaneously in different parts of the brain (Mahowald and Schenck 1992). Activity within the brain, be it electrical or metabolic, is uneven regardless of the state. Thus, cerebral blood flow has regional differences during NREM sleep and REM sleep and both are different from that observed during wakefulness (Maquet 2000). Further, human EEG slow-wave activity occurs earlier and is more intense in the frontal lobes as one enters NREM sleep (Werth *et al.* 1997). At the cellular level, some visual association cortical neurons display firing patterns characteristic of sleep even while the animal continues to perform a visual discrimination task (Pigarev 1997). Collectively such data clearly indicate that sleep is not a uniform process of the brain.

The idea that sleep is homeostatically regulated is old, however that this is a localized property dependent upon prior neuronal activity was only recently proposed

(Krueger and Obál 1993). There is evidence for this notion. Thus, in dolphins, if just one half of the brain is deprived of sleep, that half, but not the other half, demonstrates sleep rebound (Oleksenko *et al.* 1992). In humans, Kattler *et al.* (1994) mechanically stimulated one hand repeatedly during wakefulness then measured EEG-slow wave activity during subsequent NREM sleep. This measure of NREM sleep intensity was greater in the contralateral somatosensory cortex, the side receiving input from the stimulated hand, than in the ipsilateral cortex. Similarly, in rats with a unilateral whisker cut, whisker stimulation during waking enhanced EEG power in the somatosensory cortex contralateral to the intact whisker during subsequent sleep (Vyazovskiy *et al.* 2000). Other findings also suggest that sleep is targeted to specific areas depending upon their prior activity. In the developing chicken, left hemisphere sleeping is linked to the consolidation of memories developed during awake activities (Mascetti *et al.* 1999). In the developing cat, sleep deprivation blocked NREM sleep-enhanced visual cortex plasticity induced by monocular deprivation (Frank *et al.* 2001). In humans, magnetic resonance imaging (MRI) studies indicate that the localized effects after sleep deprivation depend upon the specific cognitive tasks performed during prior waking (Drummond *et al.* 1999). Positron emission tomographic (PET) studies reached similar conclusions, that the intensity of sleep is targeted to specific areas of brain depending upon prior use (Maquet 2000).

Sleep function

Our ideas concerning sleep function are presented in detail elsewhere (Krueger and Obál 1993, 2002; Krueger *et al.* 1995, 1999*a*). In its most simplified form, our hypothesis is that sleep serves to stimulate, and thereby preserve, adaptive functional networks sculpted by genetics and prior experience and simultaneously serves to integrate new network firing patterns into existing networks. The biochemical mechanisms responsible for these actions are the same as those responsible for sleep and thus, we emphasize that sleep function cannot be separated from sleep mechanisms. Further, these biochemical mechanisms directly alter input–output relationships of neural networks and thereby suggest an explanation for the separation of environmental input from organism behavior (sleep-associated unconsciousness).

Neural activation induces growth factor production (see Sections IV and V) and these growth factors act as autocrines and paracrines to alter the input–output relationships of nearby neurons. Their action thus results in two effects. First, output is divorced from prior environmental input in the sense that the same input induces a different output. Second, the pattern of activation within the affected networks changes. This latter action leads to activation of, and thus preservation of, previously inactive synapses. The same growth factors also induce genes involved in making and preserving synapses.

There is much evidence for the individual steps of our hypothesis. Thus, by way of concrete example, the production of interleukin-1β(IL1β) or tumor necrosis factor α(TNFα) is enhanced in brain by neural activity (Schneider *et al.* 1998; Albensi and Mattson 2000). In turn, IL1β or TNFα induces changes in input–output relationships within local networks. For example, IL1β and TNFα change the sensitivity of hypothalamic neurons to temperature (Shibata 1990) and within the hippocampus, IL1β and TNFα affect long-term potentiation (LTP) (Tancredi *et al.* 1992; Takagi 2000). Sleep loss inhibits LTP (Davis *et al.* in press) and increases IL1β and TNFα levels in the hippocampus (Floyd *et al.* 1997; Taishi *et al.* 1998). Both IL1β and TNFα induce sleep and are involved in sleep regulation (see Section IV). Further, IL1β and TNFα induce production of other molecules that affect network input–output relationships such as NO and adenosine (reviewed Krueger *et al.* 2001*a,b*); IL1β and TNFα also induce neurite outgrowth (Ho and Blum 1998; Munoz-Fernandez and Fresno 1998). Finally, IL1β and TNFα induce production of molecules such as matrix metalloproteinase-9 (MMP-9) (Vecil *et al.* 2000; Bevans-Nelson *et al.* 2001) and nuclear factor kappa B (NFkB) (Mattson *et al.* 2000) and NO (Stoll *et al.* 2000), which are involved in neural plasticity. Several additional sleep-promoting molecules share these types of activities with IL1β and TNFα (see Section IV). Collectively, such data support the notion that sleep is linked to synaptic plasticity.

Biochemical regulation of sleep

Several gene families are involved in the regulation of sleep (reviewed Krueger *et al.* 1999*b*, 2001*a,b*; Obál and Krueger 2000). For instance, there is extensive evidence linking the brain cytokine networks and the somatotropic axis to NREM sleep regulation. Many cytokines enhance sleep, including interleukin-1α(IL1α), IL1β, IL2, IL6, IL15, IL18, epidermal growth factor, acidic fibroblast growth factor (FGF), nerve growth factor (NGF), brain-derived neurotrophic factor (BDNF), glia derived growth factor (GDNF), interferon α(IFNα), IFNγ , TNFα, and TNFβ. In contrast, cytokines, which are inhibitory of the pro-somnogenic cytokines, inhibit spontaneous sleep; the list includes the IL1-receptor antagonist, IL4, IL10, IL13, transforming growth factor β, and insulin-like growth factor-1 (IGF-1). Many factors collectively suggest that cytokine networks operate in brain to regulate sleep : the number of different pro- and anti-somnogenic cytokines, the facts (i) that these substances are made in the CNS, (ii) that their receptors are in the CNS and (iii) that many alter firing rates of hypothalamic neurons . However, among those listed, only TNFα and IL1β have been studied extensively for their involvement in sleep regulation, though there is a growing amount of evidence implicating NGF and BDNF in sleep mechanisms.

Central or systemic injection of low doses of IL1β or TNFα enhances NREM sleep whereas high doses tend to inhibit both NREM sleep and REM sleep. If either TNFα or IL1β is inhibited using antibodies, soluble receptors, or antagonists, spontaneous sleep is reduced. These inhibitors also inhibit the excess sleep occurring after sleep loss. Substances that enhance the production of IL1β or TNFα, such as bacterial or viral products, enhance NREM sleep. In contrast, substances, which inhibit production of IL1β or TNFα, inhibit spontaneous sleep, for example, corticotropin releasing hormone (CRH; Krueger *et al.* 1999*b*, 2001*b*; Obál *et al.* 2000). Levels of the mRNAs for TNFα and IL1β and for TNF protein levels in brain vary with sleep propensity. For example, they are highest at the onset of light hours in rats (the beginning of the sleep period). They also increase after sleep loss and excessive food intake; both these stimuli enhance sleep propensity. The TNF 55 kD receptor and the IL1 type I receptor are involved in the somnogenic actions of TNF and IL1; mutant mice lacking these receptors sleep less than controls (Fang *et al.* 1997, 1998). Several downstream biochemical events leading to IL1- or TNF-induced sleep include NFκB, NO, prostaglandin D_2, and adenosine (reviewed Krueger *et al.* 1999*b*; Obál *et al.* 2000; Krueger *et al.* 2001*b*). There is also ample evidence demonstrating the involvement of the somatotropic axis in sleep regulation (reviewed Obál *et al.* 2000; Krueger *et al.* 2001*b*). Thus, injection of growth hormone releasing hormone (GHRH) enhances NREM sleep in a variety of species including humans. Growth hormone (GH) seems to enhance REM sleep. In contrast, somatostatin and IGF-1 inhibit spontaneous sleep. Inhibition of GHRH using antibodies or a GHRH peptide antagonist also inhibits spontaneous sleep; these inhibitors also reduce sleep rebound after sleep loss. Mutant rats (Obál *et al.* 2001) or mutant mice (Alt *et al.* 2001) lacking functional GHRH receptors sleep less than controls. Hypothalamic levels of GHRH and GHRH mRNA vary in phase with the sleep–wake cycle and GHRH mRNA increases during sleep deprivation. Injection of GHRH into the anterior hypothalamus enhances NREM sleep whereas injection of the GHRH peptide antagonist inhibits NREM sleep (Zhang *et al.* 1999). The somnogenic actions of GHRH are linked to the cytokines. Thus, IL1, TNF, and GHRH induce pituitary release of GH. Anti-GHRH antibodies inhibit IL1-induced NREM sleep and GH release (Obál *et al.* 1995). In cultured hypothalamic neurons IL1 receptors and GHRH receptors are colocalized in neurons; both induce enhanced intracellular Ca^{++} (De *et al.* 2002).

All of the substances thus far linked to sleep regulation have multiple biological activities. An important commonality of those actions is that most are either directly or indirectly involved in synaptic plasticity. Thus there is substantial evidence indicating the involvement of IL1β, TNFα, NO, adenosine, FGF, prostaglandins, NFκB, NGF, BDNF, GDNF, and the somatotropic axis in neurite outgrowth and/or enhanced synaptic efficacy. A fundamental hypothesis within the synaptic plasticity field is that synaptic activation results in enhanced synaptic efficacy. This enhanced efficacy is brought about by substances whose release, synthesis, or activation is promoted by synaptic activation. Many of the sleep-regulatory substances mentioned above including IL1β, TNFα, NO, adenosine, NFκB, NGF, and BDNF are released or produced in response to neural activity. Since these substances act in autocrine and paracrine fashions, this suggests that mechanistically sleep would be targeted to those brain areas with prior high activity (other evidence as outlined above supports this notion). In addition, since these substances are causative of sleep, it seems likely that sleep is related to synaptic/neural activity.

Examples of sleep and molecules involved in plasticity

NGF

We have proposed that the adaptive ability of the brain resides in the modifications of synaptic connections induced by growth factors, which accumulate as a function of neuronal activity and which promote sleep. In this section, we discuss several activity-regulated proteins thought to be involved in plasticity including the neurotrophins (Thoenen 2000), such as NGF and BDNF, and the activity-regulated cytoskeleton-associated protein (arc) (Lyford *et al.* 1995). Intracerebroventricular injections of either NGF or BDNF enhance spontaneous sleep (Kushikata *et al.* 1999; Takahashi and Krueger 1999) and microinjection of NGF into the brainstem induces REM sleep (Yamuy *et al.* 1995). Lesions or pharmacological antagonists that neutralize the effects of the neuro-trophins also alter the EEG measurements of sleep (Kapas, personal communication) and cortical plasticity (Sachdev *et al.* 1998).

Levels of NGF and BDNF mRNA in the hippocampus are sensitive to specific types of synaptic activity: excitatory transmitters using the N-methyl-D-aspartate (NMDA) receptor upregulate while the inhibitory transmitters, GABA, downregulate their mRNA levels (Zafra *et al.* 1991). Further, BDNF, NGF and arc expression are affected by sleep loss hence by neuronal activity (Cirelli and Tononi 2000; Sei *et al.* 2000; Brandt *et al.* 2001; Taishi *et al.* 2001).

A direct role for these activity-regulated proteins in sleep-related plasticity requires specific spatial and temporal regulation. Such specificity could be conferred temporally by secretion determined by activity and spatially by secretion or activation within synaptic sites. Recently, the activity-regulated upregulation of arc mRNA was shown to be targeted to the synaptic sites on the dendrites that are most active, that is, stimulation of the entorhinal cortex localizes the arc mRNA within the region of the dendrite that receives afferents from the entorhinal cortex (Steward and Worley 2001). Blocking the NMDA receptor or inhibiting the expression of arc also blocks LTP as well as learning a spatial task (Steward *et al.* 1998; Guzowski *et al.* 2000).

During sleep deprivation, both the arc and NGF protein levels are increased in layer V neurons within the cortex, a prominent projection neuron for the cortical circuitry (Cirelli and Tononi 2000; Brandt *et al.* 2001). As sleep-deprivation time increases the upregulation of arc progresses from localization within the cell body mainly to localization within the pyramidal dendrite, suggesting that these cortical cells are also transporting the upregulated growth factors or their mRNA to the sites where active stimulation occurs (Cirelli and Tononi 2001). An increase in the level of NGF-immunoreactivity within the layer V pyramidal neurons of the somatosensory cortex is also observed after sleep deprivation (Fig. 17.1; Brandt *et al.* 2001). Further, if the afferent input to the somatosensory cortex is reduced by a whisker cut, a procedure

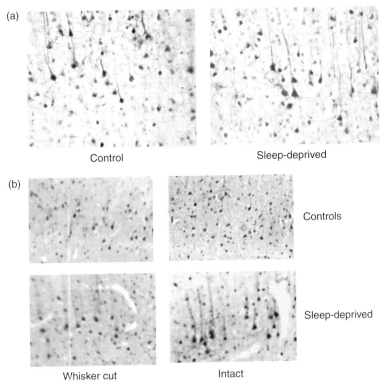

Figure 17.1 (a) NGF immunoreactivity increases in layer V of the somatosensory cortex after 6 h of sleep deprivation of rats with no whisker cut. (b) NGF-immunoreactivity in layer V of the somatosensory cortex of control (top) or sleep-deprived (bottom) that received a whisker cut (left is the contralateral cortex to the cut whiskers) 6 h prior to sacrifice. A twofold increase in the number of NGF-labeled neurons located in layer 5 occurs in the sleep-deprived cortex ipsilateral to the cut whiskers (bottom right), but not in that contralateral to the cut. (See Plate 19.)

which induces synaptic reorganization in the somatosensory barrel field, sleep loss does not affect pyramidal cell NGF expression (Fig 17.1), thereby suggesting that the sensory input is an important component of the activity-regulated expression of NGF. These data, and similar data involving the expression of glutamate decarboxylase mRNA in the somatosensory cortex (Churchill *et al.* 2001) provide strong evidence that sleep/sleep loss differentially affects the brain depending upon the nature of the ongoing synaptic reorganization.

Extracellular matrix and related molecules

Cell adhesion molecules (CAMs) are cell membrane macromolecules essential in controlling cell-to-cell adhesion during development by influencing neurite outgrowth, neural migration and adhesion, synaptogenesis, and intracellular signaling. In addition,

CAMs regulate cell-to-extracellular matrix (ECM) adhesion that appears to be critical to the processes of learning and memory. It is becoming clear that changes in membrane excitability can also influence CAMs, which in turn may regulate the neural restructuring that serves as the substrate of learning and memory.

If one function of sleep is to reconfigure and preserve the synaptic efficacy of a specific circuit that is driven by an important recent experience in the life of that individual, then candidate signaling molecules should reveal significant changes in their activity concomitant with, or soon after, the event. Measuring changes in ECM molecules would appear to be an obvious starting point. It is this matrix that permits cell-to-cell and cell-to-matrix adherence. In the late 1800s Golgi (1889) discovered inter-and peri-neuronal networks connecting cell bodies and dendrites in the adult mammalian central nervous system (CNS). More recent investigators have described this network as connections of perisynaptic astrocytic processes and extracellular scaffolding occupying the space between glial processes and neurons (Koppe et al. 1997). These ECM molecules provide physical support, regulate ionic and nutritional homeostasis of surrounding cells. They also possess ligands that interact with cell surface receptors that initiate signaling events that guide a wide range of functions including cellular proliferation, motility, differentiations, neural outgrowth, growth cone targeting, synapse stabilization, and apoptosis (Adams and Watt 1993; Juliano and Haskill 1993; Edwards et al. 1996; Nicholson and Sykova 1998; Ruegg 2001). Within the CNS, the ECM accounts for up to 20 percent of the total volume (Bignami et al. 1993), and is composed of glycoproteins and proteoglycans that are secreted into a network consisting predominantly of the proteins fibronectin, laminin, vitronectin, thrombospondin, tenascin, and collagen IV (Rutka et al. 1988; Reichardt and Tomaselli 1991; Venstrom and Reichardt 1993; Fields and Itoh 1996; Gumbiner 1996; Goldbrunner et al. 1998).

Interaction among cells and ECM molecules is dependent upon cell adhesion molecules. The CAMs are cell surface macromolecules that dictate cell-to-cell and cell-to-ECM interactions by mediating the processes of adhesion, migration, neurite outgrowth, fasciculation, synaptogenesis, and intracellular signaling (Fields and Itoh 1996; Gumbiner 1996; Schachner 1997). Cellular interactions within the ECM are highly regulated, in part, by a family of catabolic enzymes that selectively degrade ECM proteins, referred to as matrix metalloproteinases (MMPs; Fields and Itoh 1996). Collectively these molecules and remodeling enzymes create an environment of chemoattractant and chemorepulsant cues. The family of MMPs has grown to more than 20 members including collagenases, gelatinases, membrane-type MMPs, matrilysin, and stromelysins 1–3, and metalloelastase (Birkedal-Hansen et al. 1993; Kahari and Saarialho-Kere 1997; Yong et al. 1998). Normally, the ability of MMPs to degrade protein constituents of the ECM is closely regulated. This control is accomplished by three complimentary mechanisms: (i) regulation of gene transcription; (ii) modulation of pro-enzyme activation; and (iii) presence and abundance of tissue inhibitors of metalloproteinases (TIMPs). Although most MMPs are not constituitively expressed, gene transcription may be induced by such stimuli as growth factors, oncogene products, phorbol esters, as well as cell-to-ECM, and cell-to-cell, interactions. These stimuli typically result in the expression of c-fos and c-jun proto-oncogene families. This expression in turn contributes to the formation of homo- and hetero-dimeric forms of activator protein-1 (AP-1) transcription factors. AP-1 binds to specific DNA sequences that are present in the promoters of most MMP genes. The activation of these genes, however, typically is dependent on the combined effects of AP-1 proteins and other transcription factors (Mann and Spinale 1998). TIMPs are a family of secreted glycoproteins that includes at least four members, TIMP-1 through -4, possessing approximately 30–40 percent sequence similarity. The proteolytic activity of MMPs appears to be carefully regulated by TIMPs that are designed to inhibit the active forms of MMPs by forming tight noncovalent complexes with them (Bode *et al.* 1999; Skiles *et al.* 2001). Given the interrelationship among these components it appears that MMPs are pivotal in the initiation of ECM reconfiguration (Wright *et al.* 2002). In turn, MMP activity is counter-balanced by TIMPs. Our laboratories have been focusing on the relationship among changes in these molecules, duration of sleep episodes, and memory consolidation.

Initial support for the notion that ECM remodeling is a general feature of neuronal plasticity is suggested by the observation that MMP-9, a highly inducible MMP, is upregulated in various brain regions of the rat during the active phase of spatial learning (Hunter *et al.* 1999). Recent studies have expanded on the potential role of ECM restructuring in plasticity to include other CNS phenomena such as the development of cocaine sensitization (Harding and Sorg, unpublished) and sleep (Reid *et al.* 2001; Taishi *et al.* 2001) that are believed to entail changes in synaptic function. As might be expected, the cocaine studies demonstrated highly selective changes in MMP-9 limited to dopaminergic reward pathways. By contrast, the sleep studies revealed more wide-ranging alterations in MMP-9. These studies demonstrated that sleep deprivation dramatically alters the pattern and magnitude of MMP-9 changes that occur during spatial learning in a diverse set of brain regions (Reid *et al.* 2001). Together, these findings support several speculations regarding the function of sleep: (i) sleep modifies mechanisms underlying synaptic plasticity; (ii) this modification is responsible for the attenuation in cognitive function associated with sleep deprivation; and (iii) that this sleep-dependent regulation of plasticity occurs in multiple and diverse brain regions and is consistent with the proposal that sleep is a non-centralized process (Krueger and Obál 1993).

Acknowledgment

This work was supported in part by NIH grant numbers NS25378, NS27250, NS31453, HD36520 and a grant from the Sleep Medicine Education and Research Foundation, a foundation of the American Academy of Sleep Medicine.

References

Adams, J. C. and **Watt, F. M.** (1993). Regulation of development and differentiation by the extracellular matrix. *Development,* **117,** 1183–1198.

Albensi, B. C. and Mattson, M. P. (2000). Evidence for the involvement of TNF and NF-kappa B in hippocampal synaptic plasticity. *Science*, **35**, 151–159.

Alt, J. A., Obal, F. Jr., Majde, J. A., and Krueger, J. M. (2001). Impairment of the sleep responses to influenza infection in mice with a defective GHRH-receptor. *Sleep*, **24**, A144–A145.

Bevans-Nelson, S. E., Lausch, R. N., and Oakes, J. E. (2001). Tumor necrosis factor-alpha and not interleukin-1 alpha is the dominant inducer of matrix metalloproteinase-9 synthesis in human corneal cells. *Experimental Eye Research*, **73**, 403–407.

Bignami, A., Huxley, M., and Dahl, D. (1993). Hyaluronic acid and hyaluronic acid-binding proteins in brain extracellular matrix. *Anatomy and Embryology*, **188**, 419–433.

Birkedal-Hansen, H., Moore, W. G., and Bodden, M. K. (1993). Matrix metalloproteinases: a review. *Critical Reviews in Oral Biology and Medicine*, **4**, 197–250.

Bode, W., Fernandez-Catalan, C., Tschesche, H., Grams, F., Nagase, H., and Maskos, K. (1999). Structural properties of matrix metalloproteinases. *Cellular and Molecular Life Science*, **55**, 639–652.

Brandt, J., Churchill, L., Guan, Z., Fang, J., Chen, L., and Krueger, J. M. (2001). Sleep deprivation but not a whisker trim increases nerve growth factor within barrel cortical neurons. *Brain Research*, **898**, 105–112.

Churchill, L., Taishi, P., Guan, Z., Chen, L., Fang, J., and Krueger, J. M. (2001). Sleep modifies glutamate decarboxylase mRNA within the barrel cortex of rats after a mystacial whisker trim. *Sleep*, **24**, 261–266.

Cirelli, C. and Tononi, G. (2000). Differential expression of plasticity-related genes in waking and sleep and their regulation by the noradrenergic system. *Journal of Neuroscience*, **20**, 9187–9194.

Davis, C. J., Kramar, E. A., Harding, J. W., and Wright, J. W. Sleep deprivation abolishes maintenance of long-term potentiation in CA1. *Sleep* (in press).

De, A., Churchill, L., Obal, F., Jr, Simasko, S. M., and Krueger, J. M. (2002) GHRH and IL1beta increase cytoplasmic Ca(2+) levels in cultured hypothalamic GABAergic neurons. *Brain Res.* **949**, 209–12.

Drummond, S. P. A., Brown, G. G., Stricker, J. L., Buxton, R. B., Wong, E. C., and Gillin, J. C. (1999). Sleep deprivation-induced reduction in cortical functional response to serial subtraction. *Neuroreport*, **10**, 3745–3748.

Edwards, D. R., Beaudry, P. P., Laing, T. D., Kowal, V., Leco, K. J., Leco, P. A., and Lim, M. S. (1996). The roles of tissue inhibitors of metalloproteinases in tissue remodeling and cell growth. *International Journal of Obesity and Related Metabolic Disorders* **20**, S9–S15.

Fang, J., Wang, Y., and Krueger, J. M. (1997). Mice lacking the TNF 55-kD receptor fail to sleep more after TNFα treatment. *Journal of Neuroscience*, **17**, 5949–5955.

Fang, J., Wang, Y., and Krueger, J. M. (1998). Effects of interleukin-1β on sleep are mediated by the type I receptor. *American Journal of Physiology*, **274**, R655–R660.

Fields, R. D. and Itoh, K. (1996). Neural cell adhesion molecules in activity-dependent development and synaptic plasticity. *Trends in Neurosciences*, **19**, 473–480.

Floyd, R. A. and Krueger, J. M. (1997). Diurnal variations of TNFα in the rat brain. *Neuroreport*, **8**, 915–918.

Frank, M. G., Issa, N. P., and **Stryker, M. P.** (2001). Sleep enhances plasticity in the developing visual cortex. *Neuron*, **30**, 275–287.

Giuditta, A., Ambrosini, M. V., Montagnese, P., Mandile, P., Cotugno, M., Zucconi, G. G., and **Vescia, S.** (1995). The sequential hypothesis of the function of sleep. *Behavioural Brain Research*, **69**, 157–166.

Goldbrunner, R. H., Bernstein, J. J., and **Tonn, J. C.** (1998). ECM-mediated glioma cell invasion. *Microscopy Research and Technique*, **13**, 250–257.

Golgi, C. (1889). On the structure of nerve cells. *Journal of Microscopy*, **155**, 3–7.

Gumbiner, B. M. (1996). Cell adhesion: the molecular basis of tissue architecture and morphogenesis. *Cell*, **84**, 345–357.

Guzowski, J. F., Lyford, G. L., Stevenson, G. D., Houston, F. P., McGaugh, J. L., Worley, P. F., and **Barnes, C. A.** (2000). Inhibition of activity-dependent arc protein expression in the rat hippocampus impairs the maintenance of long-term potentiation and the consolidation of long-term memory. *Journal of Neuroscience*, **20**, 3993–4001.

Ho, A. and **Blum M.** (1998). Induction of interleukin-1 associated with compensatory dopaminergic sprouting in the denervated striatum of young mice: model of aging and neurodegenerative disease. *Journal of Neuroscience*, **18**, 5614–5629.

Hunter, S. E., Harding, J. W., Wright, J. W., and **Ritter, S.** (1999) Altered expression of MMP-9 in the rat hippocampus and cerebellum during the consolidation phase of spatial learning. *Society for Neuroscience Abstracts*, **25**, 882.

Juliano, R. I. and **Haskill, S.** (1993). Signal transduction from the extracellular matrix. *Journal of Cell Biology*, **120**, 577–585.

Kahari, V. M. and **Saarialho-Kere, U.** (1997). Matrix metalloproteinases in skin. *Experimental Dermatology*, **6**, 199–213.

Kattler, H., Dijk, D.-J., and **Borbély, A. A.** (1994). Effect of unilateral somatosensory stimulation prior to sleep on the sleep EEG in humans. *Journal of Sleep Research*, **3**, 1599–1604.

Kavanau, J. L. (1996). Memory, sleep, and dynamic stabilization of neural circuitry: evolutionary perspectives. *Neuroscience and Biobehavioral Reviews*, **20**, 289–311.

Koppe, G., Bruckner, G., Hartig, W., Delpech, B., and **Bigl, V.** (1997). Characterization of proteo-glycan-containing perineuronal nets by enzymatic treatments of rat brain sections. *Histochemical Journal*, **29**, 11–20.

Krueger, J. M. and **Obal, F. Jr.** (1993). A neuronal group theory of sleep function. *Journal of Sleep Research*, **2**, 63–69.

Krueger, J. M. and **Obal, F. Jr.** (2002). Function of Sleep. In *Sleep medicine* (eds T. L. Lee-Chiong, Jr., M. J. Sateia, and M. A. Carskadon), pp. 23–30. Hanley and Belfus, Inc., Philadelphia, PA.

Krueger, J. M., Fang, J., and **Majde, J. A.** (2001*b*). Sleep in health and disease. In *Psychoneuroimmunology*, 3rd edn (eds B. Ader, D. Felton, and N. Cohen), pp. 667–685. Academic Press, New York, NY.

Krueger, J. M., Obál, F. Jr., and **Fang, J.** (1999*b*). Humoral regulation of physiological sleep; cytokines and GHRH. *Journal of Sleep Research*, **8**, 53–59.

Krueger, J. M., Obál, F. Jr., and Fang, J. (1999a). Why we sleep: a theoretical view of sleep function. *Sleep Medical Reviews*, **3**, 119–129.

Krueger, J. M., Obal, F. Jr., Fang, J., Kubota, T., and Taishi, P. (2001a). The role of cytokines in physiological sleep regulation. *Annals of the New York Academy of Science*, **933**, 211–221.

Krueger, J. M., Obál, F. Jr., Kapás, L., and Fang, J. (1995). Brain organization and sleep function. *Behavioural Brain Research*, **69**, 177–185.

Kushikata, T., Fang, J., and Krueger, J. M. (1999). Brain-derived neurotrophic factor enhances spontaneous sleep in rats and rabbits. *American Journal of Physiology*, **276**, R1334–R1338.

Lyford, G. L., Yamagata, K., Kaufmann, W. E., Barnes, C. A., Sanders, L. K., Copeland, N. G., Gilbert, D. J., Jenkins, N. A., Lanahan, A. A., and Worley, P. F. (1995). Arc, a growth factor and activity-regulated gene, encodes a novel cytoskeleton-associated protein that is enriched in neuronal dendrites. *Neuron*, **14**, 433–445.

Mahowald, M. and Schenck, C. H. (1992). Dissociated state of wakefulness and sleep. *Neurology*, **42**, 44–52.

Mann, D. L. and Spinale, F. G. (1998). Activation of matrix metalloproteinases in the failing human heart, breaking the tie that binds. *Circulation*, **98**, 1699–1702.

Maquet, P. (2000). Functional neuroimaging of normal human sleep by positron emission tomography. *Journal of Sleep Research*, **9**, 207–231.

Mascetti, G. G., Rugger, M., and Vallortigara, G. (1999). Visual lateralization and monocular sleep in the domestic chick. *Cognitive Brain Research*, **7**, 451–463.

Mattson, M. P., Culmsee, C., Yu, Z., and Camandola, S. (2000). Roles of nuclear factor kappa B in neuronal survival and plasticity. *Journal of Neurochemistry*, **74**, 443–456.

McNaughton, B. L. (1998). The neurophysiology of reminiscence. *Neurobiology of Learning and Memory*, **70**, 252–267.

Moruzzi, G. (1972). The sleep–waking cycle. *Reviews of Physiology*, **64**, 1–165.

Munoz-Fernandez, M. A. and Fresno, M. (1998). The role of tumour necrosis factor, interleukin 6, interferon-gamma and inducible nitric oxide synthase in the development and pathology of the nervous system. *Progress in Neurobiology*, **56**, 307–340.

Nicholson, C. and Sykova', E. (1998). Extracellular space structure revealed by diffusion analysis. *Trends in Neurosciences*, **21**, 207–215.

Obál, F. Jr., Fang, J., Payne, L. C., and Krueger, J. M. (1995). Growth hormone-releasing hormone (GHRH) mediates the sleep promoting activity of interleukin-1 (IL1) in rats. *Neuroendocrinology*, **61**, 559–565.

Obál, F. Jr., Fang, J., Taishi, P., Kacsoh, B., Gardi, J., and Krueger, J. M. (2001). Deficiency of growth hormone-releasing hormone signaling is associated with sleep alterations in the dwarf rat. *Journal of Neuroscience*, **21**, 2912–2918.

Obál, F. Jr. and Krueger, J. M. (2000). Hormones, cytokines and sleep. In *Coping with the environment neural and endocrine mechanisms: handbook of physiology* (ed. B. S. McEwen), pp. 331–349. Oxford University Press, Oxford, UK.

Oleksenko, A. I., Mukhametov, L. M., Polyakova, I. G., Supin, A. Y., and Kovalzon, V. M. (1992). Unihemispheric sleep deprivation in bottlenose dolphins. *Journal of Sleep Research*, **1**, 40–44.

Pigarev, I. N. (1997). Neurons of visual cortex respond to visceral stimulation during slow wave sleep. *Neuroscience*, **62**, 1237–1243.

Purves, D. (1994). *Neural activity and the growth of the brain.* Cambridge University Press, New York.

Reichardt, L. F. and **Tomaselli, K. J.** (1991). Extracellular matrix molecules and their receptors: functions in neural development. *Annual Review of Neuroscience*, **14**, 531–570.

Reid, J., Meighan, S. E., Turner, G. D., Krueger, J. M., Harding, J. W., and **Wright J. W.** (2001). Paradoxical sleep deprivation impairs brain matrix metalloproteinase activity in rats trained in the circular water maze. *Society for Neuroscience Abstracts*, **27**, 315.19.

Ruegg, M. A. (2001). Molecules involved in the formation of synaptic connections in muscle and brain. *Matrix Biology*, **20**, 3–12.

Rutka, I. I., Apodaca, G., Stern, R., and **Rosenblum, M.** (1988). The extracellular matrix of the central and peripheral nervous system: structure and function. *Journal of Neurosurgery*, **69**, 133–170.

Sachdev, R. N. S., Lu, S.-M., Wiley, R. G., and **Ebner, F. F.** (1998). Role of the basal forebrain cholinergic projection in somatosensory cortical plasticity. *Journal of Neurophysiology*, **79**, 3216–3228.

Schachner, M. (1997). Neural recognition molecules and synaptic plasticity. *Current Opinion in Cell Biology*, **9**, 627–634.

Schneider, H., Pitossi, F., Balschun, D., Wagner, A., del Rey, A., and **Besedovsky, H. O.** (1998). A neuromodulatory role of interleukin-1 beta in the hippocampus. *Proceeding of the National Academy of Sciences, USA*, **23**, 7778–7783.

Sei, H., Saitoh, D., Yamamoto, K., Morita, K., and **Morita, Y.** (2000). Differential effect of short-term REM sleep deprivation on NGF and BDNF protein levels in the rat brain. *Brain Research*, **877**, 387–390.

Shibata, M. (1990). Hypothalamic neuronal responses to cytokines. *Yale Journal of Biology and Medicine*, **63**, 147–156.

Skiles, J., Gonnella, N., and **Jeng, A.** (2001). The design, structure, and therapeutic application of matrix metalloproteinase inhibitors. *Current Medicinal Chemistry*, **8**, 425–474.

Smith, C. T. (1985). Sleep states and learning: a review of the animal literature. *Neuroscience and Biobehavioral Reviews*, **9**, 157–168.

Smith, C. T. (1996) Sleep states, memory processes and synaptic plasticity. *Behavioural Brain Research*, **78**, 49–56.

Steward, O. and **Worley, P. F.** (2001). A cellular mechanism for targeting newly synthesized mRNAs to synaptic sites on dendrites. *Proceeding of the National Academy of Sciences, USA*, **98**, 7062–7068.

Steward, O., Wallace, C. S., Lyford, G. L., and **Worley, P. F.** (1998). Synaptic activation causes the mRNA for the IEG Arc to localize selectively near activated postsynaptic sites on dendrites. *Neuron*, **21**, 741–751.

Stoll, G., Jander, S. and **Schroeter, M.** (2000). Cytokines in CNS disorders: Neurotoxicity versus neuroprotection. *Journal of Neural Transmission, Supplementum*, **59**, 81–89.

Taishi, P., Chen, Z., Obál, F. Jr., Hansen, M., Zhang, J., Fang, J., and Krueger, J. M. (1998). Sleep-associated changes in interleukin-1β mRNA in the brain. *Journal of Interferon and Cytokine Research*, **18**, 793–798.

Taishi, P., Sanchez, C., Wang, Y., Fang, J., Harding, J. W., and Krueger, J. M. (2001). Conditions that affect sleep alter the expression of molecules associated with synaptic plasticity. *American Journal of Physiology*, **281**, R839–R845.

Takagi, H. (2000). Neuronal cytokine involvement in synaptic plasticity. *Nippon Yakurigaku Zasshi*, **115**, 201–207.

Takahashi, S. and Krueger, J. M. (1999). Nerve growth factor enhances sleep in rabbits. *Neuroscience Letters*, **264**, 149–152.

Tancredi, V., D'Arcangelo, G., Grassi, F., Tarroni, P., Palmieri, G., Santoni, A., and Eusebi, F. (1992). Tumor necrosis factor alters synaptic transmission in rat hippocampal slices. *Neuroscience Letters*, **146**, 176–178.

Thoenen, H. (2000). Neurotrophins and activity-dependent plasticity. *Progress in Brain Research*, **128**, 183–191.

Vecil, G. G., Larsen, P. H., Corley, S. M., Herx, L. M., Besson, A., Goodyer, C. G., and Yong, V. W. (2000). Interleukin-1 is a key regulator of matrix metalloproteinase-9 expression in human neurons in culture and following mouse brain trauma *in vivo*. *Journal of Neuroscience Research*, **61**, 212–224.

Venstrom, K. A. and Reichardt, L. F. (1993). Extracellular matrix 2: role of extracellular matrix molecules and their receptors in the nervous system. *FASEB Journal*, **7**, 996–1003.

Vyazovskiy, V., Borbély, A. A., and Tobler, I. (2000). Unilateral vibissae stimulation during waking induces interhemispheric EEG asymmetry during subsequent sleep in the rat. *Journal of Sleep Research*, **9**, 367–371.

Werth, E., Achermann, P., and Borbély, A. A. (1997). Fronto-occipital EEG power gradients in human sleep. *Journal of Sleep Research*, **6**, 102–112.

Wright, J. W., Kramar, E. A., Meighan, S. E., and Harding, J. W. (2002). Extracellular matrix molecules, long-term potentiation, memory consolidation and the brain angiotensin system. *Peptides*, **23**, 221–246.

Yamuy, J., Morales, F. R., and Chase, M. H. (1995). Induction of rapid eye movement sleep by the microinjection of nerve growth factor into the pontine reticular formation of the cat. *Neuroscience*, **66**, 9–13.

Yong, V. W., Krekoski, C. A., Forsyth, P. A., Bell, R., and Edwards, D. R. (1998). Matrix metalloproteinases and diseases of the CNS. *Trends in Neuroscience*, **21**, 75–80.

Zafra, F., Castren, E., Thoenen, H., and Lindholm, D. (1991). Interplay between glutamate and gamma-aminobutyric acid transmitter systems in the physiological regulation of brain-derived neurotrophic factor and nerve growth factor synthesis in hippocampal neurons. *Proceeding of the National Academy of Sciences, USA*, **88**, 10037–10041.

Zhang, J., Obál, F. Jr., Zheng, T., Fang, J., Taishi, P., and Krueger, J. M. (1999). Intrapreoptic microinjection of GHRH or its antagonist alters sleep in rats. *Journal of Neuroscience*, **19**, 2187–2194.

INDEX